Cardiac Surgery

Safeguards and Pitfalls in Operative Technique

Third Edition

Cardiac Surgery

Safeguards and Pitfalls in Operative Technique

Third Edition

Siavosh Khonsari, M.A., M.B., B.Ch., F.R.C.S.(C.), F.A.C.S., F.A.C.C.

Chief, Regional Department of Cardiac Surgery
Center for Medical Education
Kaiser Permanente Medical Center
Clinical Professor of Surgery
University of California, Los Angeles
Los Angeles, California

Colleen Flint Sintek, M.D.

Assistant Chief, Director of Congenital Heart Surgery
Regional Department of Cardiac Surgery
Center for Medical Education
Kaiser Permanente Medical Center
Associate Clinical Professor of Cardiothoracic Surgery
Children's Hospital of Los Angeles
University of Southern California
Los Angeles, California

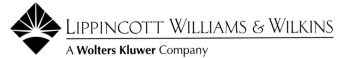

LIPPINCOTT WILLIAMS & WILKINS
A **Wolters Kluwer** Company
Philadelphia · Baltimore · New York · London
Buenos Aires · Hong Kong · Sydney · Tokyo

Acquisitions Editor: Lisa McAllister
Developmental Editor: Michael Standen
Production Editor: Erica Woods Tucker
Manufacturing Manager: Benjamin Rivera
Cover Designer: Patricia Gast
Compositor: Lippincott Williams & Wilkins Desktop Division
Printer: Maple Press

© 2003 by LIPPINCOTT WILLIAMS & WILKINS
530 Walnut Street
Philadelphia, PA 19106 USA
LWW.com

Printed in the USA

Library of Congress Cataloging-in-Publication Data

Khonsari, Siavosh.
  Cardiac surgery : safeguards and pitfalls in operative technique / Siavosh Khonsari,
  Colleen Flint Sintek. — 3rd ed.
     p. ; cm.
  Includes index.
  ISBN 0-7817-3540-8
  1. Heart—Surgery. I. Sintek, Colleen. II. Title.
  [DNLM: 1. Cardiac Surgical Procedures—methods. 2. Cardiovascular Diseases—surgery.
  WG 169 K45c 2003]
  RD598.K53 2003
  617.4'12—dc21

                                                                    2003040043

Care has been taken to confirm the accuracy of the information presented and to describe generally accepted practices. However, the authors and publisher are not responsible for errors or omissions or for any consequences from application of the information in this book and make no warranty, express or implied, with respect to the currency, completeness, or accuracy of the contents of the publication. Application of this information in a particular situation remains the professional responsibility of the practitioner.

  The authors and publisher have exerted every effort to ensure that drug selection and dosage set forth in this text are in accordance with current recommendations and practice at the time of publication. However, in view of ongoing research, changes in government regulations, and the constant flow of information relating to drug therapy and drug reactions, the reader is urged to check the package insert for each drug for any change in indications and dosage and for added warnings and precautions. This is particularly important when the recommended agent is a new or infrequently employed drug.

  Some drugs and medical devices presented in this publication have Food and Drug Administration (FDA) clearance for limited use in restricted research settings. It is the responsibility of the health care provider to ascertain the FDA status of each drug or device planned for use in their clinical practice.

                                        10 9 8 7 6 5 4 3 2 1

To our institution Kaiser Permanente Medical Center, Los Angeles, Southern California Permanente Medical Group, and to our former residents and colleagues who taught us much of what appears in this book.

Contents

Section V   Open Procedures for Congenital Heart Defects

Section VI   Miscellaneous

Preface

True wisdom consists not only in seeing what is before your eyes,
but in foreseeing what is to come.
Istuc es sapere, non quod ante pedes modest
Videre sed etiam illa quae futura sunt Prospicere.
Terence, *Aldelphi*, 1.386. (Act III, Scene 3)

The gratifying response to the previous publication, which has been translated into both Japanese and Portuguese, encouraged me to pursue and launch yet another new edition. The practice of cardiac surgery has undergone rapid progress and changes in recent years. Interventional cardiology has been aggressive and taken over some surgical procedures. With the surge of technological advances, cardiac surgeons are driven into a new era to face new challenges. The third edition of *Cardiac Surgery: Safeguards and Pitfalls in Operative Technique* has undergone extensive revision to reflect these changes. To accomplish this, I have invited my colleague, Dr. Colleen Flint Sintek, who has contributed to previous editions, to be the co-author of this work.

New material in this edition has been introduced while some obsolete sections have been deleted. A section on minimally invasive approaches has been added. A chapter on surgical management of atrial fibrillation has been introduced to reflect the currently available techniques.

Dr. Kwok Yun, who made numerous contributions to this book, reviewed all chapters devoted to adult cardiac surgery. In particular he wrote the new section on off pump coronary artery surgery and made significant changes and revisions pertaining to aortic surgery.

Dr. Gary Kochamba made numerous important suggestions regarding the format of the chapter on coronary artery disease as well as the expanded use of arterial conduits.

All chapters on congenital cardiac surgery have undergone major scrutiny. Many sections have been completely rewritten. More recent concepts dealing with the surgical management of single ventricle, including modifications of the Norwood procedure and the extra-cardiac Fontan procedure, have been incorporated into the text. A completely new chapter on surgery for coronary artery anomalies has been introduced.

This book continues to be primarily intended for younger surgeons and those in training. However, it can also serve as a handy refresher on surgical technique for senior cardiac surgeons. Pediatric and adult cardiologists as well as perfusionists, nurses, and anyone involved in the care of cardiac surgery patients should find this work useful.

The format of the book follows that of the previous editions. The emphasis on pitfalls and errors in the performance of cardiac surgical procedures is denoted by highlighted subheadings, which are preceded by a hazard sign (⃠). The reader is made aware of the mechanism of their occurrence, and appropriate recommendations are made regarding the avoidance of these complications and their surgical management. Points of particular importance are emphasized by special Nota Bene (**NB**) notations.

The text in this book does not pretend to be either encyclopedic or comprehensive. Less commonly performed procedures in cardiac surgery are excluded. The book primarily focuses on technical details. Relevant surgical anatomy is discussed in a concise and practical fashion. This has been achieved with the aid of clear "telling" illustrations by Joanie Livermore in the first edition and continued in a masterly fashion by Tim Hengst. Tim has been successful in maintaining the superb quality of the artwork which is the hallmark of the success of the book. While some illustrations from the previous edition have been deleted, ninety illustrations have been modified and 105 new ones have been added.

Siavosh Khonsari
Colleen Flint Sintek

Acknowledgments

We would like to thank Dr. Vaughn Starnes, Dr. Winfred Wells, and the cardiac surgery team at Children's Hospital of Los Angeles for their support of us and our congenital cardiac surgery service.

We would also like to thank Dr. Robert H. Anderson who was kind enough to review the plates and the descriptive text on surgical anatomy and made many helpful suggestions. We also would like to thank members of my department: Drs. Thomas Pfeffer, Manly Hyde, Jesus Torpocco, Satinder Sidhu, Kenneth Barron, Samar Hazzan, and Hui Wu who have made numerous suggestions and contributions; and the administrative members Sookie Kim, Joanne Smick, Lupe Pires, Mark Robinet, Kathy Chavez, Mark Cinque, Margarita Vargas, and Michael Graeser for their help and cooperation. Josephine Shiau has been most helpful in organizing and completing the manuscript. We are also very grateful to the Cardiac Surgery team for their dedication and hard work.

Finally we wish to thank Lisa McAllister, Executive Editor; Mike Standen, Developmental Editor; and Erica Woods Tucker, Production Editor at Lippincott Williams & Wilkins, for their support and patience.

SECTION I

General Considerations

CHAPTER 1

Surgical Approaches to the Heart and Great Vessels

PRIMARY MEDIAN STERNOTOMY

Median sternotomy is the most widely used incision in cardiac surgery because it provides excellent exposure for most operations involving the heart and great vessels.

Technique

The skin incision should extend from just below the suprasternal notch to a point equidistant from the xiphoid process and umbilicus. An electric saw with a vertical blade is most commonly used to divide the sternum. In young infants, the sternum is divided with heavy scissors. An oscillating saw, which is somewhat more cumbersome, is used for all repeat sternotomies; its use requires constant practice because only with experience can the surgeon develop a "feel" for when the blade has penetrated the posterior table of the sternum (see Repeat Sternotomy section).

Healing of the vertical median sternotomy incision may cause a prominent scar that at times gives patients, particularly young women, some concern and anxiety. This problem can be overcome by performing a median sternotomy through a bilateral submammary skin incision, as Brom recommended in 1962, which leaves a cosmetically more acceptable scar (Fig. 1-1).

Submammary Approach

Skin incisions are made 0.5 cm below and parallel with the lowest contour of both breasts. The incisions are joined in the midline across the lowest segment of the sternum (at the junction with the xiphoid process) (Fig. 1-1).

 LOWER LIMITS OF BREAST TISSUE
The precise limits of breast tissue may not be evident in the very young, making this approach cosmetically challenging. A transverse incision at the level of the xiphoid process across the chest is a prudent alternative. Otherwise, the child reaches adulthood with an ugly scar across the breasts. This must be avoided.

The breasts and skin flaps are dissected off the pectoral muscles with a cautery blade. The skin flaps are then retracted by means of one to two heavy silk sutures. To achieve secure and satisfactory traction, silk sutures are tied to a Kerlix gauze pad and attached to the anesthesiologist's crossbar.

 PRESSURE CUTS ON THE SKIN
A gauze pad placed behind the silk sutures helps to prevent the development of pressure marks from the sutures on the skin and its edges.

The sternal opening and closure are performed in the usual fashion. When the sternum is closed and hemostasis is obtained, the skin flaps are allowed to fall normally on the pectoral muscles. This position is then secured with a few absorbable sutures. Two small drains (e.g., Jackson-Pratt) are placed behind the skin flaps and brought out at the lateral extremes of the incision. They are connected to a closed suction system.

Every precaution is observed to maintain the normal contour of the breasts and the position and direction of the nipples. Otherwise, the whole purpose of this cosmetic approach would be negated.

NB The chest tube is brought out through a small curvilinear incision just above the umbilicus for aesthetic reasons.

 BLEEDING
A small vein is usually evident running transversely in the suprasternal notch. At times, however, it may be large and engorged, particularly in patients with elevated right heart pressure. Excessive bleeding may occur if this vein is inadvertently injured. It is important to be aware of its presence and to coagulate it (if tiny) or to occlude it with a metal clip. If the vein has been cut and its ends have retracted, thus making hemostasis difficult, control of bleeding can

notch and eventually into the mediastinum, leading to wound complications and mediastinitis.

 ENTRY INTO THE PERITONEAL CAVITY
During the division of the linea alba or the lower part of the pericardium, the peritoneal cavity may be entered. The opening should be closed immediately to prevent any spillage of blood or cold saline used for topical cooling into the peritoneal cavity, which may promote postoperative ileus.

 ASYMMETRIC DIVISION OF THE STERNUM
The sternotomy should be in the midline of the periosteum. By dipping the thumb and index finger into the incision and spreading them against the lateral margins of the sternum into the intercostal spaces, the proper site for sternal splitting can be located and marked by an electrocautery on the periosteum. Unequal division may leave one side of the sternum too narrow and allow the closure wires to cut through the thinner segments of bone, leading to an increased incidence of sternal dehiscence. Similarly, the costochondral junction may be damaged (Fig. 1-2).

 PNEUMOTHORAX AND HEMOTHORAX
The anesthesiologist is always asked to deflate the lungs while the surgeon is using the sternal saw so that the pleural cavities can be kept intact. This is particularly important in patients with chronic

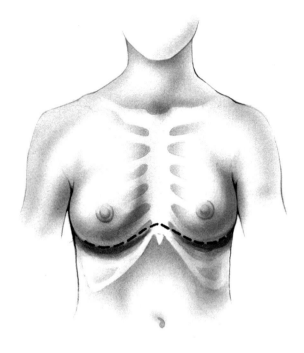
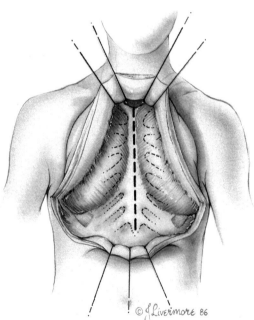

FIG. 1-1. Brom's submammary approach.

be gained by packing the suprasternal notch area and proceeding with the sternotomy. After the two sides of the sternum have been spread apart, the sites of bleeding can be easily identified and controlled.

○ ***STERNAL INFECTION***
Dissection of the suprasternal notch is not only unnecessary but also can open up tissue planes in the neck. Tracheostomy is now rarely necessary but always remains a possibility. Whenever tracheostomy is performed, a separate incision is kept as high in the neck as possible so that a superficial tracheostomy wound infection does not spread into the suprasternal

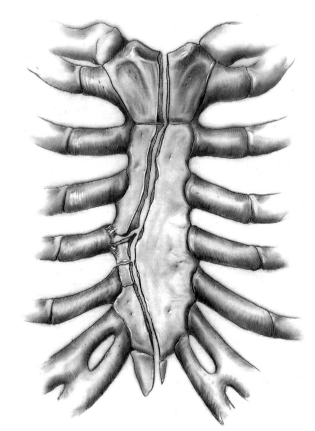

○ **FIG. 1-2.** Fracture resulting from improper division of the sternum.

obstructive pulmonary disease and hyperinflated lungs. Occasionally, however, the pleural cavities are opened by the sternal saw or during dissection of the thymus and pericardium. If the opening is small and no fluid has entered the pleural cavity, the tip of the mediastinal chest tube may be introduced for 2 to 3 cm into the pleural defect. The pleura may be opened fully, particularly in patients undergoing harvesting of internal mammary arteries. In these cases, a separate chest tube is inserted subcostally over the lateral aspect of the diaphragm for drainage of fluid and blood and evacuation of air.

USE OF BONE WAX
Excessive use of bone wax to control bleeding from the sternal marrow has gradually lost favor with many surgeons. It is sometimes associated with increased rates of wound infection, impaired wound healing, and, most serious of all, wax embolization to the lungs.

Although its routine use has been shown to have no effect on postoperative bleeding, bone wax remains a useful tool to control hemorrhage from sternal edges.

BRACHIAL PLEXUS INJURY
Brachial plexus injury has been associated with a median sternotomy. Stretching of the plexus by hyperabduction of the arm and compression of the nerve trunks between the clavicle and first rib during sternal retraction have been implicated as a cause of injury. Introduction of a Swan-Ganz catheter through the internal jugular vein can injure the brachial plexus, either directly by the introducer itself or indirectly by the formation of a hematoma in the vicinity. The most serious cause of brachial plexus injury is fracture of the first rib (Fig. 1-3). The sternal retractor should be placed with its crossbars *superiorly*, so that the blades spread apart the *lower third* of the sternal edges, and then

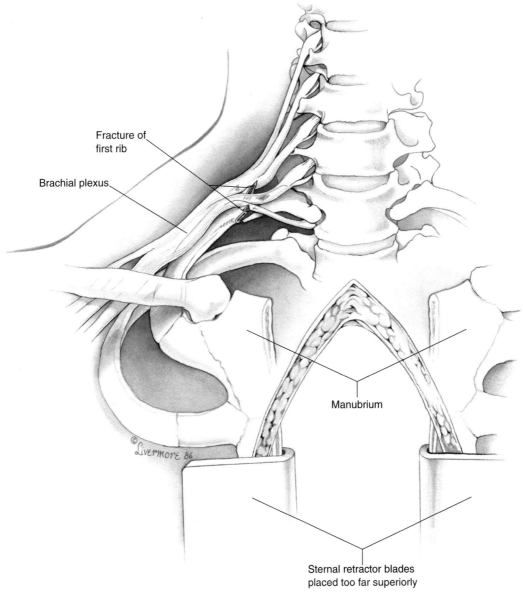

Fracture of first rib

Brachial plexus

Manubrium

Sternal retractor blades placed too far superiorly

FIG. 1-3. Mechanism of a brachial plexus injury.

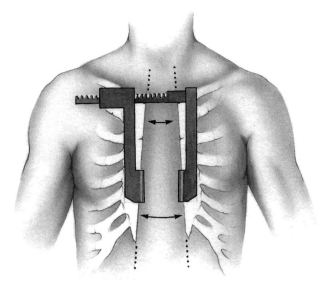

FIG. 1-4. Technique for sternal retractor placement with blades on the lower third of the sternum.

opened only gradually in a stepwise fashion (one to two turns at a time) to prevent fractures of the first rib or sternum (Fig. 1-4). If for any specific reason the crossbars of the retractor have to be placed inferiorly, it is important for the blades to be in the lower part of the sternotomy.

Retractors (e.g., Favaloro) used in harvesting the internal thoracic artery can also cause brachial plexus injury. Therefore, sudden excessive upward pull on the retractor should be avoided. The surgeon should ensure good exposure by manipulating the operating room table and his or her headlight to minimize traction of the upper sternum. Moreover, when the proximal internal mammary artery is freed, the degree of upper sternal retraction is reduced. These simple measures can often eliminate or reduce the incidence of brachial plexus injury.

 INNOMINATE VEIN INJURY
The innominate vein may be injured during dissection and division or resection of the thymus or its remnant, particularly when scarring is present from a previous operation. The scar tissue on each side of the injured vein is dissected free. Brisk bleeding can then be controlled by simple suturing. In rare instances of severe damage to the vein, it is divided and its right end is suture ligated. The other end of the vein is left open for drainage of venous return from left internal jugular tributaries until the patient is ready to come off cardiopulmonary bypass when it is similarly suture ligated.

The innominate vein is a useful channel for an additional intravenous line, which can be used to monitor central venous pressure, particularly in infants and patients with poor peripheral veins. The catheter is introduced percutaneously into the center of a 7-0 Prolene purse-string suture buttressed with fine pericardial pledgets on the innominate

vein. The purse-string suture must be tied snugly to prevent any bleeding after removal of the venous line. Sometimes a large thymic vein can be used for the same purpose.

REPEAT STERNOTOMY

An increasing number of patients requires surgical intervention a second, third, or even fourth and fifth time for replacement of prosthetic valves, definitive correction or revision of congenital heart defects, or repeat myocardial revascularization. Because it is anticipated that this trend will continue, all cardiac surgeons must acquire expertise in reoperative procedures. When making the skin incision, it is not always necessary to excise the previous scar unless it is gross and thick. The subcutaneous tissue is incised in the customary fashion, and, using electrocoagulation, the sternum is marked along the midline.

Technique

Previous wires or heavy nonabsorbable sutures are divided anteriorly but are not removed. They provide some resistance posteriorly to the oscillating saw, which helps to prevent any possible right ventricular injury (Figs. 1-5 and 1-6, inset). Only *limited*, sharp dissection adequate for the placement of a small Army-Navy retractor can be safely carried out in the suprasternal notch or around the xiphoid process.

 RIGHT VENTRICULAR INJURY
Blunt digital dissection behind the lower sternum should rarely be practiced in patients with a previous sternotomy because of possible injury to the friable right ventricular wall (Fig. 1-5).

The sternum is raised by retractors at the suprasternal notch superiorly and at the xiphoid inferiorly during sternal division with an oscillating saw (Fig. 1-6). Small rake retractors are *inserted into the marrow cavity on each side of the sternal edge* and gently lifted upward toward the ceiling, thus making the adhesions between the retrosternum and the heart slightly taut and accessible for division with the cautery or scissors (Fig. 1-7).

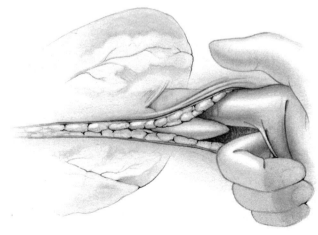

FIG. 1-5. Right ventricular injury caused by blunt digital dissection.

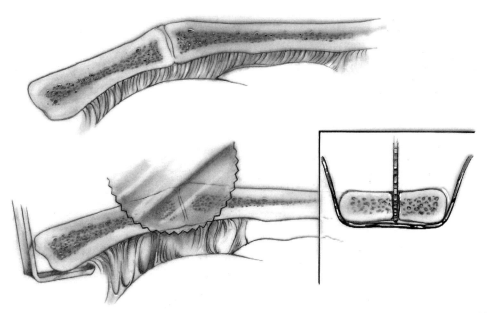

FIG. 1-6. Elevating the posterior table of the sternum to increase the distance between the saw blade and underlying structures.

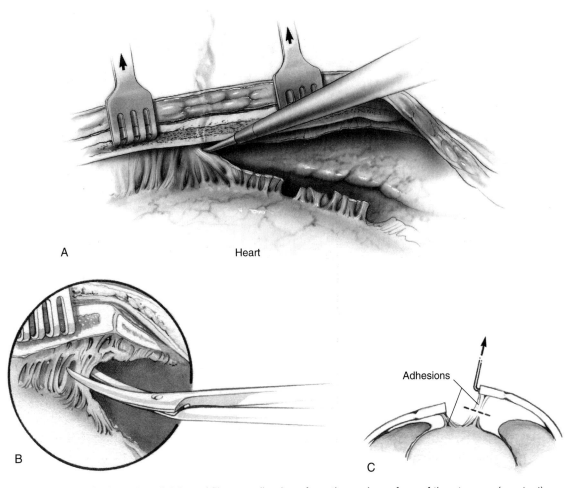

A

Heart

B

C

Adhesions

FIG. 1-7. A–C: Stepwise division of fibrous adhesions from the undersurface of the sternum (see text).

INJURY TO THE ASCENDING AORTA

Often the ascending aorta is enlarged, as in patients with poststenotic aortic dilation caused by chronic aortic stenosis or in patients with aneurysmal enlargement of the ascending aorta. In repeat sternotomy procedures, inadvertent entry into the ascending aorta is usually fatal.

A lateral chest radiograph often reveals the proximity of the right ventricle and ascending aorta to the undersurface of the sternum. However, a computed tomography scan will accurately identify the relationship between the ascending aorta and the underside of the sternum. When the ascending aorta is noted to be adherent to the undersurface of the sternum, precautions must be taken before performing a sternotomy.

Technique

Before a sternotomy is attempted, a small transverse incision is made in the second or third right intercostal space. This allows a lateral approach for dissection to free the aorta from the undersurface of the sternum. After this has been accomplished, the sternum can be divided in the manner described for repeat operation without risk of injury to the aorta (Fig. 1-8).

Our preference is femoral artery–femoral vein bypass and core cooling to 18°C before sternotomy. A long cannula with multiple side holes is ideal for satisfactory venous return. The important characteristic of this device is that it has a guidewire and a tapered dilator sheath inside the cannula. The guidewire allows easy passage over the pelvic brim.

Cardiopulmonary bypass is then established, and the patient is cooled to 18° to 20°C. Assisted venous drainage with a centrifugal pump or vacuum assist is useful. Aortic insufficiency owing to the presence of a bileaflet or a single-disc mechanical prosthesis or a disrupted aortic bioprosthesis may result in left ventricular distention. An appropriately sized vent is placed into the apex of the left ventricle through a small left

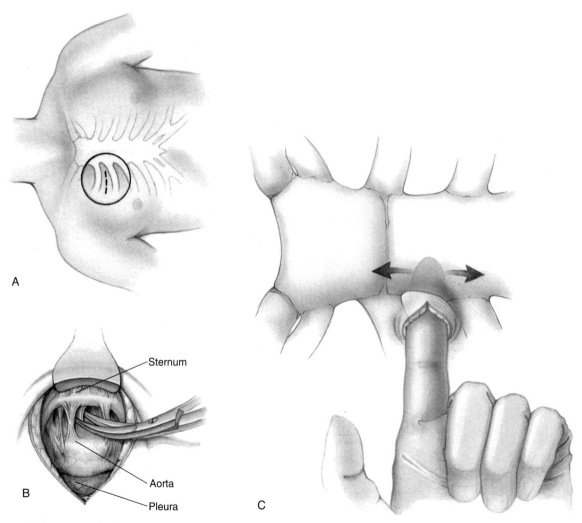

FIG. 1-8. A–C: Stepwise technique for separating the ascending aorta from the sternum in repeat procedures (see text).

anterior thoracotomy as cardiopulmonary bypass is being initiated to protect the heart from overdistention (see Left Ventricular Apical Venting section in Chapter 4). Transesophageal echocardiography is always used to monitor left ventricle volume. If left ventricular distention occurs either at the initiation of bypass or when the heart begins to fibrillate, a vent is placed immediately.

 ILIAC VEIN INJURY
Venous cannula that lack a guidewire often hang up at the pelvic brim, resulting in inadequate venous return. If an attempt is made to pass the cannula past the pelvic brim into the inferior vena cava, perforation of the iliac vein may ensue, with catastrophic consequences.

 INJURY TO THE LEFT ANTERIOR DESCENDING ARTERY
Although adhesions may obscure the precise location of the left anterior descending artery, the surgeon should place the vent in the true apex of the left ventricle (somewhat more to the left).

If the sternotomy is uneventful, the patient is then gradually rewarmed and the operation completed in the usual fashion. Conversely, if the aorta is torn or disrupted, hypothermic arrest is instituted and hemorrhage is controlled. The ascending aorta is then repaired or replaced. The conduct of the operation is then resumed to its completion.

NB This precaution may appear to be a very major undertaking with its own possible serious complications. However, it is the only way to prevent a catastrophic hemorrhage with fatal outcome.

 DIVISION OF THE POSTERIOR TABLE
The division of the posterior table of the sternum may be accomplished with heavy scissors under direct vision. This is facilitated by elevating the sternum slightly with a rake retractor. Such a maneuver is particularly important at the manubriosternal junction, where the manubrium takes a posterosuperior course (Fig. 1-6).

Fibrous adhesions to the undersurface of the sternum are mainly along the previous sternotomy. After dividing these fibrous adhesions with an electrocautery or scissors, the sternum is relatively free (Fig. 1-7). An adequate dissection is carried out so that the sternal retractor can be safely positioned and slowly opened.

By slow and careful sharp dissection along the right inferior border of the heart, the proper plane can be identified relatively easily. Some surgeons find that the use of the electrocautery blade on a low setting allows this dissection to be accomplished with less bleeding from the pericardial surfaces. The dissection can then be gradually carried upward, exposing the right atrium and aorta for cannulation in preparation for cardiopulmonary bypass.

 RIGHT VENTRICULAR TEAR
A small (Himmelstein) chest retractor can now be inserted and must be spread apart only slightly; an overzealous attempt to widen the sternal opening results in stretching of the right ventricular wall. Tearing of the right ventricle owing to saw injury or overstretching of the sternotomy is a life-threatening complication. Manual attempts should be made to control bleeding while cardiopulmonary bypass is being initiated as promptly as possible. With the right ventricle totally decompressed, the wound is repaired with multiple, fine pledgeted sutures (Fig. 1-9). In cases of saw injury, pressing the two sternal halves together and toward the heart may tamponade the bleeding while cannulation of the femoral vessels is being accomplished.

 INJURY OF THE INNOMINATE VEIN
In patients undergoing repeat sternotomies, the innominate vein is often adherent to the undersurface of the manubrium. It may be injured directly with the saw or torn as the sternal halves are being retracted (Fig. 1-9). In most cases, the bleeding can be controlled with digital pressure on the opening in the vein while the vein is carefully dissected free from the posterior aspect of both sides of the manubrium. If control of the bleeding cannot be rapidly secured, the two sternal halves should be pushed together with slight downward pressure by the assistant surgeon to minimize blood loss. Blood should be transfused as necessary and femoral arterial and venous cannulation obtained as quickly as possible. The innominate vein can then be dissected free and repaired with 5-0 Prolene suture on cardiopulmonary bypass.

If the innominate vein injury is a complex tear or transection, repair may not be feasible. Then the right side of the vein may be oversewn immediately, but the left side should be allowed to bleed freely and the blood returned to the bypass circuit by a pump sucker during cardiopulmonary bypass. Acute occlusion of venous drainage from the left subclavian and jugular veins during cardiopulmonary bypass may lead to central nervous system injury. The left-sided opening of the innominate vein may be closed just before separation from cardiopulmonary bypass.

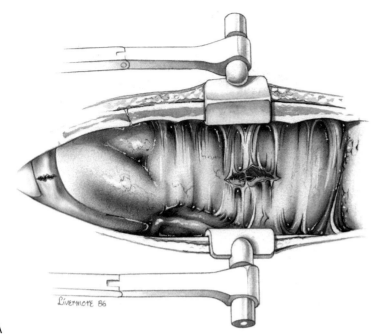

A

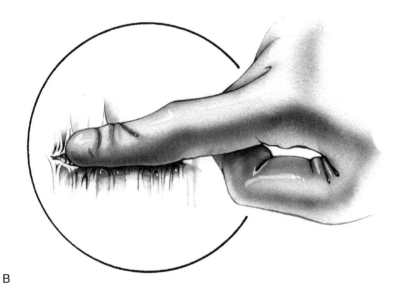

B

FIG. 1-9. A: Mechanism of a tear of the right ventricle and innominate vein in repeat procedures. **B:** Digital control of bleeding from the right ventricle.

STERNAL CLOSURE

Technique

Before sternal closure, chest tubes are placed in the mediastinal space and pericardial cavity for postoperative drainage.

 GRAFT INJURY
Chest tubes must be placed well away from arterial and vein grafts. Constant irritation and suctioning may perforate the grafts and cause brisk hemorrhage.

 MYOCARDIAL INJURY
The holes on the chest tubes must be oriented away from myocardial surface to prevent suction injury and bleeding.

The sternum is reapproximated with six to eight stainless steel wires. Generally, the wires are passed around the sternum except for the manubrium where they are passed through the bone. Care must be taken to avoid injury to the internal thoracic vessels.

In very ill patients who have difficulty being weaned from cardiopulmonary bypass, the heart and lungs become swollen and edematous. This is encountered more frequently in infants and young children. Closing the sternum in this subgroup of patients compresses the heart and compromises cardiac function. The chest is therefore left open in such cases, and the skin is closed with a patch of Esmarch Bioseal Bandage (Placentia, CA) or Silastic. When hemodynamics become stable, the patient is returned to the operating room, the Esmarch patch or Silastic is removed, and the sternotomy is closed in the customary fashion. Chest closure may be accomplished under sterile conditions in the intensive care unit.

NB The surgeon should not hesitate to use this very simple technique when indications are clear. This is a life-saving measure, and the incidence of sternal infection is surprisingly low when rigorous sterile technique is maintained.

 LOOSE WIRES
The degree of postoperative pain is partly related to the stability of the sternal closure. Movement of the sternal halves causes pain and interferes with normal respiration, resulting in postoperative pulmonary complications. If the wires are loose, normal respiratory movements

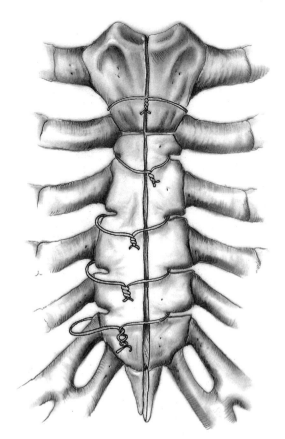

 FIG. 1-10. Loose wires sawing through the sternum.

allow the wires to saw through the sternum (Fig. 1-10).

 ROBICSEK'S MODIFICATION
When the sternum is osteoporotic and friable or the previous sternal closure has disrupted, Robicsek's modification is successful in most patients. Running wire sutures are placed parasternally on both sides followed by six to eight interrupted horizontal wire sutures, which are placed outside the longitudinal parasternal wires and tightened in the usual fashion (Fig. 1-11).

FRACTURE OF THE STERNUM
Approximation of fractured sternal edges is a difficult task. Wires are passed parasternally above and below the fracture site with the costal cartilages intervening. They are twisted tightly in the parasternal area to stabilize the fracture. These wires are then once again twisted horizontally across the sternum to close it in the usual fashion (Fig. 1-12).

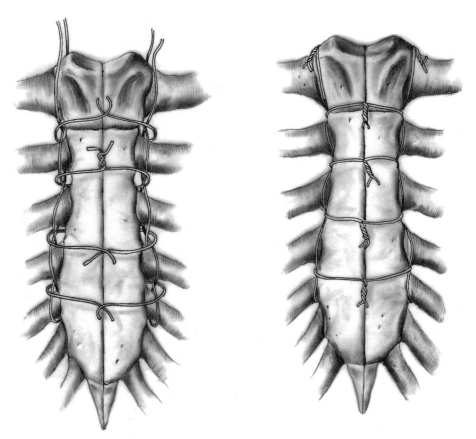

FIG. 1-11. Sternal closure with Robicsek's modification.

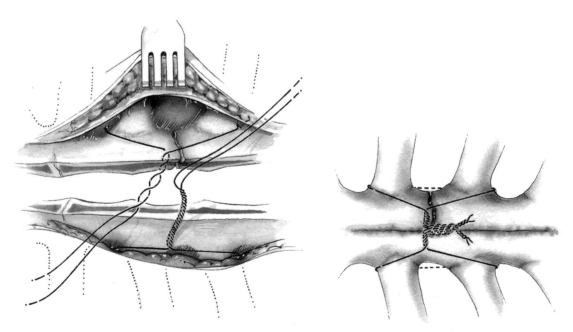

FIG. 1-12. Approximating segments of a fractured sternum.

POSTOPERATIVE STERNAL WOUND INFECTION

Sternal wound infection occurs in 1% to 2% of patients undergoing cardiac surgery and carries a very high rate of morbidity and mortality.

General Considerations

General systemic factors such as malnutrition, cardiac cachexia, renal failure, chronic obstructive pulmonary disease, obesity, diabetes, and use of corticosteroids predispose the patient to postoperative sternal wound infection. Every attempt should be made to optimize the patient's state of health before surgery. This may require a period of nutritional supplementation or an aggressive therapeutic regimen to improve cardiac function. Pulmonary toilet and breathing exercises can be beneficial in patients with a history of chronic lung dysfunction. It is a good practice to recommend weight reduction in the very obese, but not to the extent that it produces negative nitrogen balance in the immediate preoperative period. Patients with insulin-dependent diabetes who undergo bilateral internal thoracic artery dissections are at increased risk of developing postoperative sternal wound complications. It is imperative that patients with diabetes have aggressive control of their blood sugar levels in the perioperative period. Long-term use of corticosteroids is associated with poor healing, and thus careful handling of tissue is required during surgery followed by meticulous closure of the wound.

Specific Technical Considerations

Specific technical factors that require consideration include internal thoracic artery dissection, excessive postoperative bleeding, reexploration for bleeding, emergency opening of the wound in the intensive care unit, prolonged cardiopulmonary bypass, profound low cardiac output in the immediate postoperative period, and external cardiac massage. Careful control of bleeding points before heparinization ensures adequate hemostasis. After heparin has been administered, no clotting occurs; all capillary ooze must therefore be electrocoagulated and large vessels occluded with metal clips. In repeat operations when the resulting raw surfaces are great, the possibility of excessive bleeding must be contemplated. Only unhurried electrocautery dissection with step-by-step hemostasis can prevent excessive postoperative bleeding. There are times, however, when, despite all the preventive measures taken, postoperative bleeding may require exploration; occasionally, the chest may have to be opened in the intensive care unit to relieve acute tamponade. External cardiac massage may be a lifesaving measure, but it does give rise to sternal wound instability and wound complications and may be relatively ineffective in the early postoperative period. Low cardiac output

and long perfusion time also have adverse effects on wound healing. Strict adherence to aseptic surgical technique and attention to detail during operation are important measures to prevent wound complications.

Wound drainage, with or without sternal instability, is the first sign of possible sternal wound *infection*. The patient may be septic and febrile, but often he or she is otherwise asymptomatic. After the diagnosis of infection is made, the patient is promptly taken to the operating room and is placed under general endotracheal anesthesia. Then the incision is opened wide, and all the necrotic tissues are debrided and excised. The sternal edges are trimmed to ensure viable tissues. After a specimen is obtained for culture and testing for antibiotic sensitivity, the wound is irrigated with a dilute solution of 0.5% to 1% povidone iodine (Betadine) or saline solution. If the patient is not septic and the wound appears to be clean, the sternum is then brought together by means of Robicsek's modification. Otherwise, consideration is given to pectoralis myocutaneous flap (see later). Two large chest tubes are left behind the sternum and are connected to a closed drainage system (Fig. 1-13). A small, soft rubber catheter is often left in the substernal space, and through it continuous 0.5% povidone iodine or antibiotic irrigation solution is administered for 48 to 72 hours. The skin and subcutaneous tissues can be closed over a soft, flat drain connected to a closed suction system. If the quality of the subcutaneous tissues is questionable, the superficial wound should be packed open and delayed closure performed after a few days. In either case, systemic antibiotics should be continued for at least 7 days and for as long as 6 weeks in some patients.

NB *ISCHEMIC NECROSIS*
Operations are now being performed on a much older group of patients, many with multisystemic diseases. Consequently, significant instances of ischemic wound complications may be encountered. In these cases, there is no definite evidence of infection. Only necrotic bone, cartilage, and mediastinal tissues are noted and require careful debridement.

 PLACEMENT OF TUBES
Tubes should never be in direct contact with the aorta, vein grafts, or thoracic pedicle because they may cause local irritation, erosion, and serious hemorrhage (Fig. 1-14). The holes in the tubes should be oriented so that they are not in contact with the heart or the grafts to avoid suction injury and bleeding. The tubes should be placed on the thymic tissues superiorly or laterally in the gutter between pericardiopleural tissues and the undersurface of the sternum (Fig. 1-15).

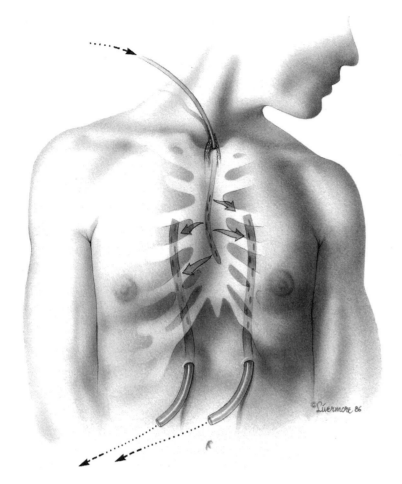

FIG. 1-13. Tube placement for retrosternal antibiotic irrigation.

If the infection is massive or there is extensive necrosis, radical debridement is performed and the sternal wound is left open. When the wound appears to be clean and relatively free of overt infection, muscle flaps are used for secondary closure.

⊘ **NECROTIC CARTILAGE**
Costal cartilages that are necrotic and contaminated must be resected because their retention almost certainly leads to chronic draining sinus tracts.

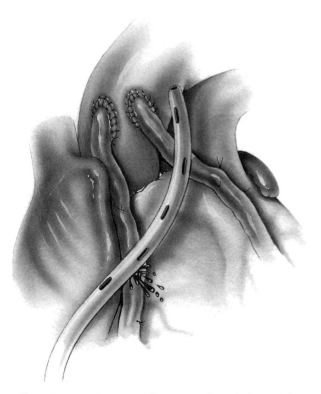

⊘ **FIG. 1-14.** Improper placement of an drainage tube.

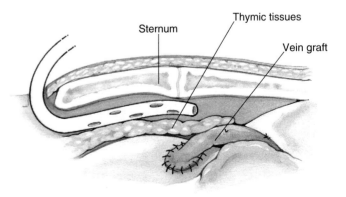

Sternum   Thymic tissues   Vein graft

FIG. 1-15. Correct placement of an irrigation tube.

Technique

Pectoralis Muscle Flap

Through the existing wound, the superficial surface of the pectoralis major muscle is exposed by elevating the overlying skin and subcutaneous tissue proceeding from the midline laterally. Dissection of the muscle off the chest wall is accomplished laterally toward the midline until the parasternal perforator arteries are encountered, usually 2 to 3 cm from the sternal border. The inferior free border of the muscle is identified, and blunt dissection is used to develop the plane deep to the pectoralis major and superficial to the pectoralis minor. A small incision is then made over the muscular insertion, being careful to preserve the cephalic vein for possible future pacemaker insertion. The humeral attachment is then divided, and the flap is advanced medially into the midline wound. The thoracoacromial pedicle must be divided to allow adequate mobility for folding the muscle into the sternotomy wound. When both pectoralis muscles are used, they are sutured together in the midline under slight tension. Occasionally, where one flap is sufficient, the muscle is sutured to the opposite sternal periosteum. The skin flaps are then advanced and closed primarily.

NB *CHOICE OF MUSCLE FLAPS*

Choice of muscle flaps should be thoroughly analyzed before beginning any procedure. The workhorse of mediastinal reconstruction is the pectoralis major muscle. The maximal bulk of muscle can be obtained using turnover pectoralis flaps based on parasternal perforating arteries from the internal thoracic artery. In most wounds of moderate to large size, bilateral flaps are necessary to fill the midline dead space. Occasionally, in narrower defects, a unilateral flap is sufficient.

 ABSENCE OF THE INTERNAL THORACIC ARTERY

The internal mammary artery is often used as a bypass conduit. In these cases, the parasternal perforator arteries have already been sacrificed, and the pectoralis flap should be based on the thoracoacromial pedicle.

 WOUND COVERAGE OF THE LOWER MEDIASTINUM

Regardless of the pectoralis flap technique, the inferior portion of the wound is the most vulnerable. Turnover flaps are not sufficient to cover the lower one-fourth to one-third of the mediastinal structures. Introducing omentum into the chest wound has been described to address such problems. Bringing omentum into the mediastinum necessitates entry into the peritoneum, a maneuver that increases the morbidity of the operation and risks introduction of infection into the abdomen.

An additional and effective technique to cover the lower mediastinal wound is the use of the superior rectus abdominus muscle as a flap.

Technique

The sternotomy incision is extended inferiorly to the umbilicus. The chosen superior rectus abdominus muscle is exposed by elevating skin and subcutaneous tissue to the lateral edge of the muscle down to the level of the umbilicus, where the muscle is divided transversely. During transection of the muscle, the superior epigastric vessels are suture ligated to prevent a donor site hematoma. The muscle is then lifted off the posterior rectus sheath up to the costal margin.

 ABSENCE OF THE INTERNAL THORACIC ARTERY

The superior epigastric artery is the continuation of the internal mammary artery. It is important to know that the internal thoracic artery is intact and patent before mobilizing the superior rectus abdominus muscle. The arteries may have been used as a conduit for myocardial revascularization or been damaged by repeat sternal closure. A selective angiogram is always indicated.

 DAMAGE TO THE EPIGASTRIC ARTERIES

Care is taken not to damage the superior epigastric pedicle that emerges from beneath the costal margin to enter the muscle.

The flap may then be folded superiorly to fill the inferior third of the mediastinum. The rectus is sutured to the pectoralis flaps and the sternal border to maintain its position, and the anterior rectus sheath is repaired with nonabsorbable sutures.

 HEMATOMA AND SEROMA

The most common complication is hematoma or seroma at the donor muscle site, whether pectoralis or rectus abdominus.

More recently, the pectoralis major muscle has been used quite successfully as a myocutaneous flap to cover the infected sternal wound.

Technique

The sternal wound is debrided and irrigated with saline and povidone-iodine solution, as described previously. Bilateral musculocutaneous flaps of the pectoralis major muscle are dissected free off the chest wall to the level of the clavicles above, anterior axillary line laterally, and posterior rectus sheath inferiorly. This is accomplished with an electrocautery and blunt dissection. Perforating arteries are sacrificed.

The myocutaneous flaps are now advanced medially and approximated to each other in the midline over two to three closed-system drainage tubes with absorbable sutures. The skin is then closed with interrupted Prolene or in two layers with absorbable sutures.

Thoracotomy

Posterolateral thoracotomy provides excellent exposure for many closed cardiac procedures, such as resection of coarctation of aorta and its repair, shunting procedures, resection of aneurysms of the thoracic aorta, ductus arteriosus surgery, and closed mitral valve commissurotomy. Anterolateral thoracotomy may be all that is needed for some procedures. In practice, we elect to perform a lateral thoracotomy and extend it anteriorly or posteriorly as needed.

The patient is stabilized securely on the operating table in a lateral position. A small pillow or a homemade roll is placed on both sides of the chest and a small roll is placed under the axilla. Another pillow is placed between the knees. Often the upper leg is extended on a pillow over the flexed lower limb. A wide strip of adhesive tape is stretched from one side of the operating table to the other across the patient's hip for additional stability.

 SCIATIC NERVE INJURY
The tape should be carefully placed so that it does not slip and compress the sciatic nerve.

A skin incision is made approximately one to two fingerbreadths below the level of the nipple, beginning at the anterior axillary line. It is extended posteriorly below the tip of the scapula, then superiorly between the scapula and the vertebral column. After the subcutaneous tissues are divided with cautery blades, the latissimus dorsi and serratus anterior muscles come into view. These muscles are divided, and the scapula is allowed to retract with the shoulder upward, thus providing exposure of the intercostal muscles. Depending on the posterior extension of the incision, the rhomboid and trapezius muscles may need to be divided.

 BLEEDING FROM MUSCULAR BRANCHES
Latissimus dorsi and serratus anterior muscles are quite vascular, particularly in patients with long-standing coarctation of the aorta, and thus their division may result in substantial blood loss. Therefore, it is essential to identify each blood vessel and ligate it securely. Although cautery coagulation may suffice in most situations, larger vessels should be controlled with suture ligatures.

NB *SPARING DIVISION OF THE CHEST WALL MUSCLE*
Often it may be possible to retract the serratus anterior muscle adequately to provide sufficient exposure for thoracotomy. This is particularly indicated in infants and children.

The desired interspace is selected by counting the ribs downward, bearing in mind that the uppermost rib that can be felt is the second rib, not the first. Excellent exposure for patent ductus arteriosus and coarctation of aorta is provided through the fourth interspace. The intercostal muscle is incised in a teasing fashion until the parietal pleura comes into view. This, in turn, is opened, taking care not to injure the underlying lung tissue. The intercostal incision is then completed under direct vision.

 INJURY TO THE LUNG
The anesthetist can attempt to deflate the lungs temporarily to protect the lung parenchyma during entry into the pleural cavity.

 INJURY TO THE INTERCOSTAL VESSELS
The neurovascular bundle is protected by the ribs. The dissection must hug the upper border of the rib to avoid injury to the intercostal artery.

The rib retractor is spread very gradually and incrementally to avoid rib fracture. If additional exposure becomes desirable, either the lower or upper rib is resected or divided posteriorly near its angle.

NB Postoperative pain owing to rib fracture could be markedly decreased if the affected segment is divided and removed to prevent the fractured bone ends from moving against each other.

One or two chest tubes should be placed in the pleural space and brought out anteriorly. The ribs are approximated with four or five interrupted heavy sutures. The serratus anterior and latissimus dorsi muscles anteriorly and the rhomboid and trapezius muscles posteriorly are then accurately and meticulously approximated with either interrupted or continuous sutures. The subcutaneous layer and the skin are then closed.

 NEEDLE (PERFORATING) INJURY TO THE INTERCOSTAL VESSELS
Care must be exercised when placing the pericostal sutures to avoid injuring the intercostal vessels.

NB Intercostal nerve block by injection of a long-acting local anesthetic agent near the intercostal nerves in the most posterior part of the incision two to three interspaces above and below the level of the incision is most effective in reducing postoperative pain.

MINIMALLY INVASIVE APPROACHES

Recently, many surgeons have adopted techniques to complete cardiac procedures through smaller incisions. The goals of these approaches are to decrease the postoperative pain, allow earlier return of the patient to normal physical activities, and achieve a better cosmetic result.

The least invasive of these procedures involves cannulation of the femoral artery and vein and endoscopic techniques to perform valve operations. Such procedures are evolving, and the addition of robotic technology and anastomotic devices will extend their applications.

Two limited incisions can be used for correction of some heart lesions: the lower ministernotomy and the submammary right thoracotomy.

Lower Ministernotomy

Various limited sternotomy approaches have been described. We have found the lower sternotomy through a limited skin incision to be an acceptable approach for atrial septal defects and some ventricular septal defects. It may also be used for off-pump coronary artery bypass graft procedures using the left internal thoracic artery.

Technique

The midline skin incision begins at the level of a line drawn between the two nipples and extends to the tip of the xiphoid process (Fig. 1-16). Dissection must be carried up to the level of the third interspace, and the pectoralis muscle is dissected off the sternum to the right or left side. (For congenital heart defects, the right side is dissected, and for left internal thoracic artery harvest, the left side is used.) A saw is used to open the sternum in the midline to the level of the third interspace. Then an angled bone cutter is used to divide the right or left half of the sternum into the third interspace (Fig. 1-17).

🚫 ***INJURY TO THE COSTAL CARTILAGE***
Every effort is made to ensure that the bone cutter divides the sternal half into the interspace between two ribs and not into the costal cartilage.

🚫 ***INJURY TO THE SKIN INCISION***
The saw may injure the skin edges superiorly. This is avoided by pulling upward with a long narrow retractor on the upper extent of the skin incision to allow the saw to reach the level of the third interspace (Fig. 1-17).

A single- or double-armed thoracotomy retractor can then be placed between the two sternal halves with the bar inferiorly and slowly opened. After opening the pericardium, traction sutures allow excellent exposure of the right atrium, inferior vena cava, lower superior vena cava, and proximal ascending aorta. Direct aortic cannulation can be achieved, but aortic cross-clamping may be difficult through this incision. Secundum and most sinus venosus atrial septal defects can be safely closed on cardiopulmonary bypass with induced ventricular fibrillation.

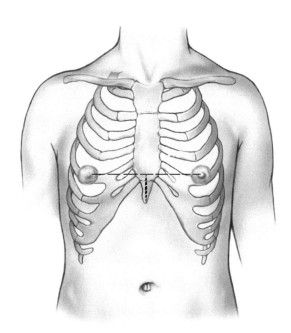

FIG. 1-16. Lower ministernotomy skin incision.

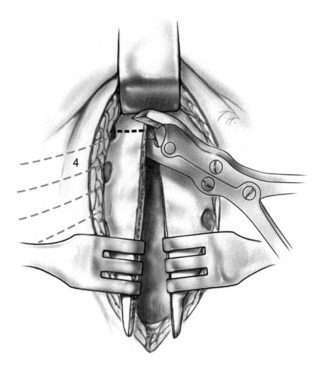

FIG. 1-17. After using a saw to divide the xiphoid and lower sternum, an angled bone cutter is used to divide the right half of the sternum into the third intercostal space.

NB *EXPOSURE OF THE SUPERIOR VENA CAVA*
A tie placed around the tip of the right atrial appendage and pulled inferiorly allows adequate exposure of the superior vena cava.

 INABILITY TO CANNULATE THE LEFT SUPERIOR VENA CAVA
If a left superior vena cava is present, this approach should not be used. Preoperative transthoracic echocardiography or an intraoperative trans-esophageal echocardiogram can usually make this diagnosis.

NB One advantage of the lower ministernotomy incision is that it can be easily extended to a full sternotomy if necessary.

Lower Ministernotomy Closure

The upper and lower portions of the right side of the sternum are reapproximated with one stainless steel wire placed vertically. The left and right halves of the lower sternum are encircled with three or four wires (Fig. 1-18). The vertical wire should not be tightened until all the wires are placed.

 MALALIGNMENT OF RIGHT SIDE OF THE STERNUM
Failure to approximate the upper and lower portions of the divided right hemisternum will result in a bony deformity at the level of the third interspace. Care must be taken to push the upper and lower portions into the same plane before tightening the vertical wire.

 DISTORTION OF THE SUPERIOR ASPECT OF THE INCISION
Tight closure of the muscle layers superiorly will create a dimpling effect. The tissue should be loosely approximated cephalad to the skin opening.

Submammary Right Thoracotomy

This incision is cosmetically very appealing for young girls and women requiring atrial septal defect closure. It may be used for mitral valve operations, although access to the ascending aorta for cross-clamping may be difficult.

Technique

The skin incision is made in the submammary fold of the right breast in an adult or the anticipated future breast fold in a preadolescent girl (Fig. 1-19). This is carried down to the chest wall, and the pectoralis major and pec-

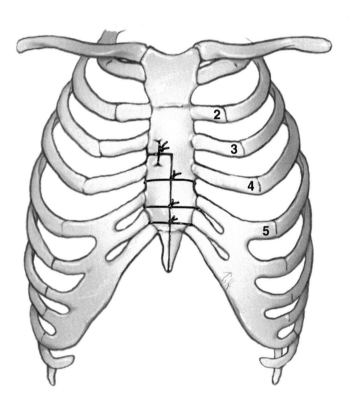

FIG. 1-18. Reapproximation of the lower sternotomy with one vertically placed wire and three horizontal wires.

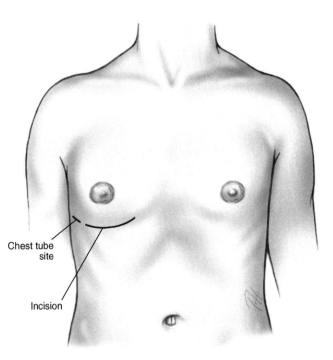

FIG. 1-19. Submammary right thoracotomy skin incision. Note the location of the chest tube.

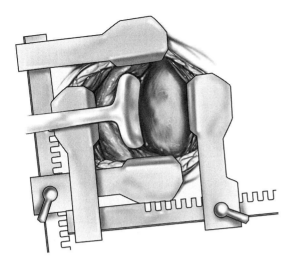

FIG. 1-20. The first single-armed retractor spreads the ribs, the second single-armed retractor retracts the muscle, and a T-shaped retractor holds the lung laterally.

toralis minor insertions onto the ribs are dissected free up to the fourth interspace. The intercostal muscle is divided just on the upper edge of the fifth rib, and the pleural space is entered.

Two single-armed retractors are placed: one between the ribs and the other at a right angle to the first retractor to spread the subcutaneous tissue and muscle. A lung retractor is then used to hold the right lung laterally (Fig. 1-20).

After opening the pericardium, traction sutures can be placed to allow exposure of the inferior vena cava, superior vena cava, and proximal ascending aorta. A tie around the tip of the right atrial appendage retracted inferiorly aids in cannulation of the superior vena cava and ascending aorta.

 INABILITY TO CANNULATE THE LEFT SUPERIOR VENA CAVA
A left superior vena cava is not accessible from this approach.

 DIFFICULT ASCENDING AORTIC CANNULATION
The ascending aorta in older children and adults may be difficult to cannulate through this incision. Femoral arterial cannulation through a small horizontal groin incision may be required.

 DAMAGE TO THE RIGHT INTERNAL THORACIC ARTERY
Injury to the right internal thoracic artery should be avoided by opening the intercostal muscle carefully toward the sternum.

Closure of Submammary Right Thoracotomy

After placing a chest tube through a small stab wound just lateral to the skin incision (Fig. 1-19), the ribs are reapproximated with heavy braided sutures. The muscle, subcutaneous layers, and skin are then closed in layers.

NB *CORRECT CHEST TUBE PLACEMENT*
The chest tube should be inserted through an incision just lateral to the skin opening. Placement of the chest tube lower than the submammary line creates an unnecessary scar that is not hidden by the usual two-piece bathing suit or tube top.

Intercostal nerve blocks with a long-acting local anesthetic in several interspaces can be administered before chest closure from within the pleural space. This decreases the need for parenteral pain medications in the postoperative period.

CHAPTER 2

Preparation for Cardiopulmonary Bypass

EXPOSURE OF THE HEART

Technique

The remnant of the thymus gland is dissected free from the pericardium. The thymic vessels are all electrocoagulated to prevent the formation of a hematoma or troublesome oozing during the operation. The larger ones should be occluded with metal clips. The pleura are peeled away from the inferior pericardium with a dry sponge, thus preventing inadvertent entry into the pleural cavities. The electrocautery blade can be used to incise the pericardium and at the same time coagulate the edges. This maneuver may trigger ventricular fibrillation if the cautery blade touches the heart. It is therefore preferable to incise the pericardium with a pair of scissors or a scalpel. The pericardium can then be opened in the usual inverted T fashion and suspended to skin edges or towels (Fig. 2-1).

The sternal retractor should be opened gradually without traumatizing the sternal edges. It should also be positioned in such a fashion that its cross-arm is in the upper part of the wound. This technique helps to prevent entanglement or overcrowding of various pump lines. The blades of the retractor should be placed as low as possible, and the sternum should be opened only to the extent that is essential for adequate exposure. This prevents possible fracture of the first rib and consequent brachial plexus injury (see Fig. 1-3).

Dissection Around the Aorta

The posterior aspect of the aorta is not always free, and therefore the cross-clamp may not include the entire wall of the aorta (Fig. 2-2). Often it helps to mobilize the aorta, particularly in reoperations, to ensure its complete cross-clamping. A large, curved or right-angled clamp is passed behind the aorta from right to left after some minor sharp dissection. Only when a clear passage is created should the clamp (with an umbilical tape) be reintroduced in exactly the same direction. The tip of the umbilical tape is then picked up by the assistant, and in this way, the aorta can be lifted out of its bed by traction on the tape (Fig. 2-3).

NB   Adventitial tissue on arteries and veins is an integral component of the vascular walls. It should not be violated but kept intact whenever possible.

Incorporation of adequate adventitial tissue in closure of aortotomy or various cannulation sites including the superior vena cava and pulmonary artery is a safe and effective technique. The adventitial component is a natural tissue that acts like a reinforcing felt pledget, adding strength to the closure.

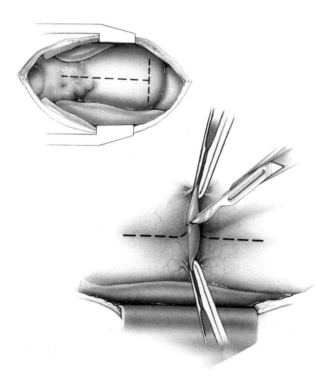

FIG. 2-1. Opening the pericardium.

20

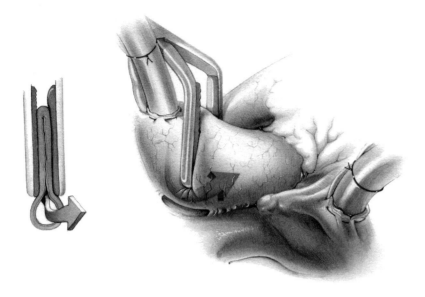

FIG. 2-2. Incomplete cross-clamping of the aorta.

⊘ **INJURY TO THE AORTA**

During dissection and passing of the clamp behind the aorta, caution must be taken to avoid injury to the aorta's posterior wall (Fig. 2-4). If such a complication occurs, it is best to control the bleeding digitally or by packing the area while preparation can be made to initiate cardiopulmonary bypass. While the patient is on bypass, the aorta is opened and the posterior wall is repaired under direct vision (Figs. 2-5 and 2-6).

⊘ **INJURY TO THE RIGHT PULMONARY ARTERY**

On rare occasions when the right pulmonary artery takes a more caudal course, it may be injured during dissection around the aorta. Again, if such a problem arises, it is best to control the bleeding by packing the area and to correct the lesion when the heart is decompressed on full cardiopulmonary bypass. The right pulmonary artery can also be injured during dissection of the superior vena cava, especially when passing a tape around this vessel (Fig. 2-7).

Dissection Around the Cava

Dissection required to pass umbilical tapes around the vena cava in preparation for total cardiopulmonary bypass may be tedious and occasionally may result in injury to the

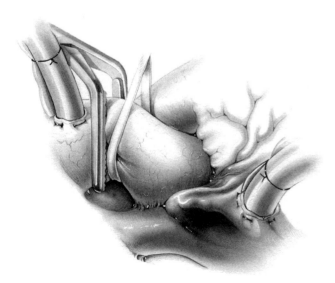

FIG. 2-3. Lifting the aorta from its bed.

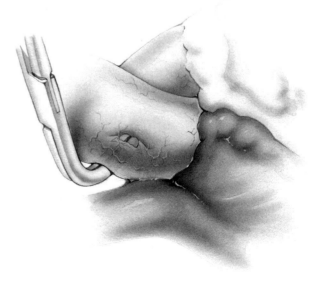

FIG. 2-4. Clamp injury to the aorta.

great veins. The parietal pericardium is divided on each side of the great veins, and a plane is established that allows an appropriate curved clamp to be passed around the cava with ease. The umbilical tapes are then introduced around each vessel with a curved clamp.

 PHRENIC NERVE INJURY
Dissection around the vena cava can be cumbersome, particularly if extensive adhesions from previous surgery are present. The right phrenic nerve coursing along the lateral aspect of the cava and the right atrium on the pleural aspect of the pericardium can easily be injured, either by sharp dissection or injudicious use of cautery. This results in paralysis of the right hemidiaphragm and complicates the ventilatory care of the patient in the postoperative period. The surgeon should therefore attempt to avoid the right phrenic nerve at all costs.

 CAVAL INJURY
Caval injury is initially controlled digitally. Cardiopulmonary bypass is established, and the problem is managed under direct vision. The site of the tear is brought into view by gently retracting the great vein with an atraumatic tissue forceps, at which time it can be sutured with fine Prolene. On rare occasions when the torn caval wall is very friable, the suturing may incorporate an adjacent segment of the intact pericardial wall for buttressing and therefore hemostasis. Tension on the suture line is relieved by means of a curvilinear incision of the pericardium (Fig. 2-8).

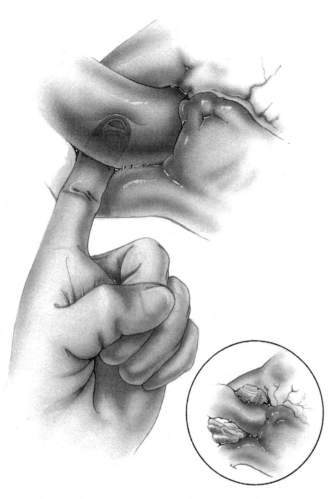

FIG. 2-5. Controlling bleeding after injury to the aorta.

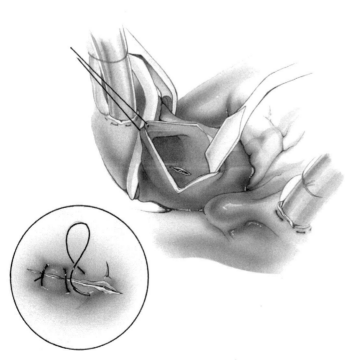

FIG. 2-6. Repair of the posterior wall of the aorta under direct vision.

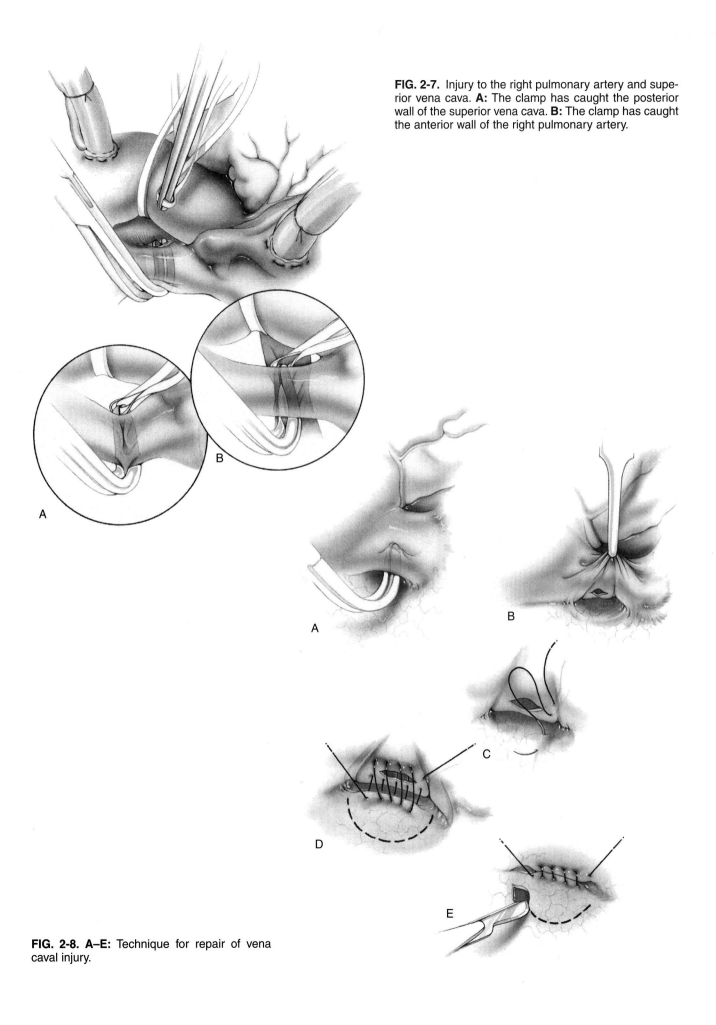

FIG. 2-7. Injury to the right pulmonary artery and superior vena cava. **A:** The clamp has caught the posterior wall of the superior vena cava. **B:** The clamp has caught the anterior wall of the right pulmonary artery.

FIG. 2-8. A–E: Technique for repair of vena caval injury.

AORTIC CANNULATION

Technique

Except in a few specific instances, the aorta is directly cannulated for arterial perfusion during cardiopulmonary bypass. Using a single or double purse-string suture technique with noncutting needles and taking small bites of the adventitia and media as high up on the aorta as feasible are perhaps the least traumatic method of aortic cannulation. A stab wound is created within the purse-string sutures. The tip of the aortic cannula is then introduced atraumatically into the opening (Fig. 2-9). The sutures can be buttressed with felt pledgets to prevent bleeding from the needle holes. The ends of the purse-string sutures, which have passed through a long, narrow rubber or plastic tube, are secured. The tubing is then tied to the aortic cannula and, if desired, further secured to the edges of the wound (Fig. 2-10). The aortic cannula is allowed to fill retrogradely with blood and is then connected to the arterial line, with attention to proper evacuation of air.

NB In patients undergoing reoperation with scarred aortic walls or pediatric patients, it may be useful to insert an appropriately sized Hegar dilator through the stab wound before inserting the aortic cannula.

 AORTIC WALL ATHEROSCLEROSIS
Although this technique of aortic cannulation is a generally safe approach, serious vascular complications may nevertheless occur. The aorta should be routinely palpated for localized thickening and calcific plaques. Transesophageal echocardiography and direct surface echocardiography of the ascending aorta are more sensitive for confirmation and localization of atheromatous changes. The site for cannulation should be disease-free if possible. Usually, the anterior aspect of the aorta just proximal to the base of the innominate artery or the segment along the inner curvature of the aorta adjacent to the pulmonary artery is relatively free of calcification.

 LEAD PIPE OR EGGSHELL AORTA
Lead pipe or *eggshell* aorta is the term used when the entire ascending aorta is calcified. Cannulation or clamping of this kind of aorta has catastrophic complications, namely, strokes and uncontrollable hemorrhage. In such cases, the femoral or axillary artery and right atrial cannulation are used to achieve deep hypothermic cardiopulmonary arrest, and the aorta is then replaced or dealt with appropriately (see Repeat Sternotomy section in Chapter 1).

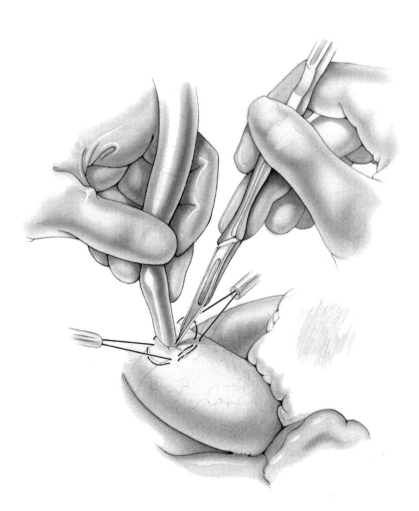

FIG. 2-9. Aortic cannulation.

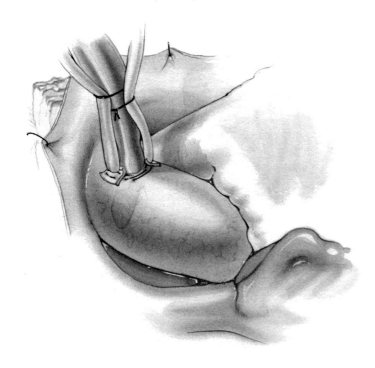

FIG. 2-10. Aortic cannulation, completed.

⊘ SIDE-BITING CLAMPS

Partial occluding clamps should be avoided, especially when aortic pressure is high, unless they are needed to control brisk hemorrhage or other complications. A clamp can crush the diseased wall and give rise to a tear in the intima, resulting in dissection of the aortic wall or disruption with massive bleeding.

⊘ THIN AORTIC WALL

Whenever the aortic wall is thin or friable, the purse-string sutures are reinforced with Teflon or pericardial pledgets on each side of the cannula to prevent any injury to the aortic wall or bleeding from the needle sites (Fig. 2-10).

⊘ LARGE AORTIC CANNULA

Aggressive introduction of too large an aortic cannula through a small aortic opening can tear the aortic wall, dislodge calcific plaques, and cause separation of the intima and dissection around the cannulation site (Fig. 2-11). An expanding adventitial hematoma may be the first sign of traumatic aortic dissection. The cannula must be removed immediately and the cannulation site excluded *carefully* with a side-biting clamp (which in itself may further the dissection) to prevent progression of the dissection. On these occasions, retrograde perfusion through the femoral artery should be established promptly and the aortic injury dealt with under controlled conditions.

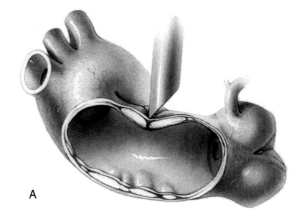

A

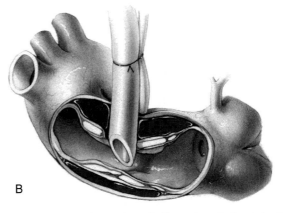

B

FIG. 2-11. Traumatic aortic wall dissection during introduction of a cannula.

SMALL AORTIC CANNULA
An excessively small cannula may create a significant gradient in the perfusion pressure. Too great a length of cannula in the aorta may interfere with perfusion of the arch vessels, especially if the tip enters one of the brachiocephalic vessels. The ideal aortic cannula should have a relatively wide but short tip. Although most commercially available cannula are manufactured with these specifications in mind, the size of the aorta varies in different individuals; therefore, the surgeon must select the appropriate length and width of the cannula judiciously.

NB *SMALL-DIAMETER AORTA*
In patients with a relatively small diameter aorta, the regular cannula may be space occupying, interfering with satisfactory perfusion. Metal- or plastic-tipped, right-angled cannula have good flow characteristics and will not hit the back wall of the aorta.

 SYSTEMIC HYPERTENSION
Whenever the systemic pressure is high, aortic decannulation may become hazardous and result in some troublesome bleeding. The systemic pressure can be lowered to a satisfactory level by temporarily removing some volume through the venous line. The arterial cannula is then removed and its aortic entry site securely sutured. The arterial line is then connected to the venous cannula, and blood is reinfused as needed.

A less effective but useful technique is transient lowering of the blood pressure by digital compression of the main pulmonary artery for decannulation purposes. This technique can also be helpful when cannulating the aorta.

NB *REPAIRING AORTIC INJURY*
If the venous lines have already been removed, the cava can be temporarily clamped, causing the systemic pressure to drop significantly. The aortic cannula is removed, and the now soft, pliable aorta is repaired. The caval clamps are then removed to allow drainage of the venous return into the right atrium. However, it is preferable to recannulate the right atrium and manipulate the blood pressure by adding or removing volume, thereby allowing safe and controlled aortic repair.

RIGHT ATRIAL CANNULATION

Technique

A single, large, dual-stage atriocaval cannula provides satisfactory venous return for most cardiac surgical procedures. This cannula is introduced through a purse-string suture in the right atrial appendage so that the tip lies in the inferior vena cava and the basket lies in the right atrium (Fig. 2-12).

 INJURY TO THE SINOATRIAL NODE
The sinoatrial node is located in the superior end of the sulcus terminalis near the cavoatrial junction (Fig. 2-13). Injury to the sinoatrial node (Fig. 2-14)

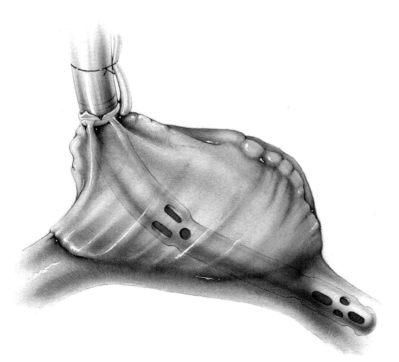

FIG. 2-12. Right atrial cannulation with a single, dual-staged cannula.

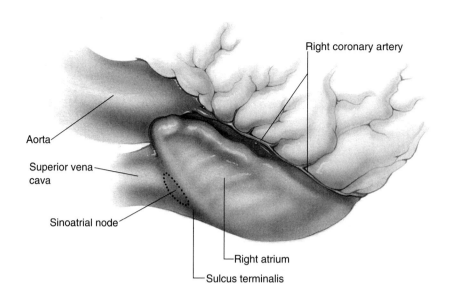

Aorta

Superior vena cava

Sinoatrial node

Right coronary artery

Right atrium

Sulcus terminalis

FIG. 2-13. Surgical anatomy of the sinoatrial node and surrounding structures.

may cause temporary conduction disturbances, which can generally be managed with a temporary atrial pacemaker wire and the infusion of isoproterenol (Isuprel) or dopamine in the immediate postoperative period. Rarely, it may be necessary to pace the atrium permanently.

 INJURY TO THE RIGHT CORONARY ARTERY
The right coronary artery follows a course in the right atrioventricular groove. Whenever the right atrial appendage is clamped, either before or after cannulation, particularly in reoperations, the sinoatrial node and the right coronary artery are at risk of injury (Fig. 2-15). Right coronary artery injury can be treated by bypassing the injured segment

with a saphenous vein graft from the aorta to the middle of the right coronary artery (Fig. 2-16).

 CANNULATION SITE
When the right atrial appendage is too friable, another site on the atrial wall is selected for cannulation. A tear of the auricle can give rise to bleeding, which can be controlled with fine Prolene sutures, sometimes reinforced with a small pledget.

 ATRIAL CANNULATION IN REOPERATION
In reoperation, the atrial wall is sometimes thin and friable, and its dissection can be tedious and hazardous. It is advantageous to leave a segment of

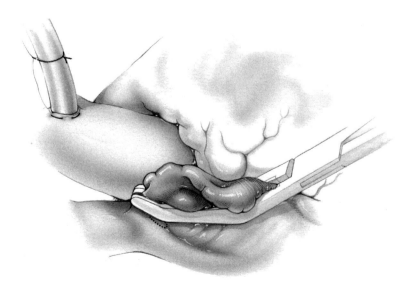

FIG. 2-14. Clamp injury to the sinoatrial node.

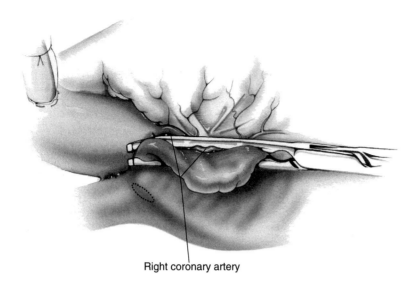

FIG. 2-15. Clamp injury to the right coronary artery.

Right coronary artery

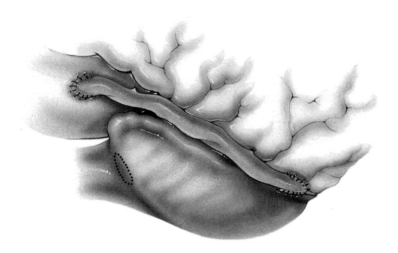

FIG. 2-16. Management of a right coronary artery clamp injury.

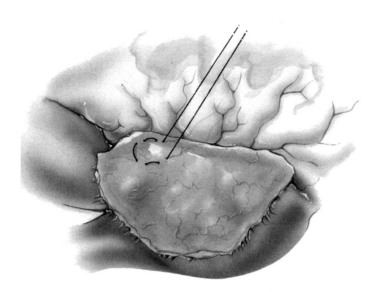

FIG. 2-17. Cannulation through a segment of pericardium left intact on the atrial wall.

pericardium intact on the atrial wall through which cannulation can be performed safely and securely (Fig. 2-17).

BICAVAL CANNULATION

Technique

Some procedures that entail exposure of the inside of the right side of the heart, such as repair of an atrial septal defect, ventricular septal defect, or tricuspid valve, require bicaval cannulation. This can be accomplished by introducing caval cannula through purse-string sutures in the right atrial appendage and lower on the right atrial wall (Fig. 2-18). At present, we cannulate each vena cava directly (Fig. 2-19). This technique provides excellent exposure of the intraatrial anatomy, which is particularly desirable in pediatric patients (see Technique of Direct Caval Cannulation section).

 LOCATION OF TAPE AROUND THE SUPERIOR CAVA

The actual site for placement of tapes around the superior vena cava should be well above (approximately 1 cm) the cavoatrial junction so as not to injure the sinoatrial node (Fig. 2-18).

 PLACING TAPES AROUND THE CAVA

Care must be taken when positioning a right-angled clamp around either the superior or inferior vena cava to avoid tearing the back wall. Sharp dissection may be necessary to create a safe passage for the clamp. In addition, the umbilical tape should be pulled around the cava slowly to avoid a sawing injury.

 EXCESS LENGTH OF THE CANNULA

Excess length of the cannula in the superior vena cava may interfere with flow from the azygos and innominate veins, thereby obstructing the venous return from the upper body. Constant monitoring of the pressure in the superior vena cava can reveal any pressure increase and thus alert the surgical team. Minor manipulation of the cannula usually relieves the obstruction, which can otherwise cause engorgement of the central nervous venous system with neurologic sequela.

NB *LEFT SUPERIOR VENA CAVA*

If a left superior vena cava is present and no innominate vein is noted, it should be directly cannulated.

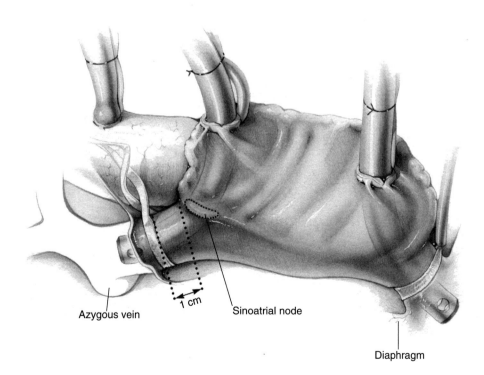

Azygous vein   1 cm   Sinoatrial node

Diaphragm

FIG. 2-18. Placement of tapes around the cava in bicaval cannulation.

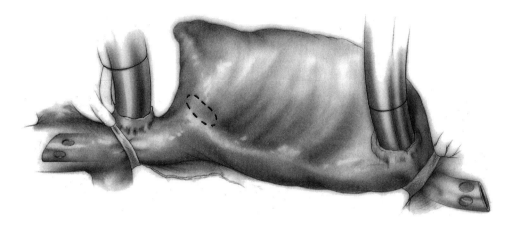

FIG. 2-19. Direct caval cannulation.

TECHNIQUE OF DIRECT CAVAL CANNULATION

Inferior Vena Cava

A 4-0 or 5-0 Prolene purse-string suture is applied at the junction of the inferior vena cava and the right atrium.

NB *FRIABLE INFERIOR VENA CAVA WALL*
Whenever the wall of the inferior vena cava appears to be friable, the purse-string suture should incorporate the parietal pericardium overlying the diaphragm for added security. However, a curvilinear releasing incision of the pericardium should be made.

A stab wound is made in the center of the purse-string suture. The opening is dilated with a straight clamp. An appropriately sized right-angled cannula is introduced, and the purse-string suture is secured around the cannula.

Superior Vena Cava

The pericardial reflection on the superior vena cava is divided to maximally free up the great vein. A rectangular or oval purse-string suture of 5-0 or 4-0 Prolene is placed in the *adventitia* of the superior vena cava close to its junction with the innominate vein. The segment of the superior vena cava with the purse-string suture is excluded with an atraumatic side-biting clamp. The adventitia within the purse-string is divided, and the vein wall is identified and incised with a knife. The opening is enlarged with a pair of Potts scissors. An appropriately sized right-angled cannula is introduced into the lumen, the side-biting clamp is removed, and the purse-string suture is secured.

Alternatively, with the inferior vena caval cannula in place, partial cardiopulmonary bypass is established and the right side of the heart is decompressed. Superior vena caval cannulation is carried out as just described but without the use of the side-biting clamp. This is particu-

larly useful in infants and patients who are hemodynamically unstable.

 SUPERIOR VENA CAVAL STENOSIS
The purse-string suture for superior vena caval cannulation should include adventitial tissue only. When it is tied after decannulation, it should not constrict the diameter of the cava. This is apt to occur when the superior vena cava is relatively small or in children and infants. If tying the purse-string suture narrows the vena cava, a side-biting clamp should be applied, the suture removed, and the opening repaired with a 6-0 or 7-0 Prolene suture.

ADEQUACY OF BYPASS

Cardiopulmonary bypass should be started gradually to avoid a drop in systemic pressure. As the arterial flow and venous return increase, the search for possible problems with the cardiopulmonary bypass is made. It is a simple matter to stop the bypass, if necessary, and rectify any complication at this stage of the operation.

Signs of Aortic Dissection

Excessive pressure in the pump line concomitant with low perfusion pressure signals aortic dissection (see Retrograde Aortic Dissection section).

Only awareness and prompt diagnosis of this complication followed by immediate cessation of cardiopulmonary bypass can ensure patient survival. The cannulation site must be switched from the ascending aorta to one of the femoral arteries, and cardiopulmonary bypass must be reestablished as expeditiously as possible. This permits the continuation of the operation. The reversal of blood flow into the lumen of the arterial system obliterates the false channel and stops the progression of aortic dissection. The problem of ascending aortic injury is then addressed in a controlled situation (see Traumatic Disruption and Dissection of the Ascending Aorta section).

Improper Positioning of Caval Cannula

A decrease in venous return causes distention of the heart. The decrease can be owing to a kink in the venous line, impaction of the basket of the dual-stage atriocaval cannula against the atrial wall, or improper positioning of the caval cannula when separate cannulations are used for the superior and inferior vena cava. The inferior vena caval cannula can be too far down, obstructing the hepatic vein drainage, which can lead to postoperative liver dysfunction. The superior vena caval cannula can be too far up, interfering with innominate and azygos vein drainage. As mentioned previously, inadequate head and neck venous return results in cerebral edema and postoperative neurologic complications. In cases of bicaval cannulation, cardiopulmonary bypass is started with only superior vena caval return, and its adequacy is ascertained by noting the volume of venous return and the central venous pressure. If the central venous pressure remains high, the superior vena caval cannula is manipulated until a near-zero central venous pressure is achieved. The inferior vena caval cannula is then unclamped, and complete venous return is accomplished (see Bicaval Cannulation section).

FEMORAL ARTERY CANNULATION

Technique

The common femoral artery (or occasionally the external iliac artery) is dissected free for a short distance above the origin of the profunda femoris branch. Umbilical tapes are placed around the common femoral artery above the prospective cannulation site *as well as the superficial and profunda arteries distally*. Vascular clamps are applied to the femoral artery both above and below the intended arteriotomy site. The profunda artery may be either clamped or snared. A small transverse arteriotomy is made where the arterial wall appears to be relatively normal. A tapered cannula of appropriate size is then gently introduced through a transverse arteriotomy into the arterial lumen and is secured in place (Fig. 2-20A).

 CANNULA SLIPPAGE
The perfusion pressure may cause the cannula to slip out. It should be secured by tying it to the umbilical tape already placed around the artery (Fig. 2-20B).

 CANNULA INJURY TO THE ARTERIAL WALL
The cannula tip may injure the arterial wall and cause separation of intimal plaque, which can result in retrograde aortic dissection (Fig. 2-21). The cannula must never be too large and should be introduced into the arterial lumen in an area that is relatively disease free.

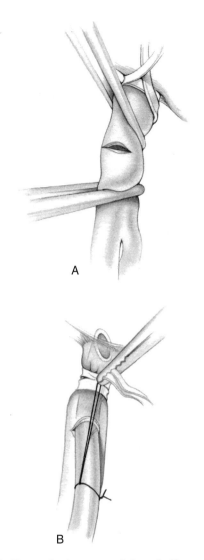

FIG. 2-20. Femoral artery cannulation. **A:** Transverse arteriotomy for introduction of the cannula. **B:** Securing the cannula to the umbilical tape.

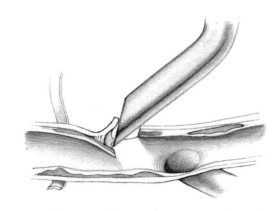

FIG. 2-21. Cannula injury to the common femoral artery causing retrograde aortic dissection.

INJURY TO THE FEMORAL ARTERY
A tourniquet or clamp used to tighten the umbilical tape around the proximal femoral artery and cannula may injure the wall of the artery. This can be avoided by placing a peanut sponge under the umbilical tape before tightening it.

 FEMORAL ARTERY DISSECTION
The surgeon should always look for a column of pulsating blood in the femoral cannula; in the absence of obvious pulsation, it is very likely that the cannula tip is not in the lumen of the vessel.

RETROGRADE AORTIC DISSECTION

Retrograde aortic dissection is indeed a catastrophic complication that may follow femoral or external iliac cannulation. A diseased artery, faulty cannulation technique, and trauma produced by a high-velocity perfusion jet are major factors that may cause a tear of the intima with medial separation. It is therefore essential to introduce an adequately sized, beveled, smooth cannula into a relatively normal vessel in an atraumatic fashion. The perfusion should be started gradually, with the surgeon being cognizant at all times of the possible occurrence of aortic dissection. Its most significant diagnostic feature is *low flow with high arterial line pressure*. The arterial return into the false lumen is responsible for excessive pressure in the arterial line while the actual perfusion pressure is quite low. This leads to a decrease in venous return. If this complication occurs, perfusion should be immediately stopped. The femoral artery or the external iliac artery on the opposite side should then be cannulated if not involved; otherwise, the ascending aorta or the subclavian artery must be cannulated.

TRAUMATIC DISRUPTION AND DISSECTION OF THE ASCENDING AORTA

Intraoperative traumatic dissection or disruption of the ascending aorta is a rare but dramatic complication of open heart surgery. The areas of aortic cannulation, the proximal anastomosis of an aortocoronary saphenous vein graft, and an aortotomy done for exposure of the aortic valve are the usual sites prone to such a complication. This is especially

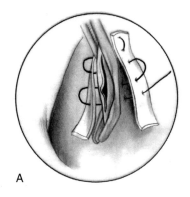

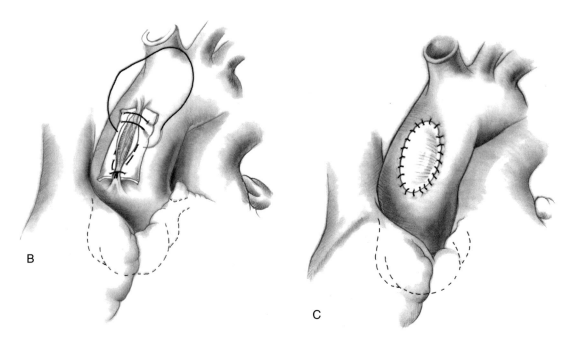

FIG. 2-22. A: Two strips of Teflon felt are sewn below the clamp. **B:** The suture line is reinforced with an over-and-over continuous suture. **C:** The torn segment of aorta is replaced with a patch of pericardium or Hemashield graft (Meadox Medicals, Oakland, NJ).

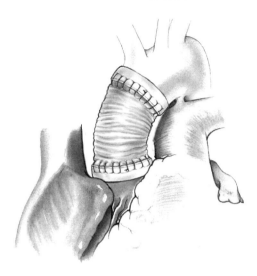

FIG. 2-23. Use of a Hemashield tube graft for aortic disruption.

so in reoperative procedures. Although faulty techniques always predispose a surgical procedure to complications, poor tissue quality and the presence of infection are most commonly the key precipitating factors in the development of aortic injury. The only preventive measure is awareness of a possibility of such complications and meticulous surgical technique in handling the tissues. In most cases, the site of the aortic injury can be excluded with an atraumatic side-biting clamp. Two strips of Teflon felt are then sewn *below* the clamp (Fig. 2-22A). The suture line is then reinforced with an over-and-over continuous suture after removing the clamp (Fig. 2-22B). Alternatively, the torn segments can be excised and replaced with a patch of pericardium or Hemashield graft (Meadox Medicals, Oakland, NJ) (Fig. 2-22C). On the rare occasions when the edges of a tear in the aortic wall are too friable to hold any kind of sutures, the ascending aorta may have to be replaced with a Hemashield tube graft (Fig. 2-23).

CHAPTER 3

Myocardial Preservation

Myocardial protection has clearly made open heart surgery a safe and reproducible technique. There continue to be many modifications of the chemical composition of the cardioplegic solution, the optimal temperature (cold or warm), and the route of infusion (antegrade or retrograde). In response to the numerous different concepts of myocardial preservation, innovative techniques, including specifically designed cannula and tubing circuits, have become commercially available to simplify delivery of cardioplegia.

AORTIC ROOT INFUSION TECHNIQUE

The cannula is introduced into the root of the aorta through a 4-0 Prolene, 1-1/2-circle purse-string suture that is then snugged down and secured to the catheter. Although any large-bore needle or catheter is satisfactory, those that can be introduced using a trocar and have a side arm for direct intraaortic pressure monitoring are preferred by some. This side arm can also function as a venting device.

⊘ *INSUFFICIENT INFUSION PRESSURE*
Distortion of, or insufficient pressure in, the aortic root may prevent adequate coaption of the aortic valve, as will aortic valve insufficiency. The cardioplegic solution therefore enters and overdistends the left ventricle, causing direct myocardial injury.

⊘ *EXCESSIVE INFUSION PRESSURE*
Excessive infusion pressure can traumatize the coronary arteries, both at their ostia and farther along their courses, resulting in ischemic myocardial injury. Accurate monitoring of infusion pressure in the aortic root can be satisfactorily accomplished from the side arm of a specifically designed cannula if desired.

⊘ *AIR EMBOLISM*
Air embolism in the coronary arteries can cause serious myocardial injury. Every effort must be made to

clear the cardioplegic line of any air bubbles. A bubble trap is now incorporated in all the cardioplegia administration systems to minimize this possibility.

⊘ *IMPURITIES IN THE CARDIOPLEGIC SOLUTION*
Impurities and particulate matter may be present in the cardioplegic solution and can occlude terminal coronary arteries, causing myocardial injury. Quality control in the preparation of the cardioplegic solution prevents such complications.

⊘ *WARM CARDIOPLEGIC SOLUTION*
Between infusions, the cardioplegic solution remaining in the tubing warms up. The warm solution should then be flushed out through the free arm of the Y connecting tube before the next infusion into the coronary system.

NB *MAINTAINING UNIFORM COOLING*
Uniform cooling of the myocardium by infusion of cold cardioplegic solution is an integral part of myocardial protection. Temperature probes in various parts of the septum and ventricular wall may be used to monitor myocardial temperature during the course of the operation.

⊘ *INADEQUATE PROTECTION OF THE RIGHT VENTRICLE*
Despite all precautions to keep the heart cool, the anterior surface of the heart tends to rewarm, probably owing to ambient air temperature and the heat radiated from the operating room lights. A gauze pad soaked with cold saline and ice placed over the heart provides additional protection for the right ventricle.

⊘ *TOPICAL HYPOTHERMIA*
Many centers use continuous topical hypothermia with good results. Despite cooling of the heart by infusion of cold cardioplegic solution, the heart's

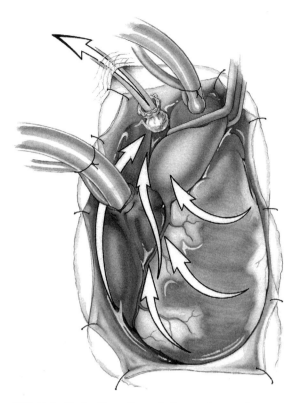

FIG. 3-1. Topical hypothermia by continuous lavage.

outer surface continues to warm. Continuous topical lavage with cold saline and dimming the overhead lights help to prolong myocardial hypothermia. A sump catheter placed in the suprasternal gutter continuously aspirates the saline from the pericardial cavity (Fig. 3-1).

A commercially available cooling "jacket" keeps the heart cold when doing valvular surgery; it is, however, cumbersome and less efficient for coronary surgery.

DIRECT CORONARY ARTERY PERFUSION

When entry into the aortic root is indicated, as in cases of aortic valve replacement, cardioplegic solution is administered directly into each coronary ostium with a cannula. This technique is equally useful in patients who have more than mild insufficiency of the aortic valve.

 CANNULA DAMAGE TO CORONARY OSTIA
Excessive pressure from the cannula against the coronary ostia can cause an intimal tear or late ostial stenosis.

 SIZE OF THE CANNULA
The cannula must be the correct size, and only a snug fit is necessary to prevent leakage. A cannula head that is too large or excessive pressure on the

coronary ostia may not only interfere with satisfactory perfusion of the coronary system but also traumatize the coronary ostia.

 SHORT LEFT MAIN CORONARY ARTERY
The cannula can also interfere with satisfactory infusion of cardioplegic solution if the left main coronary artery is short. A branching artery may have its origin very near the ostium of the left main artery and thus be obstructed by the head of the cannula itself (Fig. 3-2B). Prior knowledge of this anatomy may alert the surgeon so that preventive measures can be taken. The use of a cannula with side holes prevents this complication. A flexible, hand-held, soft-tipped cannula with a collar around the tip (e.g., a DLP cannula, Medtronic, Minneapolis, MN) can provide satisfactory infusion of cardioplegic solution directly into the coronary arteries (Fig. 3-2A). The collar around the tip presses against the aortic wall and the coronary ostium to prevent spillage of cardioplegic solution into the aorta.

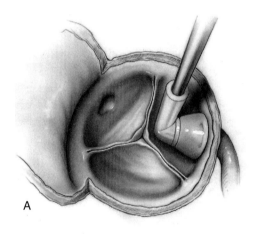

A

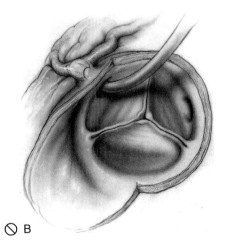

B

FIG. 3-2. A: Hand-held cannula for direct infusion into the coronary artery. **B:** Cannula advanced into the coronary artery causing obstruction at the bifurcation.

MYOCARDIAL PRESERVATION BY THE RETROGRADE PERFUSION METHOD

Retrograde infusion of cardioplegic solution into the coronary sinus is very efficient, but its effectiveness in perfusing the right atrium, right ventricle, and inferior wall of the left ventricle may not always be adequate. The technique provides retrograde perfusion of segments of myocardium that may not be equally perfused by the antegrade route in patients with severe coronary artery disease. To ensure optimal myocardial protection, an integrated method of antegrade and retrograde cardioplegia delivery is used in most centers.

Almost all retrograde cannula are dual lumen for the purpose of infusion of cardioplegic solution and monitoring of pressure in the coronary sinus. A balloon, inflatable or self-inflating, surrounds the distal body of the cannula, approximately three-eighths of an inch from the tip, proximal to the flow holes. A stylet is provided for ease of proper placement.

Technique

Through a stab wound in the center of a 4-0 Prolene purse-string suture in the mid-atrium, a special retroplegia cannula (e.g., Research Medical, Inc., Midway, UT; DLP; Sarns, 3M Healthcare, Ann Arbor, MI) is introduced and directed into the coronary sinus. The correct position of the cannula is verified by palpation. The stylet is withdrawn when the cannula is in a satisfactory position. The purse-string suture ends are snugged through a tourniquet, which is then tied to the cannula.

NB When difficulty is experienced in placing the retrograde cannula, it is often possible to elevate the decompressed heart while on bypass, visualize the course of coronary sinus, and direct the cannula tip.

⊘ PERFORATION OF THE CORONARY SINUS
The stylet and cannula must be advanced into the coronary sinus very gently and stopped if any resistance is felt. The coronary sinus wall is very thin and can be perforated by the cannula tip.

The tear in the coronary sinus must be dealt with by closing the epicardium carefully over the tear with a fine Prolene suture or patching it with a piece of autologous pericardium when the patient is on full cardiopulmonary bypass to prevent stenosis or occlusion of the coronary sinus (Fig. 3-3).

NB *MONITORING PERFUSION PRESSURE*
The pressure monitor on the cannula is monitored at all times. Perfusion pressure must be kept above 20 mm Hg and below 45 mm Hg. To accomplish

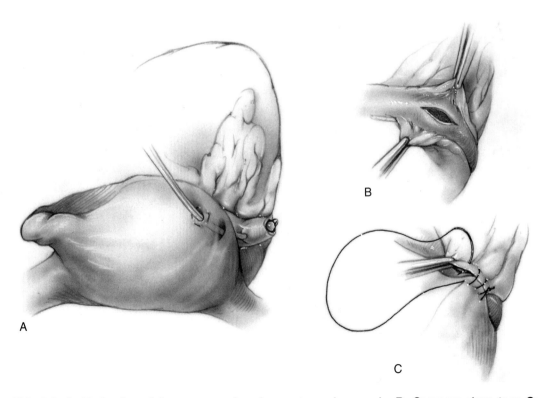

FIG. 3-3. A: Perforation of the coronary sinus by a retrograde cannula. **B:** Coronary sinus tear. **C:** Suture closure of the coronary sinus tear by epicardial tissue.

this, the position of the cannula or the perfusion flow must be adjusted accordingly.

NB *MONITORING PERFUSION TEMPERATURE*
The perfusionist monitors the temperature of the cardioplegic solution as it leaves the delivery system. The temperature can also be monitored as the solution enters the coronary sinus through specially designed retrograde cannula (e.g., Sarns).

⊘ *SPILLAGE OF CARDIOPLEGIC SOLUTION INTO THE RIGHT ATRIUM*
The balloon when inflated *should* minimize spillage of cardioplegic solution into the right atrium. This is more likely to occur when the balloon is inflated manually.

⊘ *INADEQUATE INFUSION OF CARDIOPLEGIC SOLUTION INTO THE RIGHT CORONARY VEIN*
If the cannula is advanced too far into the coronary sinus, the inflated balloon may obstruct the right coronary vein–coronary sinus junction, thus preventing any *direct* infusion of cardioplegic solution into the distribution of the right coronary vein.

Retrograde Cardioplegic Infusion by the Open Technique

When bicaval cannulation has been performed and the right atrium is opened, cardioplegic solution is administered directly into the coronary sinus. The balloon of the

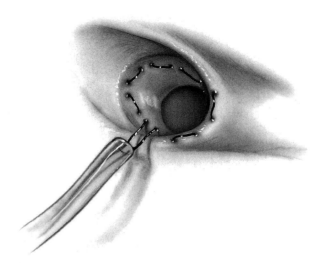

FIG. 3-4. Purse-string suture within the coronary sinus for direct placement of the cannula.

cannula is kept at the ostium of the coronary sinus with a purse-string suture of fine Prolene to prevent leakage of cardioplegic solution into the right atrium (Fig. 3-4). This technique is particularly useful in pediatric cardiac surgery. Alternatively, a catheter with a manually inflatable balloon is used. The balloon is inflated snugly to prevent backflow and to secure it in the appropriate position.

⊘ *INJURY TO THE CONDUCTION TISSUE*
Purse-string sutures must be placed on the inside of the coronary sinus ostium to prevent injury to the conduction tissue.

CHAPTER 4

Venting and Deairing of the Heart

Venting of the left side of the heart is an effective technique for cardiac decompression and air removal. It is particularly useful when a dry field is desired for precise repair of intracardiac defects.

LEFT VENTRICULAR APICAL VENTING

The apex of the left ventricle provides a satisfactory and accessible site for venting and is particularly effective for removal of air trapped in the ventricular cavity. However, it is rarely used today. Its relevance becomes important when left ventricular venting is necessary before repeat sternotomy (see Repeat Sternotomy section in Chapter 1).

Technique

The region of the left ventricular apex may be thin walled and covered by fat. The site chosen for insertion of the vent must be well away from the branches of the coronary arteries and free of loose myocardial fat. There can be bleeding from this ventricular site after removal of the vent catheter.

A double-armed, 2-0 nonabsorbable suture is passed in a U-shaped fashion through a suitable site near the left ventricular apex buttressed with rectangular Teflon felt pledgets. The distance between the stitches on the Teflon felt should be equal to the diameter of the vent catheter. The suture ends are then passed through a narrow plastic tube as a tourniquet.

With a no. 15 knife blade, a 3- to 4-mm incision is made in the center of the U-shaped stitch. This opening in the left ventricular apex is then dilated with a hemostat so that the vent catheter can be introduced gently into the left ventricle. The tourniquet is then snugged down and secured to the vent catheter. If any catheter side hole remains outside the heart, the vent will be ineffective.

When the heart is beating, gravity siphonage of the vent is usually adequate to decompress the heart and or remove trapped air bubbles. When the heart is fibrillating or motionless, particularly after the administration of cardioplegia, the vent should be connected to gentle suction with adequate negative pressure to decompress the heart. When the catheter is removed, the U-shaped stitch is tied down snugly and if necessary reinforced with a few simple sutures.

 LENGTH OF THE CATHETER
When an excessive length of the catheter is introduced into the left ventricle, its tip may traverse the aortic valve and drain much of the pump flow. This rare problem can occur particularly in infants and small children (Fig. 4-1).

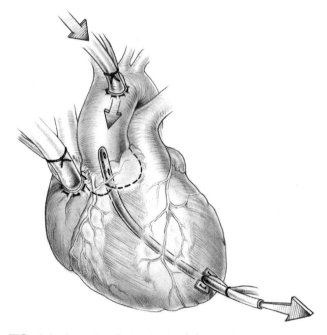

FIG. 4-1. A vent catheter in the left ventricle crossing the aortic valve; pump flow is being suctioned.

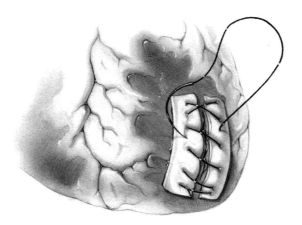

FIG. 4-2. Repair of a tear in the left ventricular apex.

○ *SUCTION INJURY*
Excessive suction can damage the left ventricular endocardium. For this reason, some vents have a double lumen and the second lumen can be left open to air. Alternatively, and probably a safer technique, the vent tubing can be vented with a one-way valve.

○ *TEARING OR BLEEDING*
When there is a tear or excessive bleeding from the left ventricular apex, the heart is decompressed. Long strips of Teflon felt with nonabsorbable sutures are used to repair the tear, as in techniques for resection of a left ventricular aneurysm (Fig. 4-2). This is probably most safely accomplished with the heart arrested with cardioplegia.

○ *AIR IN THE VENTRICULAR CAVITY*
If suction is too great or the apical opening is too large, air may be sucked into the left ventricular cavity around the vent site.

VENTING THROUGH THE RIGHT SUPERIOR PULMONARY VEIN

Venting through the right superior pulmonary vein is convenient, effective, and our technique of choice. After clamping the aorta, through a stab wound in the center of a rectangular or oval purse-string suture on the right superior pulmonary vein, the vent catheter is introduced into the left atrium and through the mitral valve into the left ventricle. The purse-string suture is then passed through a narrow rubber tube and snugged down (Fig. 4-3).

○ *DISSECTING THE ADVENTITIA WITH THE SUTURE*
The adventitia within the purse-string suture over the right superior pulmonary vein should be dissected free to prevent any obstruction to the smooth insertion of the vent catheter.

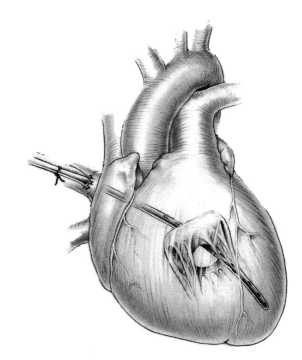

FIG. 4-3. Venting through the right superior pulmonary vein.

○ *INJURY TO THE PHRENIC NERVE*
When placing sutures on the right superior pulmonary vein, care should be taken to avoid the phrenic nerve, which runs on the parietal pericardium along the anterolateral aspect of the right superior pulmonary vein. This is more likely to occur in reoperations.

○ *REINFORCING THE SUTURE*
When tissues are thin and friable, the purse-string suture should be reinforced with Teflon felt.

○ *AIR EMBOLISM*
Air embolism can be eliminated by cross-clamping the aorta or fibrillating the heart before placing the vent catheter.

○ *VENT INJURY*
The catheter should be introduced gently and allowed to cross the mitral valve into the left ventricle without excessive force to prevent injury of the mitral valve or perforation of the left atrium or left ventricle. This complication is more likely when the heart becomes flaccid after infusion of cold cardioplegic solution. An unexplained pooling of blood in the pericardial cavity should herald the occurrence of such a catastrophe. The tear should be located and repaired with pledgeted sutures before continuing with the operation (Fig. 4-4).

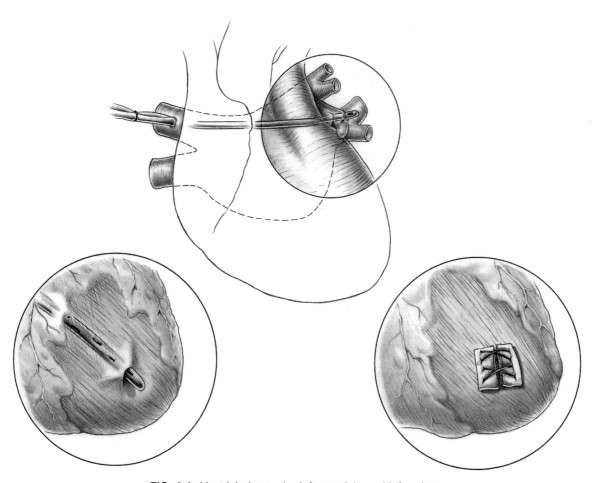

FIG. 4-4. Vent injuries to the left ventricle and left atrium.

🚫 ***DIFFICULTY PLACING VENT INTO LEFT ATRIUM***
Sometimes the vent will not pass easily into the left atrium. In these cases, the vent can be positioned after the heart is opened by passing a right-angled clamp through an atrial septal defect or patent foramen ovale into the opening on the right superior pulmonary vein. The vent is then pulled into the left atrium and positioned appropriately.

VENTING THROUGH THE SUPERIOR ASPECT OF THE LEFT ATRIUM

The left heart can also be vented through the superior aspect of the left atrium between the aorta and superior vena cava. This technique is similar to that described earlier for the right superior pulmonary vein. It is rarely used because it is cumbersome and control of bleeding from the vent site can be difficult (Fig. 4-5).

PULMONARY ARTERY VENTING

A simple but highly effective method to decompress the heart is to introduce a vent catheter through a purse-

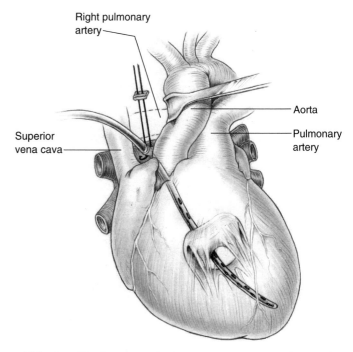

FIG. 4-5. Venting through the superior aspect of the left atrium.

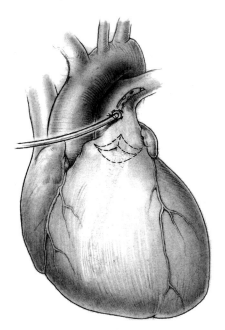

FIG. 4-6. Venting through the pulmonary artery.

string suture on the anterior surface of the pulmonary artery (Fig. 4-6). This technique prevents overdistention of both the right and left sides of the heart without the risk of systemic air embolism.

 PULMONARY ARTERY TEAR
The wall of the pulmonary artery may at times be paper thin and delicate, resulting in a tear at the vent site. This can be prevented by using pledgets on the purse-string suture. The pulmonary artery tear, if it occurs, can easily be repaired with direct suturing reinforced with pledgets.

VENTING THROUGH THE FORAMEN OVALE

We have found venting the left atrium and left ventricle through the foramen ovale in patients with congenital heart disease very useful. With this technique, a dry field is maintained for precise repair of heart defects.

Technique

With the right atrium open, a small, right-angled vent is introduced through the foramen ovale and connected to low suction. If the foramen ovale is not patent, a stab wound is made in the fossa ovalis. At the end of the procedure, the vent is removed and the opening is closed with fine suture.

DEAIRING OF THE HEART

Air embolism is indeed a serious complication of cardiac surgery, and every precaution should be taken to minimize its occurrence. A very effective way to minimize air embolism is to flood the operative field with carbon dioxide. This can be achieved by introducing a constant flow of carbon dioxide gas through sterile intravenous tubing anchored to the pericardium. The carbon dioxide displaces air (specifically nitrogen) and will dissolve in the blood when the heart is allowed to fill.

The heart usually starts to beat soon after the aortic cross-clamp is removed. When warm blood is administered in a retrograde fashion as the aortotomy is being closed in patients undergoing aortic valve replacement or as the atriotomy is being closed in patients undergoing mitral valve surgery, the heart may at times begin to beat spontaneously before the removal of the aortic cross-clamp (see Chapter 5). With each beat, the heart ejects free air bubbles that may be trapped inside it. Every cardiac surgery team has its own preference to deair the heart. We use the following technique.

The venting system, if used, is discontinued, and the heart is allowed to fill slowly by reducing the venous return. The cardioplegia administration site on the aorta or a residual opening on the aortotomy site is kept open with the tip of a right-angled clamp to facilitate venting and displacement of blood and air. At times, saline or blood can be injected slowly through the left ventricular vent, if in place, to displace air and blood through the aortic opening. The heart is shaken and the left atrial appendage is carefully invaginated into the left atrium to displace air bubbles.

 CLOTS AND THE LEFT ATRIAL APPENDAGE
Blood clots have a tendency to lodge in the left atrial appendage, particularly in patients with mitral stenosis and chronic atrial fibrillation. This can easily be detected by transesophageal echocardiography. If present, these clots must be removed.

Very gentle ventilation is begun. Often the heart has regained spontaneous rhythm and begins to eject blood through the aortic opening. A slotted vent needle is now introduced into the aortic opening and high suction is applied to it. The heart is allowed to fill and the aortic cross-clamp is removed. Transesophageal echocardiography is used routinely to monitor left ventricular function and evaluate the adequacy of valvular repair and function as well as the presence of residual air in the heart. As the left ventricular function improves, good ejection expels residual air. Occasionally, despite all these maneuvers, a pocket of air appears to be trapped in the apex of the left ventricle. By elevating the head of the table, good left ventricular contraction will often eject these trapped air bubbles out of the heart. If air still remains, the patient is placed in the Trendelenburg position, a large-bore needle is introduced into the apex of the left ventricle, and blood and air are aspirated. The right superior pulmonary vein, left atrial appendage, and roof of the left atrium in the gutter between the superior vena cava and aorta may also be subjected to needle aspiration.

 NEEDLE INJURY TO THE LEFT VENTRICLE
When the left ventricle appears to be dilated and thin, and the patient's tissues are delicate, needle aspiration of the left ventricle apex may be hazardous and cause bleeding. The needle site may require suture closure. We rarely use needle aspiration.

NB A long, 14- or 16-gauge needle passed through the anterior wall of the right ventricle and through the septum into the left ventricle near the apex is a safe and effective technique to aspirate residual air. The right ventricle entry site may need suture closure if bleeding continues after administration of protamine.

Another useful technique is to allow blood to eject from the left ventricle through the open end of left ventricular vent cannula that is buried in a pool of blood in the pericardial cavity. Any air trapped in the ventricle or atrium will gradually be ejected.

NB This technique requires the heart to be full and ejecting; otherwise, air may be sucked *into* the heart.

SECTION II

Surgery for Acquired Heart Disease

CHAPTER 5

Surgery of the Aortic Valve

Degenerative calcific change affecting the aortic valve is now the most common indication for aortic valve replacement in the United States and Western Europe. In some parts of the world, rheumatic fever continues to be the predominant cause of valvular heart disease.

Patients with congenital bicuspid aortic valve are prone to develop calcification of the valve leaflets resulting in aortic stenosis requiring surgical intervention at a younger age. However, most commonly, calcific aortic valve disease presents late in life. Consequently, other degenerative occlusive lesions, such as carotid artery disease and coronary artery disease, often coexist in these patients. Occasionally, the mitral and, rarely, the tricuspid valves may also be involved in the disease process. All these lesions may require concomitant surgical treatment. Therefore, it is essential to identify and evaluate all the relevant lesions precisely so that appropriate surgical management can be planned and performed in a systematic fashion.

MYOCARDIAL PRESERVATION

Detailed techniques for preservation of the myocardium have already been discussed in Chapter 3. A modified synchronized technique for myocardial protection has been used in our practice for valvular surgery, particularly for aortic valve disease.

Technique

With a retrograde cardioplegic cannula in place in the coronary sinus and an antegrade cannula in the aortic root, cardiopulmonary bypass is initiated and moderate hypothermia (28°–30°C) is achieved. The aorta is clamped, and 1,000 mL of cold blood cardioplegic solution (4°–8°C) is administered into the aortic root (see Chapter 3). Myocardial activity cease, and electrocardiographic monitoring reveals a flat line.

 LEFT VENTRICULAR DISTENTION
Antegrade administration of blood cardioplegic solution into the aortic root can only be satisfactorily accomplished if the aortic valve is relatively competent (see Chapter 3). Presence of significant aortic valve insufficiency results in backflow of the cardioplegic solution into the noncontracting left ventricular cavity. This causes left ventricular distention and possible myocardial injury. Thus, when the aortic valve is incompetent, the blood cardioplegic solution should be administered using a retrograde technique to achieve complete cardiac standstill. In addition, a left ventricular vent should be placed via the right superior pulmonary vein. Myocardial protection can be augmented by administering cardioplegic solution into the coronary ostia after the aorta has been opened.

 DIFFICULTY IN CANNULATION OF CORONARY SINUS
Rarely, the retrograde cannula cannot be introduced safely into the coronary sinus. Bicaval cannulation is performed, and the retrograde cannula in placed in the coronary sinus under direct vision (see Chapter 3).

Cardioplegic arrest of the heart using a retrograde technique alone may at times be slow, particularly when the heart is enlarged. Aortotomy should be performed and cardioplegic solution administered directly into the coronary arteries.

 CALCIUM DEPOSITS
The aortic leaflets may become so deformed because of calcific deposits that they physically obstruct cannulation of the coronary arteries and prevent satisfactory administration of blood cardioplegic solution. In this case, the left coronary cusp should be quickly

excised to facilitate direct cannulation and infusion of blood cardioplegic solution into the left coronary ostium. Infusion into the right coronary artery can be performed when the heart has been arrested and the diseased aortic valve has been excised.

Cold blood cardioplegia is administered (usually every 10 minutes) in a retrograde fashion to ensure the complete cessation of electrical activity of the myocardium. Between cardioplegia doses, cold oxygenated blood is continuously infused through the retrograde cannula whenever clear visualization of the aortic root is not required (such as placement of valve sutures in the sewing ring of the prosthetic valve). For optimal protection of the right ventricle, direct infusion of blood cardioplegic solution into the right coronary artery is carried out every 20 minutes, and ice wrapped with gauze is placed topically on the heart to minimize surface rewarming.

When the aortic valve has been seated and the valve sutures are being tied, the patient is rewarmed. Retrograde infusion of cold blood or cold blood cardioplegic solution through the coronary sinus is continued to ensure a com-plete cessation of myocardial activity. When the aortotomy closure is started, warm blood is infused retrogradely through the coronary sinus. Often concurrent with closure of the aortotomy, normal cardiac activity is observed. Of course, if the patient has undergone concurrent coronary artery bypass grafting, blood cardioplegia or cold blood can be infused simultaneously antegradely through the vein grafts and retrogradely through the coronary sinus.

 RIGHT CORONARY ARTERY AIR EMBOLISM
Infusion of warm blood using the retrograde technique is continued for several minutes after the cross-clamp is removed to minimize the risk of air bubbles trapped in the aortic root entering the right coronary artery.

EXPOSURE OF THE AORTIC VALVE BY TRANSVERSE AORTOTOMY

A low transverse incision is perhaps most commonly used and is preferred by many surgeons (Fig. 5-1). The epicardial fat and adventitial tissue from the right ventricular outflow tract and pulmonary artery may overlie

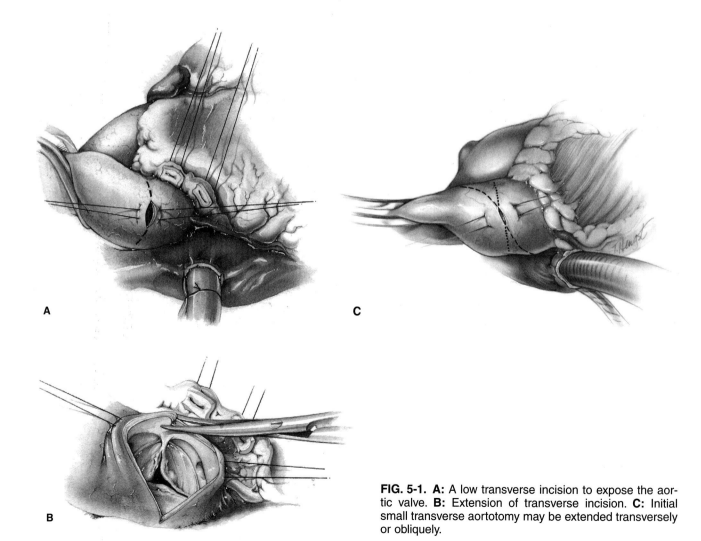

A

B

C

FIG. 5-1. A: A low transverse incision to expose the aortic valve. **B:** Extension of transverse incision. **C:** Initial small transverse aortotomy may be extended transversely or obliquely.

the desired line of aortic incision. These can be dissected free and retracted with a few pledgeted sutures (Fig. 5-1A). Fine Prolene sutures are inserted in the adventitia of the aortic wall on each side of the proposed incision line, which should be 10 to 15 mm above the origin of the right coronary artery. When the ascending aorta has been cross-clamped, the aortic wall is incised for a short distance between these sutures. A small leaflet retractor is introduced into the lumen of the aorta to expose the aortic valve.

RETRACTOR INJURY
Often the aortic wall is dilated and thinned out, particularly in elderly patients with poststenotic dilation. Aggressive traction may result in a transverse tear of the wall of the aortic root (Fig. 5-2). This may necessitate replacement of the ascending aorta or patch repair of the aortic wall.

Under direct vision, the opening is then extended on both sides; care must be taken to stay approximately 10

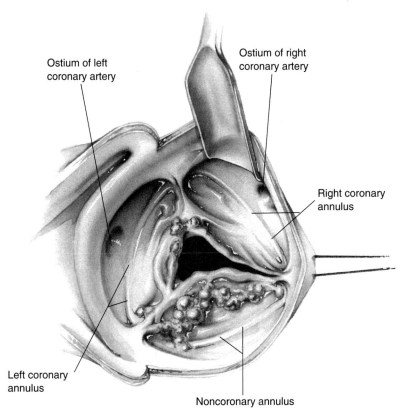

Ostium of left coronary artery

Ostium of right coronary artery

Right coronary annulus

Left coronary annulus

Noncoronary annulus

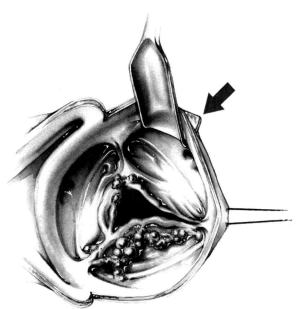

FIG. 5-2. Top: Surgical view of a diseased aortic valve. Note that the aortotomy is approximately 10 mm above the commissures. **Bottom:** Retractor injury to the aortic wall.

mm above the aortic commissures (Fig. 5-1B). Alternatively, the incision can be extended obliquely upward or downward, converting it to an oblique incision or tailoring it to provide optimal exposure (Fig. 5-1C, dashed line).

 AORTOTOMY TOO CLOSE TO THE RIGHT CORONARY OSTIUM
Poststenotic dilation, which is commonly seen in patients with aortic stenosis and congenital bicuspid aortic valve, may distort the aortic root and cause upward displacement of the ostium of the right coronary artery. The usual transverse aortotomy may then be too low and impinge on the right coronary ostium. Care must be exercised in these patients to identify the right coronary take off before making the aortotomy.

EXPOSURE OF THE AORTIC VALVE BY OBLIQUE AORTOTOMY

An oblique or hockey-stick incision is started high on the medial aspect of the aorta and is then continued diagonally downward into the noncoronary sinus to 10 mm above the aortic annulus. The aortic walls are then retracted on each side (Fig. 5-3). This incision is particularly useful in patients with small aortic roots.

 EXCESSIVE INFERIOR EXTENSION OF THE AORTOTOMY
The lower limit of the incision should be well above the aortic annulus to avoid difficulty in placing sutures in the annulus for insertion of the prosthesis. This will also facilitate the aortic closure.

 RIGHT VENTRICULAR HEMATOMA
Epicardial fat overlying the right ventricle is very friable and if traumatized can develop into a large hematoma in heparinized patients. The epicardial fat can be gently retracted away from the operative field with large felt traction sutures (Fig. 5-1A).

SURGICAL ANATOMY OF THE AORTIC VALVE

The aortic valve has three cup-shaped leaflets or cusps: the noncoronary cusp, the left cusp, and the right cusp. These spring from three crescent-shaped valvular annuli within the expanded Valsalva's sinus. The plane of the aortic annuli forms the line of demarcation between the left ventricular cavity and the aorta.

Attachments of the aortic valve to the left ventricular outflow tract are both muscular and membranous (Fig. 5-4). The three fibrous annuli are all associated with somewhat different structures. The noncoronary annulus is singular in that it does not give rise to a coronary artery and is attached to the left ventricle only by membrane. Adjoining halves of the left and noncoronary annuli and the small area beneath the intervening commissure, the fibrous subaortic curtain, are continuous with the aortic (anterior) leaflet of the mitral valve. Below the noncoronary and right coronary annuli and the intervening commissure lie the central fibrous body and the membranous septum, which are divided into atrioventricular and interventricular segments by the contiguous attachment of the nearby tricuspid valve. This membrane usually circles under the noncoronary annulus and merges with the aortic (anterior) leaflet of the mitral valve. The His's bundle passes into the muscular ventricular septum just below

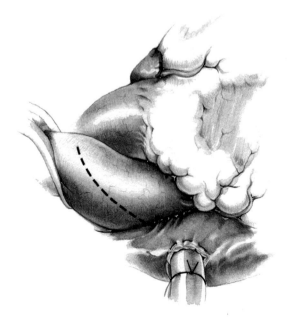
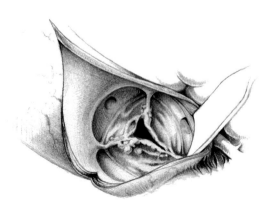

FIG. 5-3. Oblique incision to expose the aortic valve.

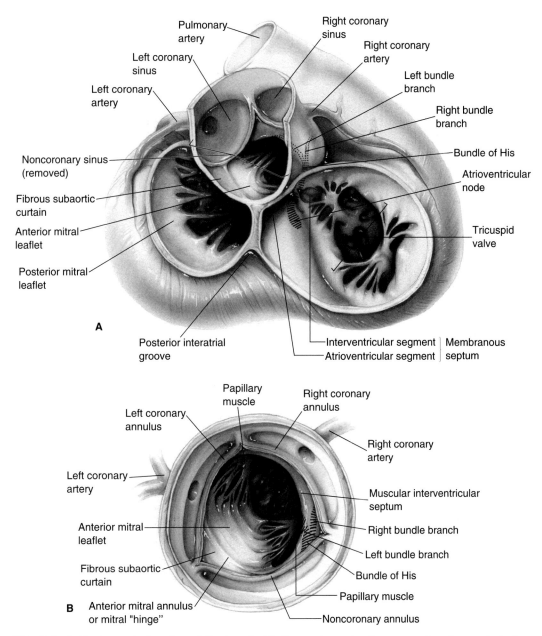

FIG. 5-4. A: Posteroanterior view of the heart with the aorta and pulmonary artery transected above the sinuses. The atria have been removed at the level of the atrioventricular valves. The noncoronary sinus has been excised at the noncoronary annulus, and the aortic leaflets have been removed. **B:** Superior view into the aortic root. The leaflets have been excised.

the membranous septum before dividing into left and right bundle branches. These travel inferiorly and downward along the medial side of the left ventricular outflow tract. This conduction tissue is, therefore, close to portions of the noncoronary and right coronary annuli. Behind the noncoronary sinus, and in direct apposition to it, are the interatrial groove and parts of the left and right atria (thus explaining the rupture of an aneurysm of the noncoronary sinus of Valsalva into these cavities).

Part of the right coronary annulus, as mentioned earlier, is directly attached through the central fibrous body to the muscular septal wall. It courses along the right ven-

tricular outflow tract, merging at its commissure with the left coronary annulus adjacent to the pulmonary valve annulus. The right coronary artery originates from the upper part of the right coronary sinus of Valsalva and courses down the right atrioventricular sulcus. The left or anterior segment of the left coronary annulus underlies the only part of the aortic root not related to any of the cardiac chambers. The right or posterior half of the left coronary annulus is in apposition to the left atrium. The left main coronary artery arises from the upper part of the left sinus and runs a short but variable distance behind it before dividing into its branches.

EXCISION OF THE AORTIC VALVE

The diseased valve leaflets are excised with scissors, leaving a 1- to 2-mm margin at the annulus (Fig. 5-5). The calcified segments of the annulus are crushed between pituitary rongeurs, and the calcium fragments are gently milked away or excised (Fig. 5-6).

 LIMITS OF EXCISION
Excision of the aortic valve too close to the annulus may disrupt the annulus and leave little tissue to hold the sutures securely. Therefore, a margin of valve leaflet must be left behind that may be trimmed away subsequently if it is deemed necessary.

DETACHMENT OF CALCIUM PARTICLES
Care must be taken not to let pieces of calcium fall into the left ventricular cavity because they can result in systemic embolization. The sucker tip is detached, and the assistant must suction all debris as the valve leaflets are being excised. A folded segment of sponge or tampon may be placed in the left ventricle after valve excision before attempting further removal of calcium from the aortic annulus (Fig. 5-7). The tampon will swell and fill the left ventricular outflow tract. Calcium particles or debris fall onto the tampon or sponge instead of being lost in the left ventricular cavity. The left ventricular cavity is flushed and irrigated with cold saline solution. The tampon or sponge is then removed.

NB Some institutions may require the tampon or the sponge to be radiopaque.

 OCCLUDING THE CORONARY OSTIA
To prevent coronary embolization during calcium removal or extraction of the sponge, the coronary ostia can be temporarily occluded with a cotton swab, a hand-held blood cardioplegic cannula, or the tip of the suction head. These precautions are especially useful for protection of the left coronary ostium; the right ostium is less likely to catch calcium particles because of its anterior position and the fact that it is often covered by the blade of a retractor.

 ANTERIOR MITRAL LEAFLET DETACHMENT
Because of the continuity of portions of the aortic and mitral valves, the aortic (anterior) mitral leaflet can become detached from its annulus during excision of the aortic valve leaflets. The surgeon should also be sensitive to this possibility during the removal of calcium and the trimming of the aortic annulus near the left and noncoronary cusps (Fig. 5-8). The aortic (anterior) mitral leaflet is especially likely to become detached with the removal of the noncoronary cusp; this results in a defect in the aortic root, which opens directly into the left atrium. This misadventure is most likely to occur when there is massive calcification of the aortic valve extending, as it often does, onto the mitral valve. The aortic (anterior) leaflet of the mitral valve must then be reattached to its annulus by means of interrupted pledgeted suture incorporating the torn peripheral edge of the mitral valve and the annulus (Fig. 5-9).

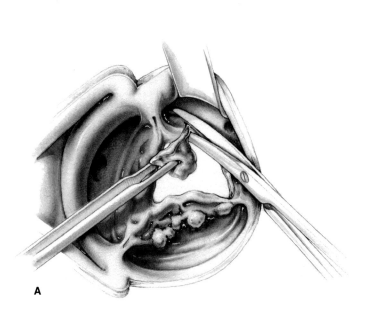
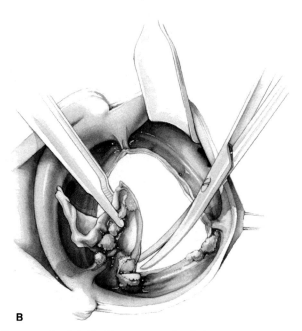

FIG. 5-5. Excising the diseased aortic valve. **A:** Right Coronary leaflet. **B:** Noncoronary leaflet.

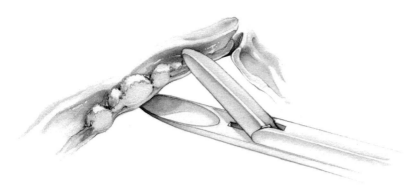

FIG. 5-6. Crushing and removing calcium fragments from a diseased annulus.

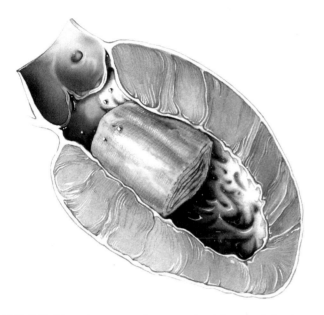

FIG. 5-7. Use of a sponge to prevent calcium particles from falling into the left ventricular cavity.

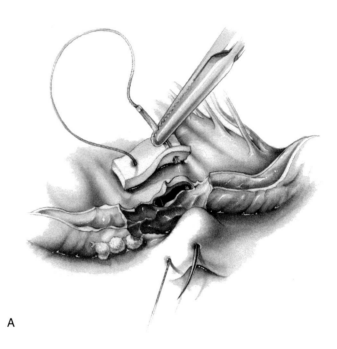

A

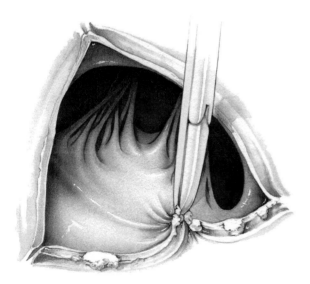

FIG. 5-8. Injudicious pulling on the calcium embedded in the aortic annulus, creating a defect through the aortic root to other chambers of the heart or the pericardium (see Fig. 5-4).

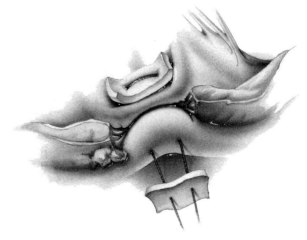

B

FIG. 5-9. A: Partial detachment of the anterior mitral leaflet, creating a defect in the left atrium. **B:** The defect is closed with pledgeted sutures, which can also be used to anchor the prosthesis.

ANNULAR WEAKNESS
Aggressive pulling on the calcium while attempting to remove it from the aortic annulus may occasionally weaken an area, which can result in perforation either outside the heart or into the other chambers of the heart. The weakened area must be recognized and approximated with pledgeted sutures (Fig. 5-9).

SIZING THE AORTIC PROSTHESIS

The prosthesis chosen for replacement of the aortic valve must fit snugly in the annulus. Three simple sutures are inserted, one in each commissure (Fig. 5-10A) or in the annulus near each commissure (Fig. 5-10B). The aortic orifice can be opened up by applying traction to these three sutures. At times, sutures placed in the nadir of the

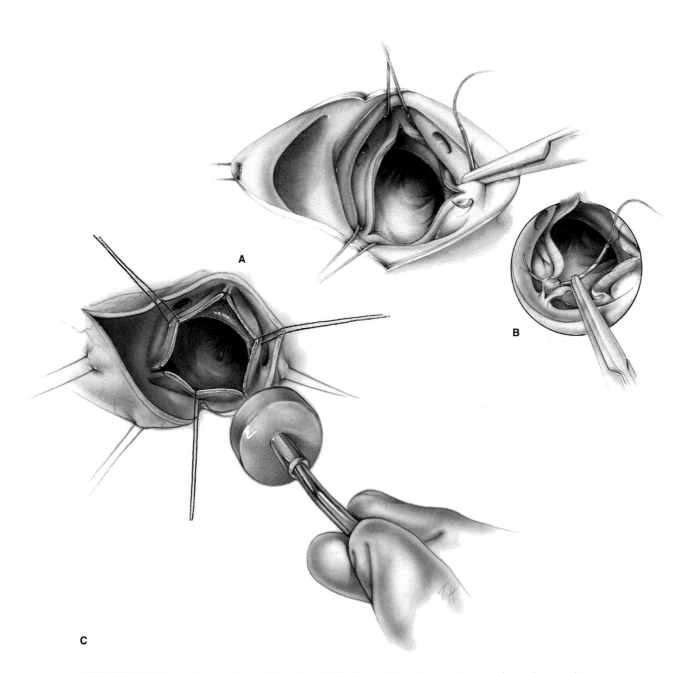

FIG. 5-10. A: Three simple sutures being inserted in the aortic valve annulus, one in each commissure. **B:** Sutures can be alternatively placed through the annulus near each commissure. **C:** Sutures placed in the nadir of the annulus for optimal sizing.

annulus between the commissures will open the left ventricular outflow tract more optimally, making sizing much easier (Fig. 5-10C). Differently sized obturators are then serially introduced into the annulus, starting with the smallest one. The correctly sized prosthesis is thus selected.

LOOSE PROSTHETIC FIT
A very loose fit indicates that the patient will not benefit from the largest possible prosthesis, which will have the optimal hemodynamics.

TIGHT PROSTHETIC FIT
A tight fit will make satisfactory seating of the prosthesis somewhat difficult. In fact, it is quite dangerous to oversize the prosthesis because it may disrupt the aortic annulus and make closure of the aortotomy difficult.

MEASURING THE ANNULUS
Because the sizers are exact replicas of the respective prostheses, the annulus must be measured with the sizer that corresponds to the specific prosthesis. This is particularly relevant when using a prosthesis designed for supraannular implantation.

It is important to distinguish the left ventricular outflow tract, aortic annulus, and sinotubular junction when sizing for an appropriate prosthesis. This may not be of much significance in patients with pure aortic insufficiency. However, in patients with severe aortic stenosis, there may be left ventricular outflow tract narrowing owing to septal hypertrophy. The poststenotic dilation may sometimes obscure or destroy the sinotubular ridge or junction. Therefore, the diameter at each level may be different, making sizing for an appropriate prosthesis somewhat demanding. It is prudent to attempt to size the left ventricular outflow tract, aortic annulus, and sinotubular junction separately so that an appropriate type of prosthesis can be selected to fit the annulus.

CALCIFIED AORTIC ROOT
When the aortic root is heavily calcified or there are calcific ridges in the wall of the aorta, the sizer cannot easily be introduced into the aortic root. The surgeon must then visually judge the size of the prosthesis.

NB ***DECALCIFICATION OF THE AORTIC ROOT***
Often there is calcification in the aortic root involving the sinuses extending into the coronary artery ostia. With experience, it is possible to decalcify the aortic root wall in specific locations to facilitate

implantation of an appropriately sized prosthesis. The technique consists of gently crushing segments of calcified intima with a rongeur and then removing them from the aortic wall to facilitate the operation. Implantation of a stentless aortic bioprosthesis or a homograft using a modified subcoronary technique will reinforce the weakened segment of the aortic wall.

AORTIC WALL TEAR
It is important not to pull away calcified segments from the wall of the aortic root to prevent a buttonhole injury. The connection of the calcified segment with the intima must be sharply divided with scissors.

TECHNIQUE FOR SUTURE INSERTION

The prosthesis is sewn into position with interrupted sutures. The most popular is 2-0 Tevdek or Ticron, double-armed with tapered needles. A deep bite of the annulus is first taken. The suture ends are then either held taut by an assistant or inserted in correct order in a circular ring (Fig. 5-11). When all the annular sutures have been placed, they are passed through the sewing ring of the prosthesis in an orderly fashion, either singly or in a vertical mattress technique. Alternatively, each suture can be passed through the annulus and the valve sewing ring in one step (Fig. 5-12). Sometimes some segments of the annulus are not in full view. Pulling on a previously placed suture will improve the exposure (Fig. 5-13). This suture can be held taut, either by the surgeon's hand or placed in the circular ring.

NB ***REMOVAL OF EMBEDDED CALCIUM PARTICLES***
The tip of the suture needle can be used to dislodge calcium particles deeply embedded in the myocardium (Fig. 5-14).

SUTURE SECURITY
The sutures must be individually tested to make certain that they include a good, secure bite of the annulus; they may tear through if they include only degenerative leaflet tissues or a narrow rim of the annulus. If the suture appears to be insecure, it is either removed or converted to a figure of eight (Fig. 5-15) and eventually passed through the sewing ring of the prosthesis in a horizontal mattress fashion.

PLEDGETED SUTURES
When the annulus is calcified or too friable to hold sutures securely, pledgeted sutures (2-0 Ethibond or

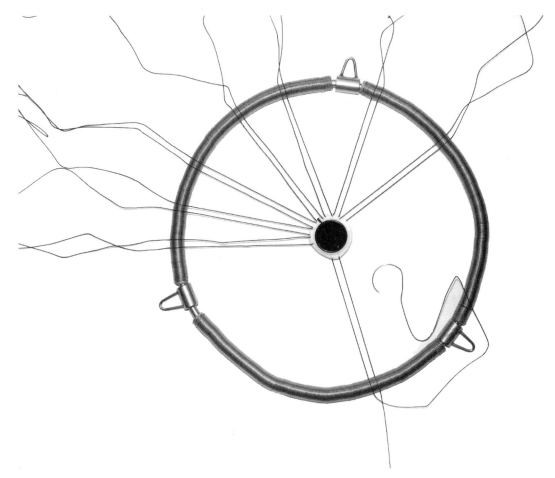

FIG. 5-11. Ring for placement of sutures in sequence.

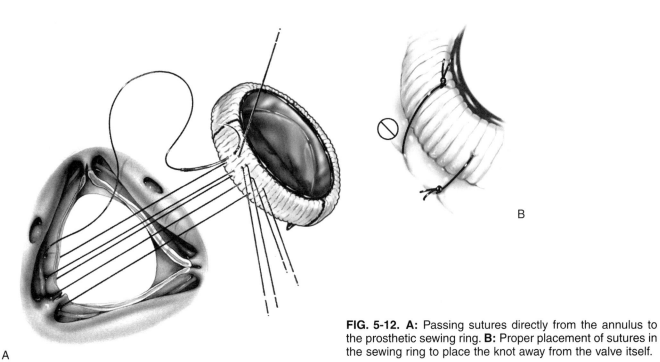

FIG. 5-12. A: Passing sutures directly from the annulus to the prosthetic sewing ring. **B:** Proper placement of sutures in the sewing ring to place the knot away from the valve itself.

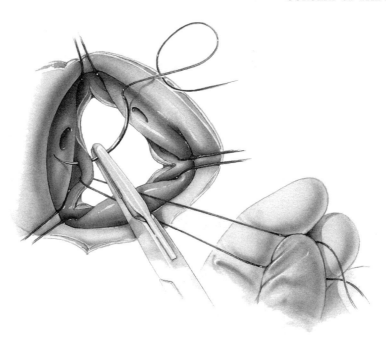

FIG. 5-13. Exposure for placement of sutures in the aortic annulus.

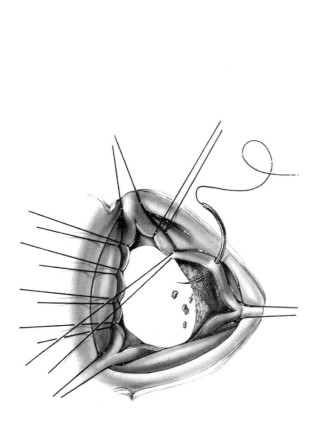

FIG. 5-14. Using the tip of the needle to dislodge calcium embedded in the myocardium.

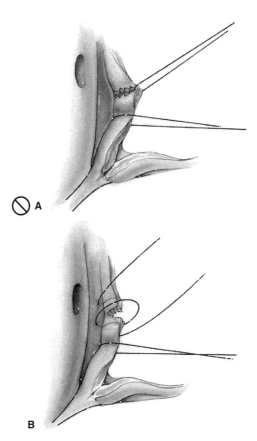

FIG. 5-15. Converting an insecure suture **(A)** to a figure-of-eight suture **(B)**.

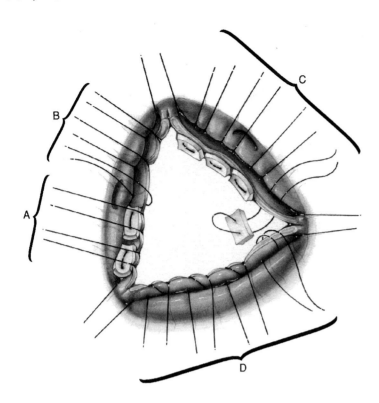

FIG. 5-16. **_A:_** Inserting the sutures in an everted fashion, with the pledgets lying above the annulus in the aorta. **_B:_** Simple sutures. **_C:_** Inserting the sutures from below allows the pledgets to remain subannular. **_D:_** Figure-of-eight sutures.

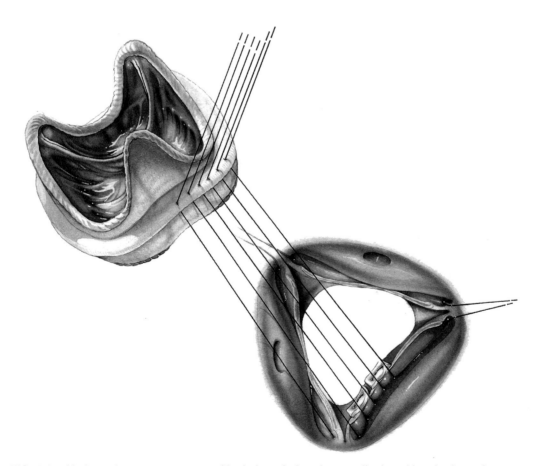

FIG. 5-17. Horizontal mattress sutures, with pledgets below the annuli, placed in a horizontal mattress fashion in the prosthetic ring.

Ticron) are satisfactory alternatives. It is technically easier to insert the sutures in an everted fashion, with the pledgets lying above the annulus in the aorta (Fig. 5-16A). The alternative technique for placing sutures from below, which allows the pledgets to remain subannular in the left ventricle, provides a secure and satisfactory buttressing effect (Fig. 5-16C). In our practice, we use this technique only in specific situations; we fear that the pledgets may at times interfere with normal movement of a disc prosthesis. Also, if a suture breaks, the loose pledgets must be retrieved. The prosthesis is removed to find the loose pledget and then replaced. Therefore, pledgets should only be used on the ventricular aspect of the annulus in very specific situations, e.g., endocarditis. The sutures are then inserted in the prosthetic ring in a horizontal mattress fashion (Fig. 5-17). The routine use of pledgets has markedly reduced the occurrence of paravalvular leaks.

HEART BLOCK

Deeply placed sutures near the noncoronary and right coronary annuli can injure the conduction tissues and give rise to various forms of heart block (Fig. 5-18). When there is massive calcification extending onto the ventricular septum or when the tissues are friable because of endocarditis or abscess formation, this complication may be inevitable. Temporary ventricular wires are recommended for all patients undergoing aortic valve surgery. If the patient is still in complete heart block at the completion of the procedure, temporary atrial wires should be placed to allow for atrioventricular sequential pacing. A permanent pacemaker may need to be implanted before the patient's discharge if atrioventricular conduction has not been reestablished.

INJURY TO THE LEFT CORONARY ARTERY

The precise site of suture placement in the aortic annulus is often obscured by pathologic changes, calcifications, and deformities. Deep sutures placed near the left coronary annulus may puncture the left main coronary artery as it passes behind the aortic root (Fig. 5-19). This is indeed a very grave error, and the surgeon must always be sensitive to this possibility and take every precaution to avoid its occurrence; otherwise, massive myocardial infarction will ensue. This error should be rectified by immediate removal of the inflicting suture. If the structural or functional integrity of the left main coronary artery is in any way jeopardized, bypass grafting of all its major branches must be performed.

DRYING OF THE TISSUE PROSTHESIS

Tissue prostheses tend to lose moisture when in a dry field, a process accelerated by heat generated from the operating room overhead lights. The valvular tissue will be permanently damaged, which may result in premature prosthetic failure. As a precaution, the prosthesis must be kept moist by intermittently rinsing it with normal saline solution at room temperature.

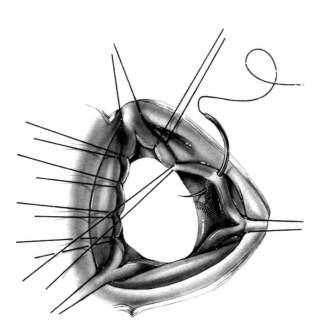

FIG. 5-18. Injury to the conduction tissues caused by deeply placed sutures.

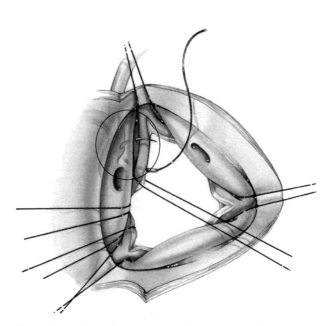

FIG. 5-19. Left main coronary artery punctured by a deep suture near the left coronary annulus.

SUTURE PLACEMENT IN PROSTHETIC SEWING RING

Suture needles are passed through the prosthetic sewing ring from below upward, with the needle exiting at the junction of the outside half with the inside half of the sewing ring (Fig. 5-12B).

Sutures placed in such a fashion in the sewing ring of a bioprosthesis are well away from the tissue–sewing ring interface and avoid traumatizing or perforating the tissue leaflets. Similarly, the suture knots will face away from the orifice of a mechanical valve, preventing contact with the disc or leaflets.

BIOPROSTHETIC STRUTS POSITION

Before placing sutures in the prosthesis, every precaution should be taken to ensure that the tissue prosthesis is oriented so that the struts do not obstruct the coronary artery ostia.

SEATING THE PROSTHESIS

When all sutures have been accurately placed in the sewing ring, the prosthesis is gently lowered and fitted snugly in the annulus. It is customary with many surgeons to rinse the sutures with saline solution for its lubricating effect, which will allow the sutures to be pulled through the sewing ring more smoothly.

NARROW SINOTUBULAR JUNCTION

When the sinotubular junction of the ascending aorta is narrower than the aortic annulus, the appropriate size prosthesis will be too large to pass through it. In such situations, the holder is removed and the prosthetic low-profile valve [e.g., St. Jude Medical (Minneapolis, MN) or Medtronic Hall prosthesis] is turned on end, then lowered and seated safely in the aortic annulus (Fig. 5-20).

CHEMICAL OR THERMAL INJURY TO A BIOPROSTHESIS

Antibiotics or other chemical solutions may react with glutaraldehyde and produce irreversible damage to the tissue prosthesis. Therefore, these valves should be rinsed only with room temperature physiologic saline solution.

PROSTHETIC DISTORTION

Some tissue prostheses, notably the Baxter Carpentier-Edwards porcine, Baxter Edwards bovine pericardial, and Hancock II bioprostheses, have flexible

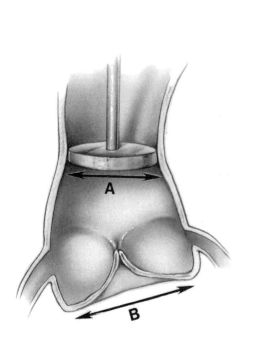

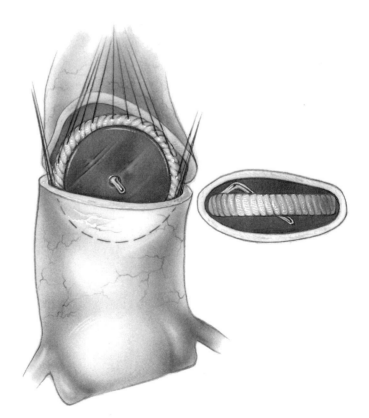

FIG. 5-20. Technique for implantation of the optimal size prosthesis through a narrow ascending aorta. **A:** Sinotubular diameter. **B:** Annular diameter.

SURGERY OF THE AORTIC VALVE / 59

rings. The surgeon should not attempt to manipulate and push a large prosthesis down into a relatively small aortic annulus because such force could distort the flexible rings and the valve leaflets causing incompetence.

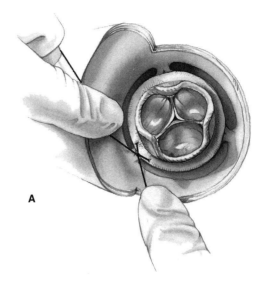

 OBSTRUCTIVE ELEMENTS
No redundant tissue fragment, calcium, or subannular pledgets should protrude into the left ventricular outflow tract in such a way as to prevent satisfactory opening and closing of the valve (Fig. 5-21). Normal valve function must be ensured and any obstructing element removed before final anchoring of the prosthesis.

After the prosthesis has been satisfactorily seated, the sutures are tied down securely and cut short.

 DIRECTION OF TYING
The direction of tying the sutures should always be parallel to the curve of the sewing ring (Fig. 5-22). Any deviation from this principle may traumatize the leaflet tissue or the prosthetic valve through contact with the suture material or the surgeon's finger tip.

 LONG SUTURE ENDS
Sutures, when tied, must be cut short; and the direction of the knot must be leaning toward the periph-

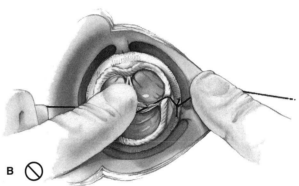

A

B

FIG. 5-22. Tying sutures down parallel with the direction of the sewing ring **(A)**, not across the prosthetic leaflets **(B)**.

ery of the sewing ring of the prosthesis. A long suture end will scratch the leaflet tissue, resulting in chronic irritation, injury, and, finally, perforation of the tissue leaflets. A long suture end can also protrude into the prosthetic orifice and interfere with the normal closure of the occluding mechanism of the mechanical valve.

 ABNORMAL LOCATION OF THE CORONARY ARTERY OSTIUM
Occasionally the orifice of the left main coronary artery is located next to the commissure of the aortic annulus. It is important to orient the tissue prosthesis so that the struts do not face the coronary ostium (Fig. 5-23).

UNOBSTRUCTED PROSTHESIS FUNCTION
Before closure of the aortotomy, it is imperative that normal, unobstructed opening and closing of the prosthesis be visually verified.

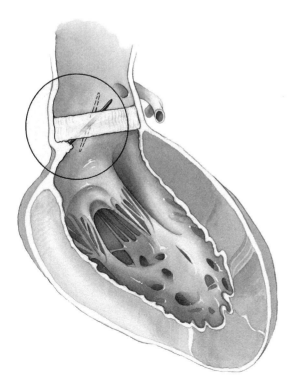

FIG. 5-21. Subannular projection of a bit of calcium or a pledget, which may limit motion of the valve.

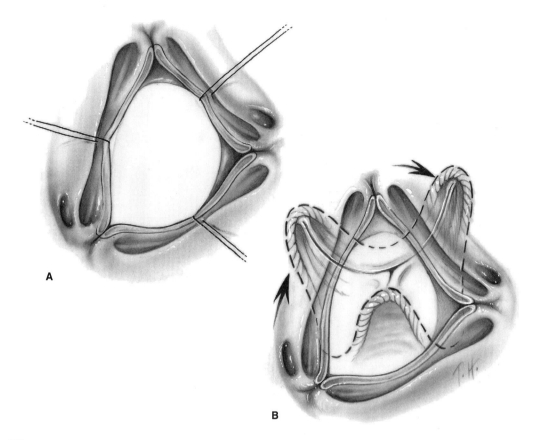

FIG. 5-23. A: Aberrant location of coronary artery ostia at the commissures. **B:** Rotation of the bio-prosthesis to prevent coronary artery flow interference by the struts.

 SEPTAL HYPERTROPHY
Patients with long-standing aortic stenosis will have marked septal hypertrophy. Similarly, hypertensive heart disease causes concentric hypertrophy of the left ventricle, including the septum. The surgeon must be cognizant of the discrepancy in size of the left ventricular outflow tract and the aortic annulus. Special technical details should be considered when implanting prostheses of different design.

The single-disc group of prostheses, exemplified by the Medtronic-Hall mechanical valve, has the advantage of rotatability. The surgeon should take advantage of this design feature and fine-tune the rotation of the prosthesis to ensure free movement of the disc. The smaller part of the disc that descends into the left ventricle must be well away from the septum for fear of its becoming stuck against it.

The bileaflet group of prostheses, exemplified by the St. Jude Medical, which can also be rotated, is subject to the same principle of free movement of the leaflets. The leaflets are often positioned parallel to the septum. In extreme cases of septal hypertrophy, there may be relatively decreased flow across the leaflet close to and parallel with the septum. This possible theoretical disadvantage probably has no hemodynamic consequence.

When the left ventricular outflow is markedly limited by septal hypertrophy, some septal muscle mass can be excised, e.g., in patients with idiopathic hypertrophic subaortic stenosis (see Fig. 6-4 in Chapter 6). At times, multiple vertical myotomies allow the left ventricular outflow tract to dilate and open up.

AORTOTOMY CLOSURE

The aortotomy closure is usually accomplished with continuous 4-0 Prolene sutures in a double-layer fashion starting at each end of the incision. The sutures are then tied to each other anteriorly (Fig. 5-24).

 BLEEDING FROM THE AORTOTOMY ENDS
Troublesome bleeding from the aortotomy ends can be prevented to some extent by suturing back and taking a bite of undivided aortic wall before continuing forward along the incision (Fig. 5-24, inset).

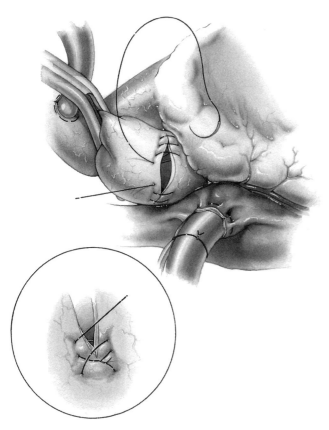

FIG. 5-24. Aortotomy closure with a special precaution to prevent bleeding from the ends of the incision.

delicate aortic tissue as easily. The aortotomy suture line can be reinforced with strips of autologous pericardium initially if the aorta is noted to be thin walled or friable (Fig. 5-25).

 CONTROLLING BLEEDING FROM THE AORTOTOMY ENDS
To control bleeding from either end of the aortotomy, it is prudent to cross-clamp the aorta temporarily or to reduce the perfusion flow considerably; this will provide good exposure of the bleeding sites and facilitate satisfactory placement of pledgeted sutures to obtain absolute control of bleeding.

NB ***AUGMENTATION OF THE AORTOTOMY***
Sometimes the struts of the tissue prosthesis protrude into the aortotomy and could result in tension along the suture line. Patch enlargement of the aortotomy with autologous pericardium treated with glutaraldehyde or bovine pericardium allows ample room for the prosthetic struts and ensures a safe closure (Fig 5-26).

 AORTIC WALL INJURY
Sometimes the aortic commissures are asymmetric and abnormally located. This is seen in patients with calcified bicuspid valves. In these cases, the seated bioprosthesis may be tilted a little anteriorly. Very rarely the strut of the bioprosthesis may perforate the aortic root during closure of the aorto-

CORONARY AIR EMBOLISM
Air embolism in the coronary arteries, particularly the right coronary artery, probably does occur during the evacuation of air from the left ventricle. Every precaution must be taken to prevent or reduce air embolism in the coronary arteries. The pump flow is first reduced considerably, and the right coronary artery is occluded digitally by the assistant. The surgeon then partially unclamps the aorta and allows blood mixed with air trapped in the aortic root to flow freely from the vent opening on the aortotomy. High suction is applied to a slotted vent needle in the aortic root to continuously remove any air bubbles that may be ejected as the heart is filled and ventilation is begun (see Chapter 4). Only when all air has been evacuated can the vent needle be removed and the vent suture tied down.

FRIABLE AORTIC WALL
A friable aortic wall may necessitate the placement of additional reinforcing pledgeted sutures. Occasionally, when the aortic wall has been denuded of its adventitia, fine Tevdek suture material is preferable to Prolene because it tends not to cut through

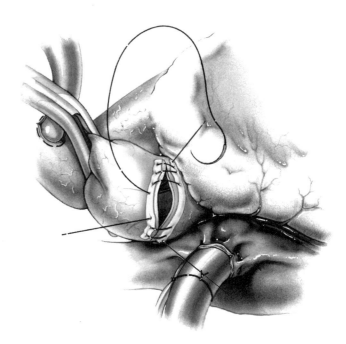

FIG. 5-25. Reinforcement of the aortotomy with strips of pericardium.

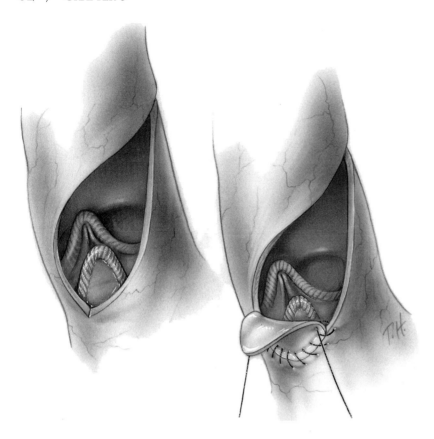

FIG. 5-26. Patch enlargement of the aortotomy.

tomy secondary to tenting of the anterior aorta over the strut (Fig. 5-27). This may necessitate resection of the damaged ascending aorta and replacement with an interposition tube graft.

Technique

The aorta is again clamped, retrograde cold blood cardioplegic solution is administered, and cardioplegic arrest of the heart is established. A right superior pulmonary vein vent is placed, and the heart is decompressed. The torn and diseased aorta is resected. If the quality of the aortic wall is good, the defect can be closed with a patch of glutaralde-

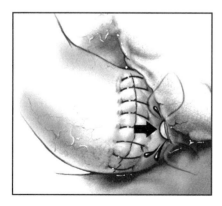

FIG. 5-27. Perforation of the aortic wall by a bioprosthetic strut.

hyde-treated pericardium. Conversely, if the aortic wall is very thin, dilated, and friable, then the aorta is dissected free from pulmonary artery and transected just above the commissures. The aortic wall is reinforced with a strip of felt and anastomosed to an appropriately sized tube graft (see Chapter 9). The distal end of the tube graft is then reapproximated to the distal aorta in a similar fashion.

HOMOGRAFT, AUTOGRAFT, AND PORCINE STENTLESS AORTIC ROOT IN AORTIC VALVE REPLACEMENT

The mechanical and bioprosthetic valves used in clinical practice have reached a very high level of sophistication and proven to be very effective valve substitutes. Nevertheless, the inconvenience and risk of lifelong anticoagulation therapy for mechanical valves and limited longevity of bioprostheses are of concern.

Donald Ross of London and Sir Brian Barrat-Boyes of Auckland, New Zealand, introduced the aortic homograft for aortic valve replacement more than four decades ago. Ross extended the concept and used a pulmonary autograft in the aortic position. The superior hemodynamics, freedom from the need for anticoagulation, and longevity of both the aortic homograft and the pulmonary autograft have been well substantiated over the years.

More recently stentless porcine aortic valves have become available. The Freestyle aortic root bioprosthesis (Medtronic, Minneapolis, MN) has been treated with an anticalcification agent that may extend its longevity to 15 to 20 years. The stentless porcine valves have been shown to have hemodynamics similar to those of aortic homografts. The porcine aortic root thus may have hemodynamic and longevity benefits similar to those with the aortic homograft but with the advantage of having all sizes available in the operating room.

PULMONARY AUTOGRAFT REPLACEMENT OF THE AORTIC ROOT: THE ROSS PROCEDURE

Through a median sternotomy approach, the aorta is cannulated as distally as possible. A single atriocaval cannula is usually sufficient, but bicaval cannulation is equally satisfactory. A left ventricular vent through the right superior pulmonary vein will decompress the heart and keep the field relatively dry. After initiation of cardiopulmonary bypass, systemic cooling is started. The aorta is clamped, and antegrade blood cardioplegic solution is administered. This is complemented by continuous retrograde cold blood followed by cold blood cardioplegic solution (see previously).

Of course it is of paramount importance that the pulmonary valve be absolutely normal. All patients who are to undergo aortic valve replacement with a pulmonary autograft undergo extensive evaluation preoperatively. Nevertheless, it is necessary for the surgeon to visualize and ascertain the normality of the pulmonary valve at the outset before committing to this procedure.

A transverse incision is made on the anterior aspect of the pulmonary artery near the confluence of the right and left pulmonary arteries. The pulmonary valve is visualized. It must be a normal-appearing trileaflet valve, free of any disease.

 ABNORMAL PULMONARY VALVE
If there is any evidence of pulmonary valve disease, such as previous endocarditis, bicuspid leaflets, or the presence of perforations in the leaflet, the valve is left intact and the pulmonary artery opening is closed with 4-0 Prolene suture. The aortic valve should then be replaced with another alternative such as a homograft, stentless porcine, or any other appropriate prosthetic valve.

After satisfactory inspection of the pulmonary valve, a low transverse aortotomy is made. Cold blood cardioplegia is administered directly into the coronary ostia, in particular, the right coronary artery, for better protection of the right ventricle.

 CONGENITAL ANOMALY OF THE CORONARY ARTERIES
Abnormal take off of the coronary arteries from the aortic root may complicate the procedure and requires some technical modifications.

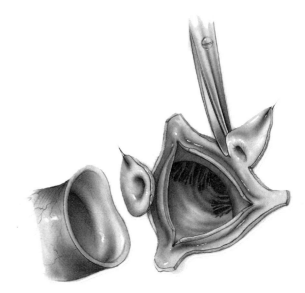

FIG. 5-28. Aorta has been transected. Coronary ostia are removed as large buttons of the aortic wall.

The aortic valve is removed and the annulus debrided of calcium as described previously. The aorta is transected, and the left and the right coronary artery ostia are both removed with a large button of aortic wall. The buttons are dissected free along the course of the coronary arteries to ensure their full mobility (Fig. 5-28).

 ABERRANT BRANCHES OF CORONARY ARTERIES
Special care must be exercised not to injure any aberrant coronary arteries.

The pulmonary artery is now completely transected at the confluence of its branches (Fig. 5-29). The dissection

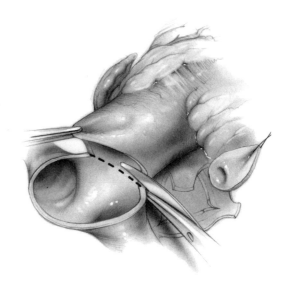

FIG. 5-29. Pulmonary artery is transected at the confluence of right and left pulmonary arteries.

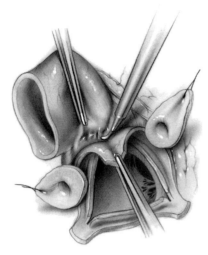

FIG. 5-30. Pulmonary artery is dissected free of the aortic root with a low-current electrocautery.

is continued with a low-current electrocautery, freeing the pulmonary artery and its root from the root of the aorta down to right ventricular muscle (Fig. 5-30). All small bleeding vessels are electrocoagulated.

 INJURY TO THE LEFT MAIN CORONARY ARTERY
The course of the left main coronary artery is intimately related to the pulmonary artery and its root. Dissection in this area must be carried out with utmost care.

NB Retrograde perfusion of blood through the coronary sinus identifies small bleeding vessels that otherwise would have gone unnoticed. Hemostasis at this stage of the operation can be accomplished effectively and easily compared with when the procedure is completed and the aortic clamp removed.

When the pulmonary artery is well mobilized, a right-angled clamp is introduced into the right ventricle through the pulmonary valve. An incision is made on the right ventricular outflow tract down onto the right-angled clamp 6 to 8 mm below the pulmonary valve annulus (Fig. 5-31A).

 INJURY TO THE PULMONARY VALVE
The previous precaution is most important to prevent any injury to the pulmonary valve that is to be used in the aortic position (Fig. 5-31B).

This incision is then extended transversely across the right ventricular outflow tract (Fig. 5-32). The endocardium on the posterior aspect of the right ventricular outflow tract is incised with a knife 6 to 8 mm below the pulmonary valve annulus (Fig. 5-33). The pulmonary artery is now enucleated using Metzenbaum scissors with the blade angled in such a way so as to not injure the first septal branch of the left anterior descending coronary artery (Fig. 5-34).

 INJURY TO THE FIRST SEPTAL CORONARY ARTERY
The first septal branch of the left anterior descending coronary artery has a variable course and may at times be very large. The enucleating technique described allows detachment of the pulmonary artery root atraumatically. In our unit, all patients who are possible candidates for the Ross procedure undergo coronary angiography preoperatively for the specific delineation of coronary artery anatomy. If the first septal artery take off is very high and its size is significant, we may decide not to perform the Ross procedure for fear of developing massive septal infarction.

The pulmonary autograft is now freed from the right ventricular outflow tract and is trimmed of excess fatty tissue.

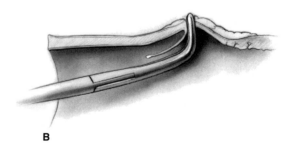 **BUTTONHOLE IN THE PULMONARY ARTERY**
To prevent buttonhole injury to the pulmonary artery wall, a finger is carefully placed inside it

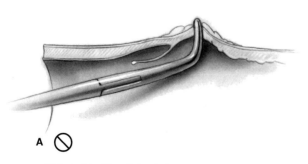

FIG. 5-31. Tip of the right angle should be 6 to 8 mm below the pulmonary annulus. **A:** The optimal site for detachment of the pulmonary root from the right ventricle. **B:** Pulmonary valve can be injured if the ventriculotomy is too high.

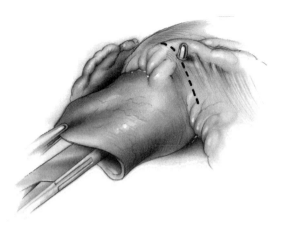

FIG. 5-32. The tip of the right-angled clamp depicts the site of a right ventricular incision along the dotted line.

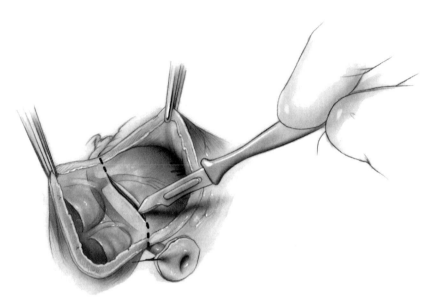

FIG. 5-33. The endocardium on the posterior right ventricular outflow tract is incised 6 to 8 mm below the pulmonary annulus.

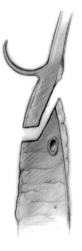

FIG. 5-34. Pulmonary root is enucleated without injury to the first septal coronary artery.

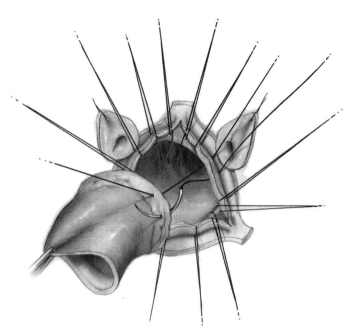

FIG. 5-35. Interrupted sutures are placed in the annulus and pulmonary autograft (see text).

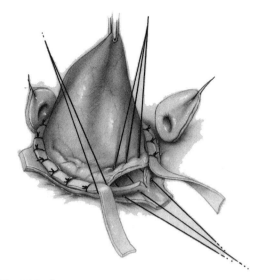

FIG. 5-36. Sutures are tied over a strip of pericardium.

across the pulmonary valve while removing epicardial fatty tissue.

The pulmonary autograft is then placed in a pool of blood alongside the right atrium, keeping the tissue alive in a blood milieu for its possible theoretical advantage.

Simple interrupted 4-0 Ticron sutures are now placed very closely together at the level of the annulus and below the level of the commissure to create a circle of stitches in a single plane (Fig. 5-35). This entails taking bites of the subaortic curtain, the membranous and muscular segment of the left ventricular outflow tract. The aortic annular sutures are now passed through the pulmonary autograft just below its annulus.

Alternatively, the pulmonary autograft can be anastomosed to the aortic root with a continuous suture of 4-0 Prolene. The suture line should begin at the commissure between the left and right coronary sinuses, passing the needle inside out on the aortic annulus and outside in on the pulmonary autograft. The posterior suture line is completed, and then the second needle is used to complete the anterior anastomosis. A nerve hook may be used to ensure that the suture line is tight before tying the two ends together.

 ORIENTATION OF THE PULMONARY AUTOGRAFT
The correct orientation of the pulmonary autograft is of great importance. It should be placed in such a fashion so that its sinuses overlie the sinuses of the native aorta to facilitate left main coronary artery implantation.

 INJURY TO THE PULMONARY AUTOGRAFT LEAFLET
When placing sutures in the pulmonary autograft, care must be taken not to pass the needle through the pulmonary valve leaflet.

The pulmonary autograft is lowered into position, and the sutures are tied over a strip of autologous pericardium previously treated with glutaraldehyde (Fig. 5-36). With continuous suture technique, a strip of pericardium may be incorporated into the anastomosis.

An incision is then made in the area of the proposed implantation of the left main coronary artery button. A 4.0-mm punch is used to enlarge the opening. The left main coronary button is attached to the pulmonary autograft with 5-0 or 6-0 continuous Prolene suture (Fig. 5-37).

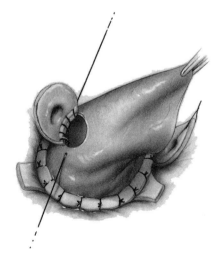

FIG. 5-37. Anastomosing the left coronary button to the pulmonary autograft.

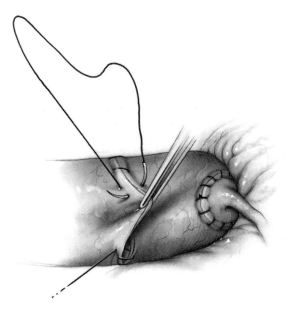

FIG. 5-38. Attachment of the pulmonary autograft to the aorta.

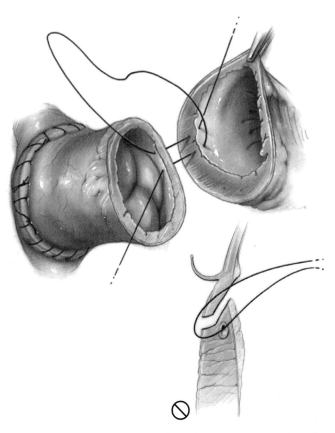

FIG. 5-39. Top: Approximating the cryopreserved pulmonary artery homograft to the right ventricular outflow tract. Bottom: Full-thickness sutures may occlude the septal artery.

 KINKING OF THE LEFT MAIN CORONARY ARTERY
There should be no kinking of the left main coronary artery. An appropriately sized probe must be passed into the left main coronary artery to ensure its unobstructed course.

Similarly, the right coronary artery button is now attached to the pulmonary autograft in the same fashion.

NB It is often prudent to perform the right coronary attachment after completion of the distal aortic anastomosis. The aortic clamp can be removed for a moment to distend the aortic root and the precise location of the right coronary anastomosis can be noted. The aorta is clamped again, and the right coronary artery anastomosis is completed.

The pulmonary autograft is now trimmed to meet the transected distal ascending aorta with ease. They are then anastomosed using 4-0 or 5-0 continuous Prolene suture (Fig. 5-38).

An appropriately sized, cryopreserved pulmonary homograft is selected and oriented with one sinus posteriorly and two sinuses anteriorly in an anatomic fashion. Its correct length is tailored, and the distal anastomosis is carried out with 4-0 or 5-0 Prolene suture (Fig. 5-39).

 KINKING OF THE PULMONARY HOMOGRAFT
Leaving the pulmonary homograft too long may result in kinking of the distal suture line when the heart is filled with blood.

 GRADIENT ACROSS DISTAL SUTURE LINE
There is a tendency for a gradient to develop across the distal anastomosis. This may be owing to immune reaction. It may also be owing to the purse-string effect of a continuous suture line. To prevent this complication, sutures should be spaced close together.

Using 4-0 Prolene, the proximal anastomosis is started on the posterior aspect of the incision on the right ventricular outflow tract. After taking the tension off the suture line on the medial aspect, the lateral aspect of the posterior suture line is continued, taking shallow bites of the endocardium to avoid the septal branches of the left anterior descending coronary artery (Fig. 5-39 bottom).

 SEPTAL ARTERY INJURY
Full-thickness suture in this area is apt to cause injury to the septal artery (Fig. 5-37, inset). The remainder of the anterior suture line is now completed.

The procedure is now completed (Fig. 5-40).

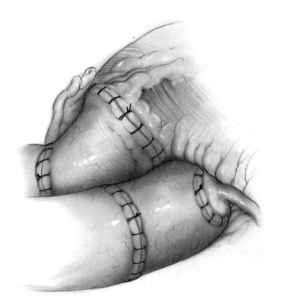

FIG. 5-40. Completed pulmonary autograft replacement of the aortic root.

NB The surgeon may elect to complete the right ventricular to pulmonary artery confluence connection with a pulmonary homograft interposition before implanting the pulmonary autograft in the aortic root.

Recent experience with pulmonary autograft replacement of the aortic root reveals possible root dilation with time. Therefore, many institutions now prefer to implant the pulmonary autograft in older children and adults using a modified subcoronary technique, as was originally performed by both Ross and Barrat-Boyes. The technique is similar to that described for the implantation of stentless bioprostheses.

AORTIC VALVE REPLACEMENT USING STENTLESS AORTIC BIOPROSTHESIS OR AORTIC HOMOGRAFT

It is clear that the normal geometry of the aortic root can be better maintained if the whole root is replaced with an aortic allograft or stentless aortic bioprosthesis. This technique is described in detail in the section on pulmonary autograft replacement of the aortic root (Ross procedure). Nevertheless, a modified subcoronary technique for the replacement of the aortic valve with an aortic homograft has been practiced since its introduction four decades ago with excellent results. We have employed a similar technique when implanting the stentless aortic root bioprosthesis.

Technique

Three traction sutures are placed on the anterior surface of the aorta (Fig. 5-41). A small transverse aortotomy is made and then extended both upward and downward under direct vision to provide good exposure of the aortic root. The aortic valve is examined and removed (see Aortic Valve Replacement section). Three 4-0 Ticron simple sutures are placed in the nadir of each annulus. Traction on these sutures opens the aortic annulus and

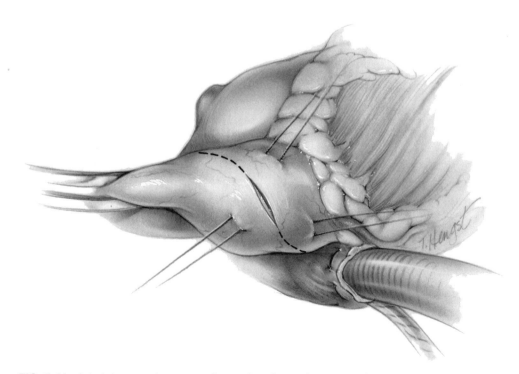

FIG. 5-41. Arteriotomy and exposure for aortic valve replacement with a stentless bioprosthesis.

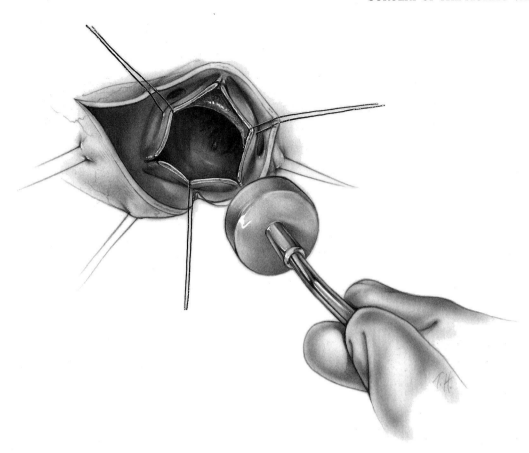

FIG. 5-42. Sizing the left ventricular outflow tract.

left ventricular outflow tract maximally, allowing accurate sizing (Fig. 5-42).

 TOO LOW AORTOTOMY
If the aortotomy is too proximal, it will be impossible to resuspend the commissures of the prosthetic valve or homograft high enough (see later). A small transverse aortotomy is made initially at least 1 cm above the right coronary ostium. The aortic root should be visualized through this opening. If the incision is too close to the valve commissures, it should be closed and a new incision made more distally on the aorta.

 UNDERSIZING THE VALVE
The valve sizer should fit snugly in the aortic annulus. It is advisable to oversize the valve 1 to 3 mm. The larger surface area of the cusps allows greater apposition of the leaflet tissue, thus reducing the possibility of valvular insufficiency.

 DISCREPANCY BETWEEN THE SINOTUBULAR AND AORTIC ANNULUS DIAMETER
If the diameter of the sinotubular junction is more than 2 mm greater than that of the annulus, the modified subcoronary technique should not be used. Some patients with poststenotic dilation of the aorta will demonstrate this finding. Performing a subcoronary implant of a stentless prosthesis or homograft valve in these patients will result in valvular insufficiency when the aortic root is pressurized and the commissures of the implanted valve are pulled outward. Some surgeons have advocated reducing the size of the sinotubular junction in such patients. However, it is probably safer to perform the implant as a root replacement (see previously) or select a stented prosthesis.

NB ***TYPE OF AORTOTOMY***
In patients with good-sized aortic roots, the aortotomy should be made transversely several millimeters above the native commissures. This allows precise sizing and resuspension of the prosthetic commissures. In patients with small aortic roots, an oblique aortotomy extended downward into the noncoronary sinus allows better visualization and easier placement of sutures. However, the oblique incision does distort the anatomy of the aortic root so that resuspending the commissures is more challenging.

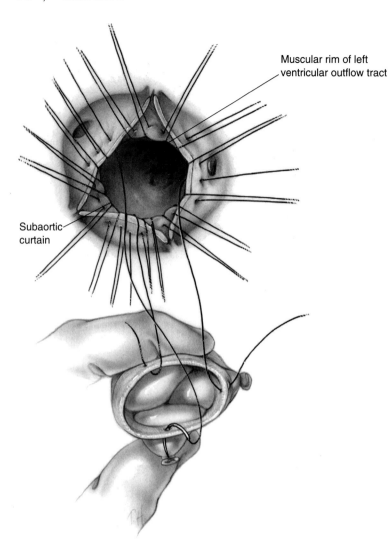

Muscular rim of left
ventricular outflow tract

Subaortic
curtain

FIG. 5-43. Simple interrupted suture placement in the annulus, subaortic curtain, and muscular segment of the left ventricular outflow tract and bioprosthesis.

Simple interrupted sutures of 4-0 Ticron are now placed 2 to 3 mm apart at the level of the annulus and below the level of the commissures to create a circle of stitches in a single plane. This entails taking bites of the subaortic curtain, the membranous and muscular segment of the left ventricular outflow tract. The three sutures that were originally placed in the nadir of the aortic annulus are now passed through the Dacron skirt of the appropriately sized stentless bioprosthesis just below the lowest aspect of the leaflet cusps (Fig. 5-43).

 LEAFLET INJURY
It is important to place the needle well away from the margin of the leaflet attachment. Needle perforation of the leaflet tissue of the bioprosthesis results in irreparable injury (Fig. 5-44).

The remaining sutures are placed in the skirt of the device in a similar fashion. The prosthesis is lowered into position, and the sutures are tied snugly and cut short.

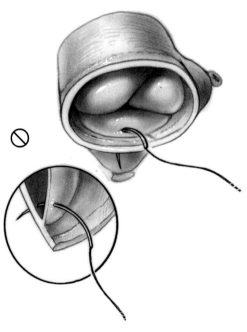

FIG. 5-44. Incorrect needle position causing leaflet injury.

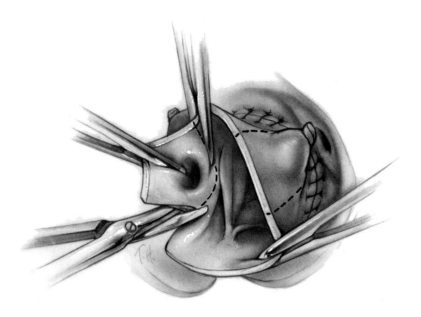

FIG. 5-45. Removal of the coronary sinuses of a prosthesis.

NB Many surgeons using homografts prefer to invert the device into the left ventricle and attach the homograft to the annulus with a continuous suture. This technique takes less time and can be accomplished with very good results. However, the porcine aortic root bioprosthesis is not as pliable as a homograft and may be damaged during the process of its inversion into left ventricular outflow tract followed by being pulled up into the aorta. The use of multiple interrupted simple sutures allows a precise proximal suture line without distortion or purse stringing.

With the prosthesis seated within the aortic root, the right and left coronary sinus portions of the stentless bioprosthesis are scalloped to fit beneath the patient's own coronary ostia, leaving a 4- to 5-mm rim of prosthetic tissue behind (Fig. 5-45). All excess tissue is cut away, leaving the noncoronary sinus portion below the sinotubular junction intact (Fig. 5-46). The three commissures are now pulled upward 2 to 3 mm above the native commissures and attached to the aorta at equidistant points with 4-0 Prolene sutures buttressed with pledgets. These sutures need not be tied down at this stage. They are placed there to allow proper orientation of the device and its secure attachment to the aortic wall in a precise fashion (Fig. 5-47). Alternatively, the surgeon may frequently check the positioning of the bioprosthetic commissures while performing the distal suture line (Fig. 5-48).

NB The importance of resuspending the commissures of the bioprosthesis as high as feasible cannot be overemphasized. This maneuver stretches the device upward and allows a larger segment of the leaflets to coapt during diastole, preventing any central aortic leak.

The scalloped portion of the device is sutured to the native aortic wall parallel with the native annulus. This technique ensures a precise, waterproof suture line well away from the coronary ostia. The suture line starts at the nadir beneath each coronary artery ostium and progresses upward to the top of the commissure on each side (Fig. 5-49). The sutures are tied together at the top of the com-

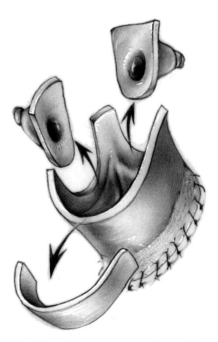

FIG. 5-46. Excision of the coronary artery ostia and excess noncoronary prosthetic wall.

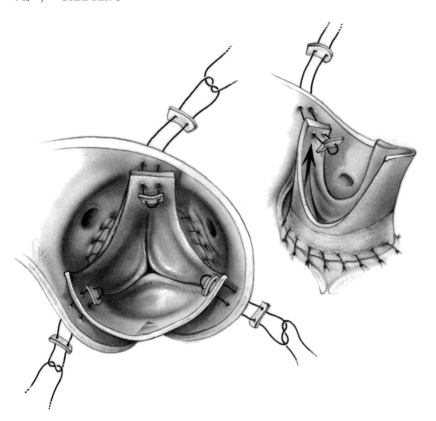

FIG. 5-47. Suspension of the prosthetic commissures above the native aortic commissures.

missure between the left and right coronary sinus outside the aorta. If pledgeted commissural sutures have been used, they are now tied outside the aorta buttressed by another pledget.

 LOW-LYING RIGHT CORONARY OSTIUM
The right coronary sinus portion of the stentless porcine bioprosthesis has a muscle bar that is covered by an extension of the Dacron skirt. This

should not be cut. Therefore, the distal suture line along the right coronary sinus must be performed several millimeters above the annulus so as not to buckle the muscle bar of the prosthetic valve. If the patient's right coronary ostium is particularly low, the prosthetic valve should be rotated 120 degrees to place the muscle bar in the patient's noncoronary sinus. All three prosthetic sinuses are then scalloped.

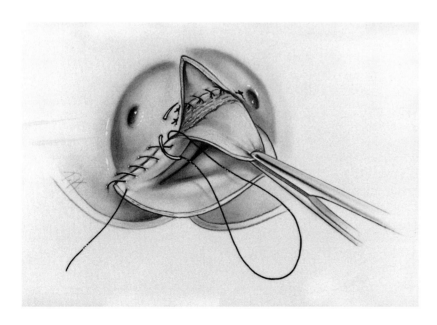

FIG. 5-48. Distal suture line beneath the left coronary ostium with frequent assessment of commissure placement.

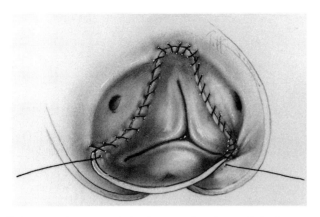

FIG. 5-49. Completed distal suture line beneath both coronary artery ostia.

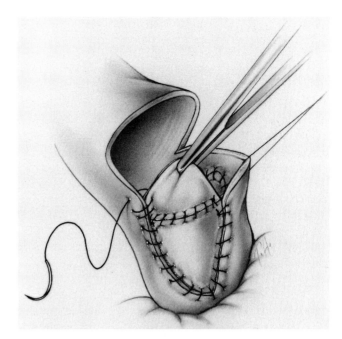

FIG. 5-51. Using a portion of the noncoronary sinus of a stentless valve to enlarge an aortotomy in such a way as to correctly align commissures. Aortic closure completed with a patch of GORE-TEX or pericardium.

 DISTORTION OF COMMISSURES WITH CLOSURE OF AN OBLIQUE AORTOTOMY

If closure of the native aortic wall over the retained noncoronary sinus portion of the prosthetic valve brings the commissure between the left and noncoronary sinus and the commissure between the right and noncoronary sinus too close together, the noncoronary sinus of the prosthesis is used to enlarge the aortic root (Fig. 5-50). This is accomplished by interposing the noncoronary sinus of the device in the aortotomy closure in such a way to realign the commissures correctly (Fig. 5-51). A small, triangle-shaped piece of pericardium or GORE-TEX is then used to complete the aortic closure.

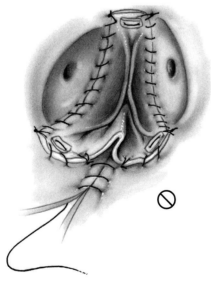

FIG. 5-50. Primary closure of an oblique aortotomy may distort commissural alignment.

 BULGING OF THE RETAINED NONCORONARY SINUS WALL INTO THE LUMEN OF THE AORTA

If closure of the aortotomy results in protrusion of the prosthetic noncoronary sinus into the aorta and the commissures are appropriately located, the noncoronary sinus should be scalloped and reattached to the aortic wall as was done for the right and left coronary sinuses. Alternatively, the bulge, if not excessive, can be approximated to the native aortic wall with separate sutures (see later).

NB *CLOSURE OF A TRANSVERSE AORTOTOMY*

When a transverse aortotomy has been made, the rightward aspect of the closure will often include the top of the retained noncoronary sinus of the prosthetic valve. Taking two to three bites behind (posterior to) the rightward extent of the aortic opening results in a nearly circumferential aortic suture line. This reinforces the sinotubular junction, which may help to prevent later dilation and resultant valvular incompetence.

The noncoronary sinus segment of the bioprosthesis is secured to the native aortic wall with another 4-0 Prolene suture. The intervening dead space can be obliterated with one or two 4-0 Prolene sutures placed inside to outside and tied over a Teflon pledget. The aortotomy is then closed with continuous 4-0 Prolene sutures. If an oblique aortotomy has been used, the proximal portion of the opening must be closed before suturing the retained prosthetic noncoronary sinus to the native aortic wall.

ENDOCARDITIS

Endocarditis of the native aortic valve or affecting a previously placed prosthesis may cause such erosion and destruction of the annulus so that valve replacement may become a challenging and dangerous undertaking. All infected tissue should be removed. Complete debridement of all necrotic material is essential. In areas where the aortic annulus is destroyed, the left ventricular outflow tract and aorta are reapproximated with bovine pericardium or glutaraldehyde-treated autologous pericardium. Aortic valve replacement is then carried out in the traditional manner.

 SUBANNULAR NECROTIC CAVITIES
Removal of necrotic tissue from the subannular area can create small cavities. The surrounding friable tissue will not hold sutures well. Deep bites with pericardial pledgeted sutures are taken to occlude these cavities. When tied, the sutures may later be used to anchor the new prosthesis into position.

Extensive infection and abscess formation involving the aortic annulus is a serious condition. The tissues may be too necrotic to hold sutures well, thus precluding placement of a prosthetic valve into the native annulus. A very effective technique is to replace the aortic root or aortic valve, depending on the degree of tissue necrosis, with either an aortic homograft or possibly a stentless bioprosthesis as described previously (aortic root replacement with homograft or autograft). These devices conform to the damaged aortic root much better.

LATE PARAVALVULAR LEAKS

In most patients, paravalvular dehiscence resulting in leaks around the aortic prosthesis is owing to imperfect surgical technique. Some of the predisposing factors, such as a calcified or degenerative annulus (which allows the sutures to cut through the tissues), have already been referred to previously. Paravalvular leaks tend to occur more commonly along the noncoronary annulus and the adjacent half of the left coronary annulus. Massive calcification affecting the aortomitral leaflet continuity may obscure the annulus and interfere with correct placement of anchoring stitches. In addition, the exposure of the

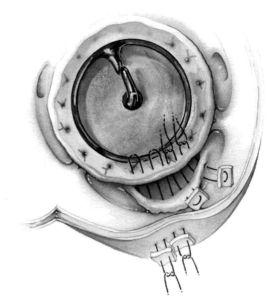

FIG. 5-52. Technique for repair of a paravalvular leak (see text).

noncoronary annulus is sometimes difficult from the surgeon's side (patient's right side). Often the annular sutures are inadvertently placed in the less ideal aortic wall above the annulus. In time, these sutures may cut through the aortic wall and produce a paravalvular leak. It is therefore important for the surgeon to be aware of all these details so that all the necessary precautions can be taken.

Technique for Repair

The paravalvular defect is identified under direct vision. The tissue margin of the defect commonly becomes fibrous during the period since the operation. Pledgeted sutures are passed deeply through the tissue margin of the defect and then through the sewing ring of the prosthesis before tying (Fig. 5-52).

When the tissue margin of the defect is not satisfactory, sutures are passed through the sewing ring of the prosthesis before taking a deep bite near the annulus through the full thickness of the aortic wall to the outside of the aorta. The sutures are then tied over Teflon felt pledgets (Fig. 5-52).

When there are multiple paravalvular leaks or the site of the leak is not quite distinct, it is necessary to explant the prosthesis and implant a new one, taking all the necessary precautions.

CHAPTER 6

Management of the Small Aortic Root

It is clear that no prosthetic valve is hemodynamically equal to the patient's own heart valves. Therefore, whenever valve replacement is done, the patient receives a less optimal valve substitute. This is particularly exemplified in patients with small aortic roots. The problem is even more relevant in patients with large body stature.

Fibrosis, calcification, or simply a very small aortic root can limit the maximal orifice of the aortic annulus. Therefore, a prosthesis that fits in the annulus comfortably may be unacceptable hemodynamically. Many ingenious techniques have been developed to overcome this mismatch between patient and prosthesis.

TILTED PROSTHESIS TECHNIQUE

Depending on the type of prosthesis, by tilting the plane of implantation by 5 to 10 degrees, it is often possible to implant a larger valve into the aortic root. The technique is similar to that described for aortic valve replacement (see Chapter 5). However, simple interrupted sutures are used to attach the prosthesis to the left and right coronary annuli. Starting from either end of the noncoronary annulus and arching upward to a central point 5 to 8 mm above its nadir, sutures, double-armed with needles (2-0 Ticron), are passed first through the sewing ring in a horizontal fashion downward from above and then through the aortic wall. The needles are finally passed through small pledgets or strips of Teflon felt outside the aorta (Fig. 6-1). The prosthesis is then lowered in this tilted position, and the sutures are tied as described previously. The sutures on the noncoronary side are tied outside the aorta over the Teflon felt pledgets.

 LOCATION OF THE AORTOTOMY
The right margin of the aortotomy should be at a higher level than usual, 1.5 to 2 cm above the noncoronary annulus, to facilitate sewing the prosthesis in a tilted fashion and, at the same time, to allow satisfactory closure of the aortotomy.

 BUTTRESSING OF THE SUTURES
All sutures anchoring the prosthesis onto the aortic wall above the annulus must be buttressed with Teflon pledgets or a strip of Teflon felt or pericardium. The aortic wall requires reinforcement to be strong enough to hold the prosthetic valve in position.

 OPENING ANGLES OF DISC PROSTHESES
The opening angles of discs differ by manufacturer. The Medtronic-Hall disc opens maximally to a 75-degree angle. This is an important point of concern. The combined tilting angle and disc opening angle should not be more than 80 to 85 degrees. Otherwise, there is the risk that when the disc opens, it may not close!

The concept of the tilting technique allows the implantation of a larger prosthesis in the supraannular position along the noncoronary annulus.

 ORIENTATION OF SINGLE-DISC PROSTHESES
The Medtronic-Hall and other tilting-disc prostheses should have the larger of their two openings facing the noncoronary sinus, resulting in a nearly central flow (Fig. 6-2A). The line of the flow is thus nearly parallel with the disc in the open position. If the prosthesis is sewn into place with the smaller opening facing the noncoronary sinus, then the disc is obstructive to forward flow (Fig. 6-2B).

 USE OF BILEAFLET PROSTHESES
Bileaflet prostheses have excellent hemodynamics and are preferred by many surgeons for use in patients with the small aortic roots. When used in the tilted position, the leaflets may stick to the aortic wall. Free mobility of the leaflets must be ensured by proper orientation of the prosthesis.

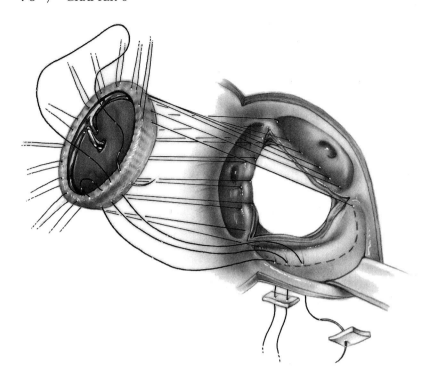

FIG. 6-1. Technique of securing a disc prosthesis (Medtronic-Hall) in the tilted position.

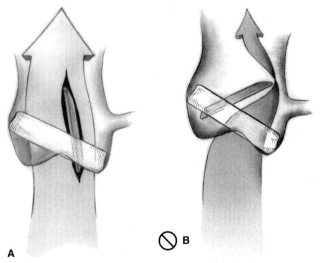

FIG. 6-2. A: The Medtronic-Hall prosthesis in the tilted position with the disc in the correct orientation. **B:** The disc in the incorrect orientation, obstructing the flow.

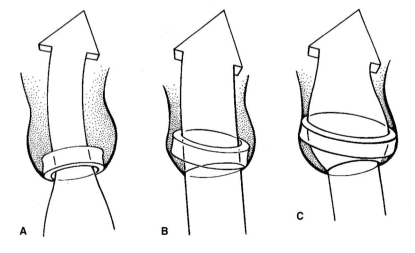

FIG. 6-3. A: Obstruction of the flow owing to an aortic root that is larger than the internal orifice of the prosthesis. **B:** Maximal possible flow in an aortic root of the same size as the internal orifice of the prosthesis. **C:** No increase of flow in an aortic root that is smaller than the internal orifice of the prosthesis.

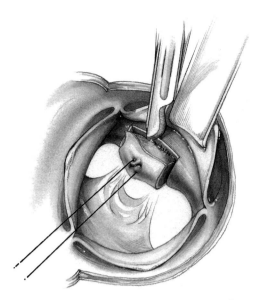

FIG. 6-4. Myectomy for septal hypertrophy.

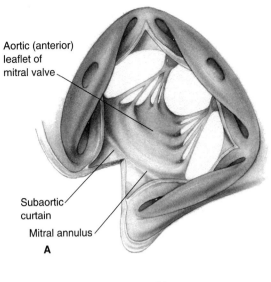

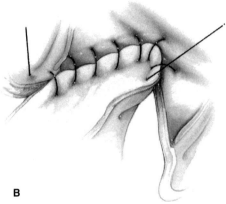

FIG. 6-5. A: Aortotomy is extended onto the subaortic curtain. **B:** Enlargement of the aortic root with a patch of pericardium.

🚫 *INAPPROPRIATE SIZE OF THE PROSTHESIS*
It is pointless to attempt to insert a prosthesis whose internal orifice is larger than the orifice of the left ventricular outflow tract or aortic annulus. If the left ventricular outflow tract is too narrow, the tilting technique of valve replacement obviously will not be very rewarding (Fig. 6-3).

NB *SEPTAL MYECTOMY*
Septal hypertrophy may be most marked in patients with severe aortic stenosis. At times, the left ventricular outflow tract may become narrower than the aortic root. The hypertrophied septal mass may interfere with the normal function of mechanical prosthetic valves. A limited myectomy or shaving off excess septal muscle bulging into the left ventricular outflow tract may allow a wider lumen and ensure normal function of the valvular prosthesis (Fig. 6-4).

PATCH ENLARGEMENT TECHNIQUE

It is always preferable to use the largest possible prosthesis whenever valve replacement is contemplated. A prosthesis larger than the aortic annulus, however, does not abolish the obstructive gradient across the left ventricle and the aorta (Fig. 6-3). Therefore, if the aortic annulus is a dominant obstructive factor, it must be enlarged to accept a larger prosthesis. Often the subaortic curtain is long enough to allow satisfactory enlargement of the aortic root. The oblique aortotomy is extended downward through the commissure between the noncoronary and the left coronary aortic annuli onto the subaortic fibrous curtain up to, but not including, the mitral annulus (Fig.

6-5A). A patch of glutaraldehyde-treated autologous pericardium or bovine pericardium is cut to shape and sewn into place with a continuous 3-0 Prolene suture (Fig. 6-5B).

When further enlargement is warranted, the incision is extended farther from the subaortic curtain through the mitral annulus and for a variable distance onto the anterior (aortic) leaflet of the mitral valve. This necessarily entails incision of the left atrial wall to a similar extent from the mitral annulus (Fig. 6-6A). A patch of glutaraldehyde-treated autologous pericardium or bovine pericardium of appropriate size and shape is then sewn into place with 3-0 continuous Prolene suture incorporating the left atrial wall and the anterior mitral leaflet (Fig. 6-6B). Rarely, this approach may distort the mitral valve particularly in patients with a small left atrium. The atrial opening may be enlarged by incorporating a second patch of pericardium (Fig. 6-6C). These techniques of aortic root enlargement have the added advantage that the left ventricular outflow tract, as well as the aortic annulus, can be enlarged considerably. The aortic prosthesis of

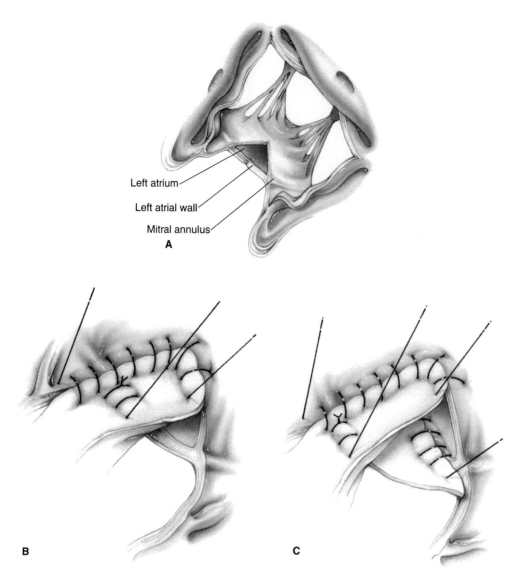

Left atrium

Left atrial wall

Mitral annulus

A

B   **C**

FIG. 6-6. A: Aortotomy is extended onto the mitral annulus and anterior leaflet of the mitral valve. Note entry into the left atrium (see text). **B:** Enlargement of the aortic root with a patch of pericardium. Note the incorporation of the left atrial wall and mitral leaflet (see text). **C:** Separate patch closure of a left atrial opening.

choice is then inserted into place by the technique described previously (Fig. 6-7).

 HAZARDS OF AORTIC VALVE REPLACEMENT
All the pitfalls discussed in relation to routine aortic valve replacement pertain when using these techniques.

 TILTING THE PROSTHESIS
The prosthesis should be sewn in with a slight tilt, as described earlier, so that the anchoring sutures that cross the patch can be tied on the outside wall of the patch 4 or 5 mm above the annulus. This patch is then used to augment the aortotomy clo-sure with a continuous 4-0 Prolene suture. If autologous pericardium appears to be thin and insecure, it can be reinforced by a patch of GORE-TEX or Hemashield (Medox Medical, Oakland, NJ).

 HEMOLYSIS
If a GORE-TEX patch or Hemashield graft is used, it may be lined with autologous pericardium to prevent possible hemolysis in the postoperative period.

 NARROW LEFT VENTRICULAR OUTFLOW TRACT
The previously discussed techniques enlarge the aortic annulus quite effectively. If the left ventricular outflow tract is too narrow, however, it remains

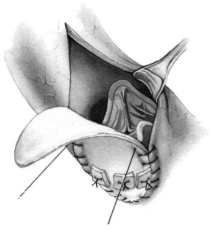

FIG. 6-7. Insertion of the prosthesis into the enlarged aortic root.

a limiting factor. Placement of a larger prosthesis or enlargement of the aortic annulus will not relieve the basic hemodynamic problem.

These techniques are useful and not too difficult to perform. However, it must be pointed out that aortic root or aortic valve replacement with a homograft or a stentless aortic bioprosthesis is very effective and is the procedure of choice when an optimal result is to be obtained (see Chapter 5).

The obstruction usually associated with a small aortic root can be satisfactorily relieved in most patients using one of the techniques described previously. The Rastan-Konno aortoventriculoseptoplasty (see Chapter 22) is rarely indicated in patients with a simple, small aortic root.

CHAPTER 7

Surgery of the Mitral Valve

Degenerative, myxomatous changes are probably the most common cause of mitral valve disease in North America and Western Europe. However, rheumatic fever continues to be the major cause of acquired valve disease worldwide.

Rheumatic fever results in a pancarditis, but the pathologic effects are noted predominantly on the endocardium and cardiac valves, particularly the mitral valve. During the acute phase of myocarditis, the left ventricle dilates, which causes stretching of the annulus of the mitral valve. The mitral insufficiency thus produced is temporary and disappears when the left ventricle regains its normal function. Rheumatic heart disease is a chronic and progressive condition.

The earliest permanent change is the fusion of the commissures, followed by thickening and fibrosis of the valve leaflets. These pathologic events are responsible for the creation of the turbulent flow that, together with the continuing rheumatic process, further enhances the progression of the disease and eventual involvement of the subvalvular apparatus. The chordae and papillary muscles become thickened, shortened, and fused to each other and to the mitral leaflets; all these events augment the turbulence of flow. A continuous cycle of progression of pathologic changes and increasingly disturbed flow is thus created, eventually leading to severe mitral valve disease, calcification, and hemodynamic embarrassment.

Ischemic heart disease and myocardial infarction can result in asynchronous left ventricular contraction and papillary muscle dysfunction. This often interferes with normal coaptation of mitral valve leaflets, which are usually free of any significant disease. The resultant mitral valve insufficiency allows the left ventricle and mitral annulus to dilate, which in turn increases the degree of mitral insufficiency.

Bacterial endocarditis can affect both normal and abnormal heart valves. It can destroy the mitral valve leaflet configuration, resulting in gross mitral valve insufficiency.

SURGICAL ANATOMY OF THE MITRAL VALVE

The mitral valve forms the inlet of the left ventricle. It consists of two leaflets: the aortic (anterior) and mural (posterior) leaflets, which are attached directly to the mitral annulus and to the papillary muscles by primary and secondary chordae tendineae. A series of chordae tendineae originates from the fibrous tips of the papillary muscles and inserts into the free edges and the undersurfaces of the mitral leaflets, thus preventing the prolapse of the leaflets into the left atrium during systole and contributing to the competency of the mitral valve. The attachments of the leaflets to the annulus meet at the anterolateral and posteromedial commissures. One-third of the mitral valve annulus provides attachment for the aortic (anterior) leaflet, and the mural (posterior) leaflet arises from the remaining two-thirds of the annulus.

When the mural annulus is studied from a strictly anatomic standpoint, it is attached to the left ventricular myocardium through the interposition of a narrow membrane and thus is actually slightly elevated above the opening of the left ventricle. This subannular membrane extends underneath the mural annulus to the region of both commissures and merges with the fibrous skeleton of the heart. The aortic (anterior) leaflet is continuous with the adjoining halves of the left and noncoronary annuli of the aortic valve and also with the small area beneath the intervening aortic commissure, the fibrous subaortic curtain (Fig. 7-1).

The annulus of the mitral valve is surrounded by many important and vital structures. The nearby left circumflex coronary artery traverses around the mitral annulus in the posterior atrioventricular groove. The coronary sinus also runs in the more medial segment of the same groove. The atrioventricular node and its artery, usually a branch of the right coronary artery, runs a course parallel and close to the annulus of the aortic (anterior) leaflet of the mitral valve near the posteromedial commissure. As mentioned earlier, the remainder of the aortic (anterior) leaflet annulus is contiguous with the aortic valve. These relation-

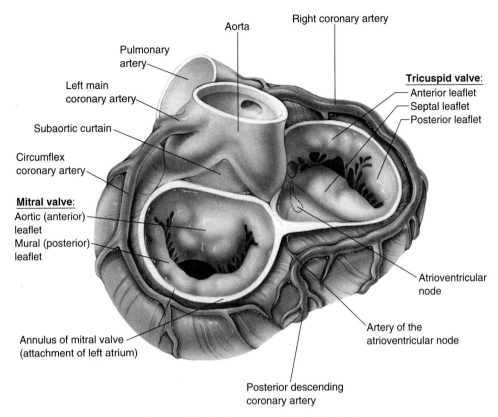

Aorta

Right coronary artery

Pulmonary artery

Left main coronary artery

Subaortic curtain

Circumflex coronary artery

Mitral valve:
Aortic (anterior) leaflet
Mural (posterior) leaflet

Annulus of mitral valve
(attachment of left atrium)

Posterior descending coronary artery

Tricuspid valve:
Anterior leaflet
Septal leaflet
Posterior leaflet

Atrioventricular node

Artery of the atrioventricular node

FIG. 7-1. Surgical anatomy of the mitral valve.

ships have significant clinical implications during mitral valve surgery (Fig. 7-2).

TECHNICAL CONSIDERATIONS

Incisions

A median sternotomy is the incision most commonly used, although left and right thoracotomy also affords good access to the mitral valve (Fig. 7-3).

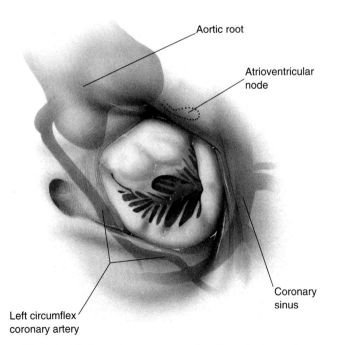

Aortic root

Atrioventricular node

Left circumflex coronary artery

Coronary sinus

FIG. 7-2. Vital structures surrounding the mitral annulus.

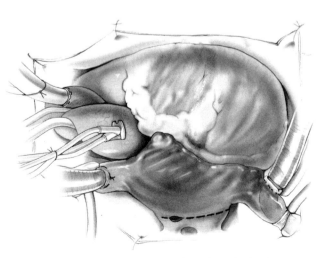

FIG. 7-3. Surgical approach to the mitral valve.

Myocardial Preservation

When satisfactory cardiopulmonary bypass has been established, the aorta is cross-clamped and cold blood cardioplegic solution is administered into the aortic root (see Chapter 3) to bring about prompt diastolic cardiac arrest.

AORTIC INSUFFICIENCY

Satisfactory administration of cardioplegic solution into the aortic root can only be accomplished if the aortic valve is competent. Aortic insufficiency, if present, directs the cardioplegic solution into the left ventricular cavity. The perfusion pressure causes distention and stretch injury to the myocardium. This complicating factor can be prevented by administering cardioplegic solution using the retrograde technique, an equally effective method in arresting the heart (see Chapter 3).

Exposure of the Mitral Valve

There are many different approaches for exposure of the mitral valve. Bicaval cannulation is preferred for all patients undergoing mitral valve surgery (see Chapter 2).

Interatrial Groove Approach

The left atrium is opened with an incision just posterior to the interatrial groove (Fig. 7-3). The opening can be enlarged inferiorly extending to the back of the heart.

FATTY FRAGMENTS

If the left atrium is opened with an incision into the interatrial groove, care must be taken to prevent fragments of fatty tissue in the groove from entering the left atrial cavity. Similarly, when the atriotomy is being closed, fatty fragments may invaginate through the closure into the atrium.

EXTENSION OF THE INCISION

Upward extension of the incision behind the superior vena cava should be avoided because subsequent closure may become somewhat tedious. Generous inferior extension to the back of the heart provides satisfactory exposure of the mitral valve in most cases (Fig. 7-4). Closure of this posterior extension of the incision is facilitated by suturing from inside the left atrial cavity under direct vision.

DRAINAGE OF CARDIOPLEGIC SOLUTION

At least one of the caval snares must be loosened during administration of cardioplegic solution to allow it to drain into the oxygenator. If both snares

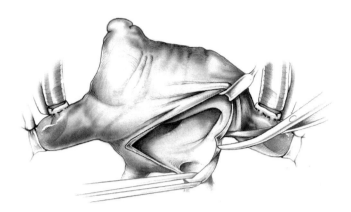

FIG. 7-4. Extension of the incision inferiorly to the back of the heart.

are down, cardioplegia may distend the right heart unnecessarily. If the right atrium is not opened at any time, the cava do not necessarily require snares around them because venous drainage may be adequate.

AIR EMBOLISM

The aorta must be cross-clamped before opening the left atrium to avoid possible air embolism.

Specially designed retractors are introduced into the left atrium. Optimal exposure is obtained when the retractor held by the assistant pulls the atrial wall at least 1 cm from the mitral annulus upward and slightly to the patient's left. Many self-retaining retractors are available to improve exposure of the mitral valve. They may be particularly helpful if there is a shortage of assistants in the operating room.

RETRACTOR INJURY

Because the atrial wall may be somewhat friable, excessive pull on the retractor may produce a shearing tear of the atrial wall edges, thus complicating closure. On many occasions, two smaller retractors provide better and safer exposure than a single large one because the assistant is able to divert the pulling force from one retractor to the other to accommodate the surgeon's view (Fig. 7-5).

Transatrial Oblique Approach

If the left atrium is small, exposure of the mitral valve through the interatrial groove may be suboptimal. In reoperative procedures, massive adhesions may make dissection hazardous on the back of the heart, particularly near the region of the interatrial groove. In such cases, an oblique transatrial approach provides excellent exposure

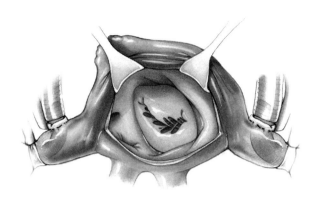

FIG. 7-5. Use of two small retractors to avoid tearing the atrial wall edges.

of the mitral valve (Fig. 7-6). The aorta is cross-clamped, and cardioplegic solution is administered as before. After the aorta is clamped, an oblique incision is made in the right superior pulmonary vein with a long-handled no. 15 blade. Warm blood will gush out to decompress the left atrium. This will allow expeditious cooling and arrest of the heart.

The vena caval snares are secured. The opening in the right superior pulmonary vein is extended obliquely across the right atrial wall. By gently retracting the right atrial wall edges, the incision can now be extended across the interatrial septum and through the fossa ovalis just

inferior to the limbus (Fig. 7-6). At this time, a retrograde cardioplegic cannula can be introduced into the coronary sinus under direct vision. It can be immobilized with a fine purse-string suture of Prolene placed on the inside of the coronary sinus ostium, away from the conduction tissues (see Chapter 3, Fig. 3-4). In this manner, infusion of cardioplegic solution can supplement the antegrade technique.

 OVEREXTENDED SEPTAL INCISION
Extension of the septal incision far beyond the anterior limbus of the fossa ovalis may divide the mitral valve annulus, making mitral valve replacement insecure. It could also create a passage outside the atrium into the transverse sinus. The septal incision should therefore terminate just distal to the anterior margin of the fossa ovalis. The septal incision can be extended inferiorly on the fossa ovalis if additional exposure is required (Fig. 7-6C).

The septal edges are retracted with two small retractors. This provides excellent exposure of the mitral valve without distorting it, an important advantage when mitral valve reconstruction is being contemplated (Fig. 7-7).

Transatrial Longitudinal Septal Approach

When there are excessive adhesions from previous surgery, excellent exposure of the mitral valve can be obtained through a longitudinal septal approach. Depending on the size of the right atrium, an oblique or longitu-

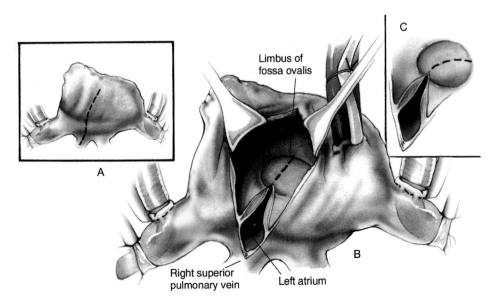

FIG. 7-6. A: Incision on the right superior pulmonary vein extends across the right atrium. **B:** Transatrial incision. Extension of the incision across the interatrial septum just to the limbus of the fossa ovalis. **C:** For additional exposure, the septal incision is extended along the fossa ovalis.

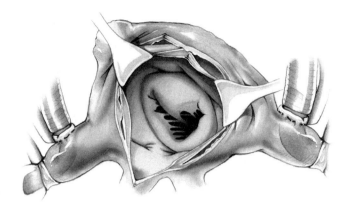

FIG. 7-7. Retraction of the septal edges to provide exposure of the mitral valve without distorting it.

dinal incision is made on the right atrial wall. Excellent exposure of the right atrial cavity and interatrial septum is thus obtained. A longitudinal incision is made along the posterior margin of the fossa ovalis and extended both superiorly and inferiorly to provide good exposure of the mitral valve (Fig. 7-8).

 PROXIMITY TO THE MITRAL ANNULUS
The annulus of the mitral valve is at the muscular septal wall most anterior to the fossa ovalis. Therefore, the longitudinal septal incision should be made posterior to the fossa ovalis, leaving a good margin of septal wall between the opening and the mitral annulus. This segment of the septum is retracted to provide excellent exposure of the mitral valve.

OPEN MITRAL COMMISSUROTOMY

Mitral commissurotomy can be accomplished safely and precisely under direct vision. With the availability of cardiopulmonary bypass, the closed technique is rarely used.

A median sternotomy is the incision of choice, although the mitral valve can be approached through either a right or left thoracotomy.

The left atrium is incised by one of the techniques described earlier for exposure of the mitral valve. The mitral leaflets are identified and, by means of two fine Prolene traction sutures, gently pulled upward toward the left atrial cavity. At times, use of nerve hooks can also provide the same effect. Often this maneuver will stretch the valve leaflets apart and show the line of commissural fusion as a furrow extending between them. If visibility through the valve ostium is adequate, the chordae and papillary muscles are examined for evidence of shortening and fusion to each other and, especially, fusion to the undersurfaces of the valvular leaflets.

A right-angled clamp is introduced through the mitral valve opening and placed directly below the fused commissures. It is then opened gently beneath the leaflets to facilitate incision with a no. 15 blade into the commissures without severing the chordal attachments (Fig. 7-9). Occasionally, the papillary muscles are fused to the undersurface of the leaflet, making commissurotomy hazardous. With the opened right-angled clamp in place, the commissure is first incised near the annulus; this incision is extended inward over the clamp, cutting vertically into the papillary muscle and the thickened, fused chordae. A papillary muscle may become weakened or partially severed when obliquely divided, necessitating its repair or reimplantation or even mitral valve replacement.

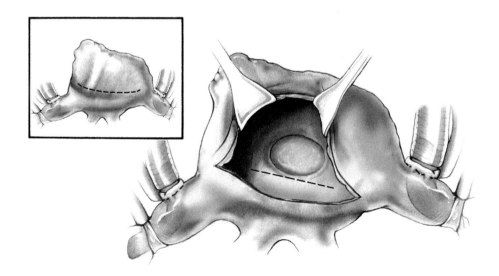

FIG. 7-8. Transatrial longitudinal septal approach.

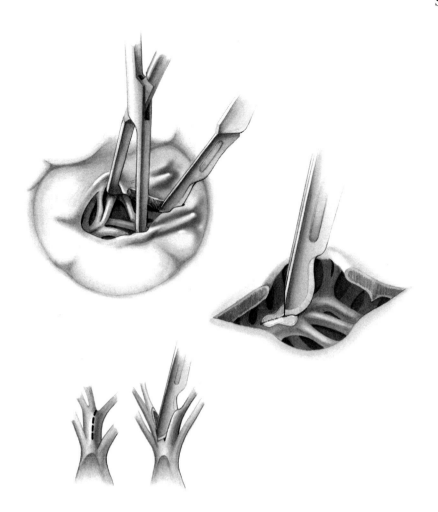

FIG. 7-9. Technique for a open mitral commissurotomy (see text).

🚫 *OVEREXTENSION OF COMMISSUROTOMY*
The extent of commissurotomy must be as complete as possible without producing valvular incompetence. If the incision is extended too far toward the annulus, annuloplasty may become necessary (see Mitral Valve Reconstruction section).

MITRAL VALVE RECONSTRUCTION

Mitral valve incompetence can be the result of chordal elongation or rupture, leaflet abnormality, annular dilation, or any combination thereof. Ischemia may lead to papillary muscle dysfunction, infarction, or even rupture, thus producing mitral regurgitation. For this reason, it is necessary to examine and evaluate every aspect of the mitral valve complex in detail so that efforts at valvular reconstruction will be fruitful. A simple pathophysiologic classification of the mitral valve complex may be helpful.

Type I: The presence of annular dilation *only*. The leaflets, chordae, and papillary muscles are intact.
Type II: The presence of ruptured or elongated chordae and/or papillary muscles.

Type III: The presence of ventricular or papillary muscle dysfunction causing asynchronous closure of the mitral valve (owing to an ischemic or infarcted papillary muscle and left ventricular wall). The leaflets, chordae, and papillary muscles are intact.

All techniques described previously for approaching the mitral valve provide excellent exposure. The transseptal approach, however, has the added advantage of allowing the valve to be evaluated in its normal anatomic configuration without being distorted by excessive retraction. This is a point of importance when contemplating reconstructive procedures (Fig. 7-7).

Mitral Valve Annuloplasty

Commissuroplasty

In a subgroup of patients, the cause of mitral insufficiency is annular dilation only; therefore, reducing the enlarged annulus is all that is required. This can be accomplished by successive figure-of-eight sutures at both commissures, incorporating only the posterior annulus.

The needle of an atraumatic 2-0 Tevdek suture is passed through the annulus at the commissure and then again 1 cm farther along on the posterior annulus. The same suture is then placed through the annulus 0.5 cm from the commissure (or midway between the first two stitches). Finally, it is passed through the annulus 1 cm farther away before it is tightened and securely tied. If indicated, another figure-of-eight suture, similarly placed, can decrease the annular size even more (Fig. 7-10). Good judgment dictates the appropriate size of each stitch so that a good repair can be accomplished without overcorrection. These sutures may be buttressed with Teflon felt pledgets for added security.

SYMMETRIC ANNULUS
It is important to have an anatomically symmetric annulus. Therefore, the procedure should include both the anterolateral and posteromedial commissural aspects of the annulus in exactly the same fashion.

RESIDUAL MITRAL VALVE INCOMPETENCE
Inadequate reduction of the annulus may not correct the valvular insufficiency. The mitral valve must be evaluated after annuloplasty for incompetence by injecting saline into the left ventricle looking for an insufficient jet.

MITRAL STENOSIS
Overcorrection will result in mitral stenosis. The orifice may be examined digitally, and an appropri-

ately sized obturator may be introduced into the valve to ascertain the presence of an adequately sized orifice.

DEGENERATIVE DISEASE
When the pathologic entity is degenerative disease, the tissues are thin and weak, and sutures may tear through. The use of Teflon felt or pericardial pledgets may help to prevent this complication.

EXCLUSION OF THE ANTERIOR ANNULUS
Annuloplasty should incorporate only the *mural annulus* and not the *anterior annulus* because it is usually the mural portion that has dilated. Incorporation of the anterior segment of the annulus may distort the mitral configuration and thus result in valvular insufficiency.

SUTURE PLACEMENT
The sutures should be placed in the fibrous annulus, rather than into the leaflet itself, or into the atrial wall beyond the annulus.

This technique is quite satisfactory for a small group of patients who are in heart failure and have developed *mild* mitral insufficiency owing to left ventricular and mitral annular dilation. In patients with ischemic disease, myocardial revascularization may improve left ventricular function, which can decrease dilation of the mitral annulus.

Most patients with mitral insufficiency will require mitral valve reconstruction in conjunction with mitral

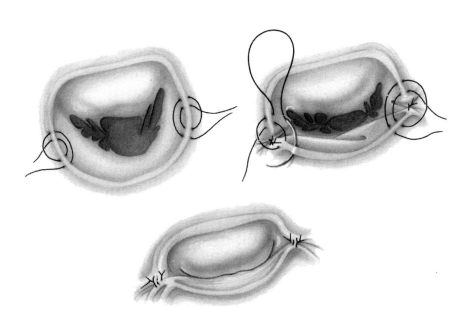

FIG. 7-10. Figure-of-eight technique for a mitral valve annuloplasty.

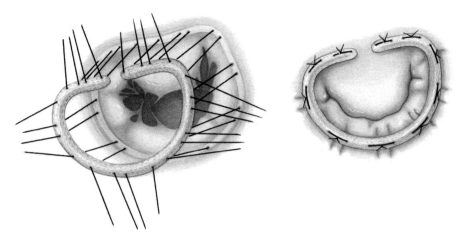

FIG. 7-11. Carpentier ring annuloplasty.

annular remodeling with specially designed annuloplasty rings. Many rings and bands are now available.

Carpentier-Edwards Ring

This is a rigid, *incomplete* ring that is very efficacious in approximating the anterior and posterior annulus closer together and allows the mitral annulus to regain its normal form. This rigid ring has the systolic configuration of the mitral valve, which will retain its shape also during diastole (Fig. 7-11). A modified model of the Carpentier ring (Fig. 7-12) is a complete ring that has some flexibility in the area of the posterior annulus (Carpentier-Edwards Physio Annuloplasty Ring, Baxter Healthcare Corporation, Santa Ana, CA).

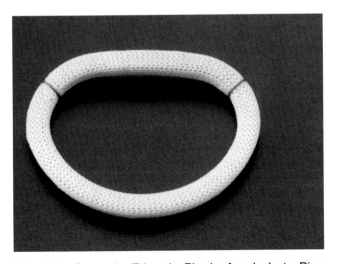

FIG. 7-12. Carpentier-Edwards Physio Annuloplasty Ring (Baxter Healthcare Corporation, Edwards CVS Division, Santa Ana, CA).

Technique

After satisfactory repair of the mitral valve, sutures of 2-0 Ticron are passed through the annulus at each *trigone*. With the aid of a right-angled clamp placed behind the chordae, the anterior leaflet is very gently stretched to expose its surface area. The sizer must correspond to the area of the anterior leaflet and the distance between the trigones. In this manner, the appropriate-size ring is selected. Approximately seven to 10 simple sutures are placed evenly in the posterior annulus approximately 3 to 4 mm apart; similarly, two to four sutures are placed in the anterior annulus between the trigonal stitches. All sutures are then evenly passed through the ring, which is then lowered into position and the sutures are securely tied (Fig. 7-11).

 SUTURE PLACEMENT
The sutures should be appropriately spaced on both the annulus and the ring, taking into account their different sizes. This may entail taking wider bites on the posterior annulus to ensure correct seating of the ring.

 DELICATE, FRIABLE TISSUE
Often, left atrial and annular tissue is edematous and friable. In these cases, horizontal mattress sutures with soft felt pledgets may be used instead of simple sutures. This will prevent tearing of the suture through the tissues.

Cosgrove-Edwards Annuloplasty System

This is a silicone rubber band covered with polyester velour cloth (Fig. 7-13). It is implanted as a reinforcement band for annuloplasty of the posterior annulus. The Cosgrove-Edwards Annuloplasty System (Baxter Healthcare

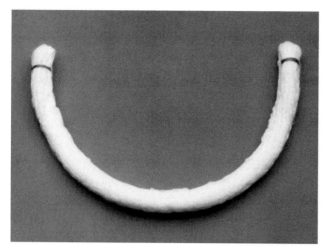

FIG. 7-13. Cosgrove-Edwards annuloplasty band (Baxter Healthcare Corporation, Edwards CVS Division, Santa Ana, CA).

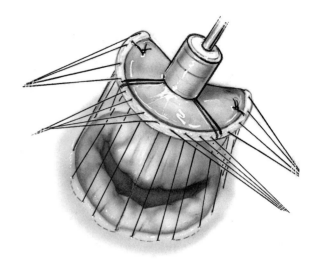

FIG. 7-15. Sutures are placed in the annuloplasty band.

Corporation, Edwards CVS Division, Santa Ana, CA) provides a measured correction of the dilated annulus.

Technique

After satisfactory repair of the mitral valve, sutures of 2-0 Ticron are passed through the annulus at each trigone. With the aid of a right-angled clamp placed behind the chordae, the anterior leaflet is very gently stretched to expose its surface area. The sizer must correspond to the area of the anterior leaflet and the distance between the trigones. In this manner, the appropriate size ring is selected. Approximately seven to nine simple sutures are placed evenly in the posterior annulus approximately 3 to 4 mm apart (Fig. 7-14). All sutures are then evenly passed

through the ring, which is then lowered into position (Fig. 7-15). The sutures are tied securely over the template to allow precise annular reduction. The template is then removed (Fig. 7-16).

NB Sutures must be deep enough to include a substantial bite of good strong annular tissue. At times, sutures can be passed from the ventricle into the atrium through the posterior annulus, taking care not to interfere with the chordal attachments (Fig. 7-14).

NB It is important that the distance between the simple sutures be the same on the mitral annulus and annuloplasty ring. Redundant posterior annulus is reduced by taking larger simple bites on the annulus than on the ring, thereby folding the annulus into the ring.

🚫 *HEMOLYSIS*
An adequate repair may have very mild residual insufficiency. Even a small jet of blood against a

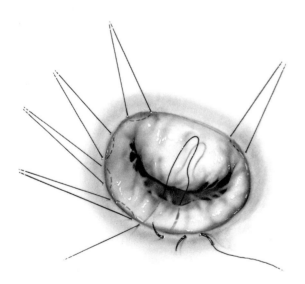

FIG. 7-14. Sutures are placed in the trigones and the posterior annulus.

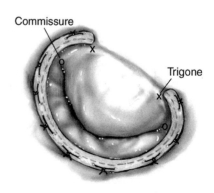

FIG. 7-16. Completed posterior annuloplasty band.

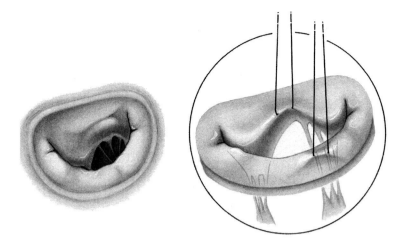

FIG. 7-17. Estimating the degree of elongation of the chordae by measuring the distance between the plane of the mitral valve annulus and the attachments of the lengthened chordae to the elevated leaflet.

foreign material may produce significant hemolysis. The surgeon must take all precautions to prevent this complication.

In children, we prefer not to use any ring. However, we place multiple sutures in the posterior annulus buttressed with pericardial pledgets to reduce the size of the posterior annulus. This technique allows growth of the mitral valve annulus. Alternatively, a fine Prolene double-armed suture is run along the posterior annulus from commissure to commissure and tied over a dilator equal to the appropriate mitral valve size for that patient. The expectation is that the Prolene suture will fracture as the child grows, allowing growth of the annulus.

NB It is generally prudent to choose a smaller size ring or band. It is important for the length of the posterior mitral annulus from trigone to trigone to be as short as possible without creating mitral stenosis.

In fact, the mitral leaflet should appear redundant and generously fill the mitral orifice when the left ventricle is full for optimal results.

Shortening of the Chordae Tendineae

Sometimes the chordae become elongated and allow the leaflets to prolapse into the left atrium during systole, causing mitral incompetence. Before chordal shortening can be initiated, the amount of abnormal lengthening must be established. To do this, the leaflets must be pulled gently into the left atrium with two fine Prolene traction sutures or nerve hooks. The degree of elongation of the chordae can be closely estimated by measuring the distance between the plane of the mitral valve annulus and the attachment of the lengthened chordae to the elevated leaflet (Fig. 7-17). This excess length can be sewn to the undersurface of the leaflet (Fig. 7-18). Alternatively, GORE-TEX sutures can be used as artificial chordae to

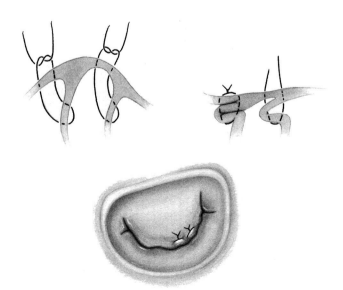

FIG. 7-18. Attachment of the elongated chordae to the mitral leaflets.

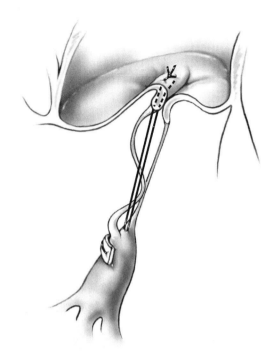

FIG. 7-19. Replacement of elongated or ruptured chordae with a GORE-TEX chord.

provide a precise and fixed length for the ideal distance between the papillary muscle and the leaflet (Fig. 7-19).

Attachment of the Chordae to the Mitral Leaflets

A double-armed, 5-0 Prolene suture is used to shorten each elongated chorda. The first needle is passed through the chordae at or slightly below the plane of the mitral annulus. The second needle is then placed midway between the first suture and the undersurface of the leaflet. Both needles are then passed upward through the

leaflet, very close to one another, and tied snugly on the atrial side. This draws up the excess length of chordae underneath the leaflet and pulls it down to the level of the plane of the mitral valve to reestablish apposition with the other leaflet (Fig. 7-18).

🚫 *LEAFLET TEAR*
The leaflet must be somewhat thickened or fibrous. The chordae-shortening sutures may injure or tear an otherwise normal leaflet, thus interfering with a satisfactory repair and culminating in leaflet tear.

NB Chordal shortening procedures are performed only in children for growth potential possibilities. In adults, we have adopted the much simpler technique of using GORE-TEX artificial chords (see later).

Mitral Valve Prolapse

Mild asymptomatic mitral valve prolapse (Barlow syndrome) may progress to clinically significant mitral insufficiency. It is the result of myxomatous and degenerative changes in the leaflet tissues with subsequent elongation or even rupture of the chordae. Acute rupture of a chord or a trunk of chordae gives rise to prolapse of a segment of mitral leaflet into the left atrium, resulting in severe mitral regurgitation.

Posterior Leaflet Resection with Annuloplasty

A quadrangular portion of the posterior leaflet that encompasses the prolapsed segment of leaflet is resected. The posterior annulus in the area of the quadrangular resection is reduced with two to three interrupted sutures of 2-0 Ticron. The leaflets edges are reapproximated with 5-0 Prolene sutures tied on the ventricular or atrial aspect of the leaflets (Fig. 7-20). The posterior annulus is rein-

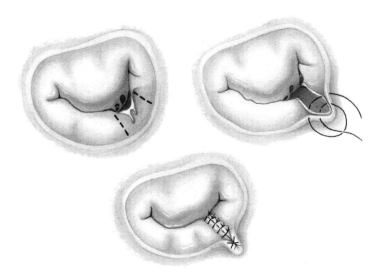

FIG. 7-20. Leaflet resection with an annuloplasty.

forced with one of the annuloplasty support systems as described previously.

 EXCESSIVE EXCISION OF LEAFLET TISSUE
Good judgment is needed when excising redundant prolapsed leaflet tissue. Too large an excision may compromise adequate repair. In cases in which a relatively large segment has been removed, leaflet approximation is markedly facilitated by sliding the remaining leaflet segments toward each other. This can be accomplished by detaching the remaining posterior leaflet segments from the annulus, commissure to commissure, and reattaching them back to the annulus after reduction annuloplasty. The posterior annulus must be reinforced with one of the annuloplasty systems to avoid any tension on the repair (Fig. 7-21).

 MITRAL INSUFFICIENCY FROM IMPROPER LEAFLET APPOSITION
Taking too wide a bite in the posterior mitral leaflet for reapproximation may decrease the surface area and produce mitral insufficiency by preventing proper apposition of the leaflets to one another.

 THIN LEAFLET TISSUE
The leaflet tissue may be very thin and friable and sutures may cut through it, resulting in the return of mitral valve insufficiency. Pledgets of pericardium can be used to buttress the sutures; care must be taken to avoid deforming the leaflet.

 SUTURE UNTYING
Fine Prolene sutures may come untied if they have not been tied properly. This can result in disruption of the repair and significant valvular regurgitation. In this context, it should be borne in mind that fine GORE-TEX sutures tend to untie and therefore should be avoided in leaflet repair.

COEXISTENT MITRAL ANNULAR DILATION
There is always coexistent mitral annular dilation. It is therefore necessary to reinforce the posterior annulus with one of the annuloplasty support systems as described previously.

CHORDAL ABNORMALITY AFFECTING THE ANTERIOR MITRAL LEAFLET

Chordal rupture or markedly elongated chords affecting the anterior leaflet of the mitral valve can result in significant mitral valve incompetence. The affected chordae can be reinforced by transposing the corresponding posterior leaflet attachment to the anterior leaflet of the mitral valve, often referred to as the flip-over procedure.

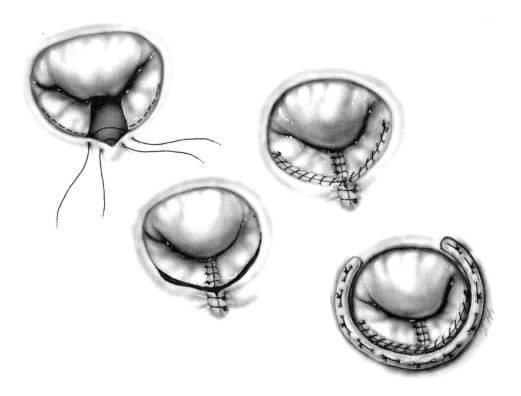

FIG. 7-21. Sliding technique for posterior leaflet repair with reinforcement of the posterior annulus.

Technique

A quadrangular segment of the posterior leaflet, with normal primary chordae facing the ruptured or markedly elongated chorda of the anterior leaflet, is detached from the posterior leaflet and posterior annulus. It is then flipped over and attached to the anterior leaflet of the mitral valve with multiple interrupted sutures of fine Prolene sutures. All secondary chordae from the transposed segment are detached to allow full mobility. The defect in the posterior leaflet is reconstructed as described previously (Fig. 7-20).

A much simpler technique is to replace the ruptured or elongated chorda with a single GORE-TEX suture without disrupting the posterior leaflet or posterior annulus of the mitral valve.

GORE-TEX Chordal Replacement

Technique

A 5-0 GORE-TEX suture, double-armed with a tapered needle, is used to replace the ruptured or elongated chorda of the anterior leaflet. The needle is passed through the tip of the papillary muscle from which the diseased chorda originates. The suture is then *locked* on itself.

One of the needles of the GORE-TEX suture is then passed through the anterior leaflet at the site of attachment of the ruptured chorda. The anterior leaflet is then pulled upward into the left atrium with the aid of nerve hooks, placing tension on the rest of the chorda. The length of the GORE-TEX suture is adjusted to approximate the length of the other normal chordae. The GORE-TEX suture is then *locked* on itself. This will fix the length of the replaced (GORE-TEX) chorda. The other arm of the GORE-TEX suture follows precisely the same route, its length similarly adjusted, and locked on itself. The two arms are then tied together (Fig. 7-19 and 7-28D).

PAPILLARY MUSCLE
The tip of the papillary muscle is usually fibrotic and quite strong. The GORE-TEX suture is buttressed by pericardial pledgets for added security when the papillary muscle tip is muscular.

NB *IMPORTANCE OF LOCKING*
It is absolutely essential for the GORE-TEX suture to be locked on itself, both at the tip of the papillary muscle and at the leaflet attachment, to ensure that the correct length of the replaced (GORE-TEX) chorda is fixed.

SHORTENED ARTIFICIAL CHORD
If the GORE-TEX suture is not securely locked on itself, it will be pulled up when being tied. This will result in a shortened new artificial chorda tethering

the anterior mitral leaflet and creating valvular incompetence.

This technique can be modified and applied in the management of elongated as well as ruptured chordae.

MITRAL VALVE REPLACEMENT

Increasing experience with mitral valve repair has allowed many patients with degenerative mitral valve disease or mitral annular dilation to undergo reconstructive procedures as previously described quite successfully. However, when reparative procedures do not appear to provide a lasting successful outcome, mitral valve replacement should be considered.

In recent years, experimental and clinical studies have established the importance of the subvalvular apparatus in retaining the normal geometry of the left ventricle and its function. Therefore, whenever the mitral valve has to be replaced, every attempt should be made to preserve the native subvalvular apparatus or replace native chordal structures with GORE-TEX sutures to maintain the mitral annular papillary muscle continuity.

Technique

The diseased anterior leaflet is detached from the annulus between the two commissures. If the anterior leaflet is not extensively diseased, an ellipse of tissue is excised and the rim of the leaflet tissue containing primary chordae is reattached to the anterior annulus using pledgeted mattress sutures to be used subsequently for valve implantation (Fig. 7-22). If the leaflet is thickened or calcified, it is divided into two to four segments, depending on the size of the valvular leaflet. Each segment then is trimmed to create a button of leaflet tissue with attached chordae. These buttons are reattached to the anterior annulus with the valve sutures in an anatomic fashion (Figs. 7-23 and 7-24). The normal geometry probably is maintained better if the anterior leaflet is not subdivided.

The posterior leaflet, when pliable, usually can be retained completely together with the attached chordae tendineae. Redundant leaflet tissue is folded up into the annulus by placing the valve sutures through the annulus and bringing them through the leading edge of the leaflet tissue (Fig. 7-24b). Alternatively, incisions or small wedge resections of leaflet tissue between the chordal attachments are performed if the posterior leaflet is thickened and fibrotic to allow implantation of the larger valve.

At times, the mitral valve leaflet and the subvalvular apparatus are grossly diseased and calcified and must be totally resected. The diseased leaflets are then pulled and stretched slightly with a heavy suture or an Allis forceps

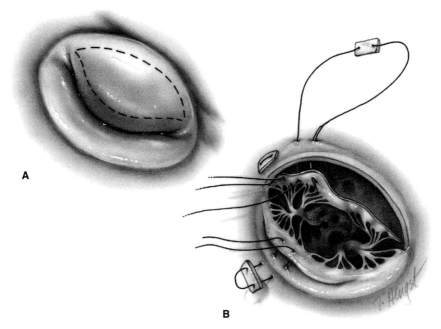

FIG. 7-22. A: An ellipse of the anterior leaflet is removed. **B:** The rim of the anterior leaflet is attached to the anterior annulus.

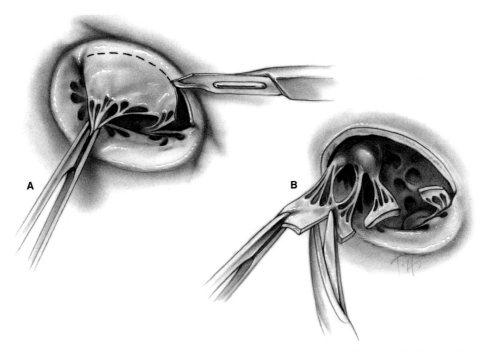

FIG. 7-23. A: Anterior leaflet is detached. **B:** The anterior leaflet is divided into buttons with chordal attachments.

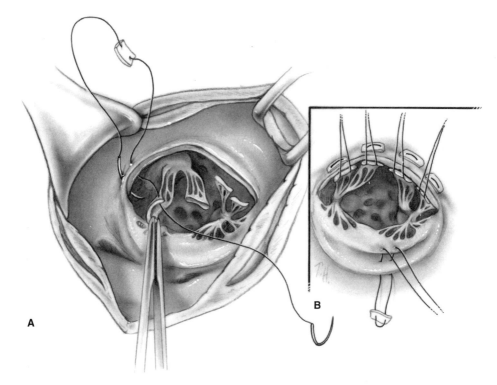

FIG. 7-24. A: Each chordal button is reattached to the anterior annulus, retaining its normal geometric position. **B:** The posterior leaflet is kept intact. Redundant tissue is folded into the left atrium.

to bring their annular attachments into view (Fig. 7-25A). With a long-handled no. 15 blade, the mitral leaflets are divided circumferentially 4 to 5 mm from the annulus (Fig. 7-25B). A traction suture in the annulus adjacent to the posteromedial commissure allows better exposure and provides countertraction for the complete removal of the diseased valve (Fig. 7-25C). This suture can subsequently be used in anchoring the prosthesis. The diseased chordae tendineae are then excised with scissors (Fig. 7-25D).

 EXCESSIVE LEAFLET EXCISION
A good margin of leaflet tissue should always be left with the annulus to allow secure anchorage of sutures for subsequent placement of a prosthesis. Overzealous excision of leaflets may leave a weakened annulus, making valve replacement insecure or even resulting in detachment of the left atrium from the left ventricle.

 PAPILLARY MUSCLE EXCISION
Only the calcified and diseased chordae should be excised, leaving the fibrous tips of the papillary muscles untouched. Removal of an excessive amount of papillary muscle may weaken the ventricular wall, which may result in hematoma within the wall and possible rupture (see later).

⊘ ***EXCESSIVE PULL ON PAPILLARY MUSCLE***
During the process of leaflet excision, the valve tissue should never be pulled overzealously. The heart arrested with cardioplegia is flaccid, and any excessive pull on the papillary muscle may tear a buttonhole defect through the weakened left ventricular wall (Fig. 7-26A, B). If such a catastrophe occurs, it must be detected immediately and repaired with pledgeted mattress sutures (Figs. 7-26C, D). The posterior descending coronary artery is likely to be in close proximity to this type of ventricular wall tear. Precautions must therefore be taken to avoid occluding the coronary artery in the process of repairing the defect. Pledgeted, double-armed, atraumatic sutures are passed deeply, well away from the coronary artery, and tied snugly over another pledget. If bleeding continues after the application of several well placed sutures, the whole area of the defect should be covered with a patch of bovine pericardium, meticulously sewn to the surrounding normal myocardium with continuous 3-0 Prolene sutures. Some coronary artery branches may have to be sacrificed within the continuous suturing process. This is inevitable and must be borne in mind when dealing with this potentially lethal problem.

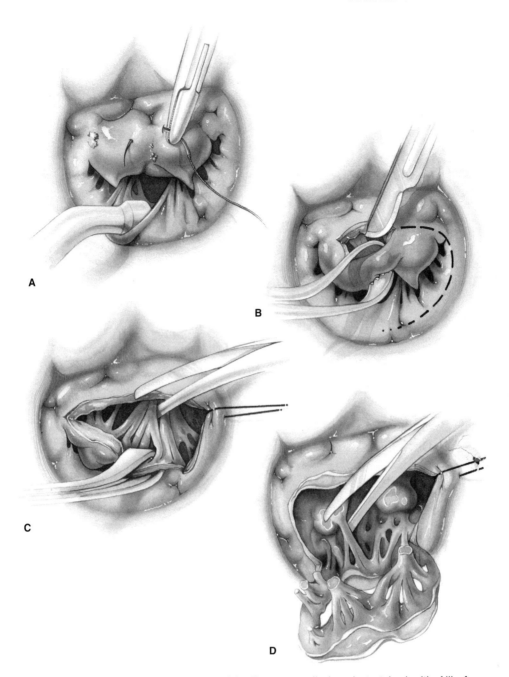

FIG. 7.25. Mitral valve excision. **A:** Diseased leaflets are pulled and stretched with Allis forceps or heavy suture to expose their annular attachments. **B:** The mitral leaflets are divided circumferentially with a long-handled no. 15 blade 4 to 5 mm from the annulus. **C:** A traction suture in the annulus adjacent to the posteromedial commissure allows better exposure and provides countertraction for the complete removal of the diseased valve. **D:** The chordae tendineae and fibrotic tips of the papillary muscles are then removed with scissors.

MITRAL VALVE CALCIFICATION

Calcification of the mitral valve and annulus is quite common. Care should be taken to remove as much calcium as possible without weakening the annulus. Occasionally, removal of calcium or degenerative material may leave a hollow cavity in the annulus. This should be immediately irrigated and closed securely with soft tailor-made pledgeted sutures. These sutures may or may not be used to help anchor the prosthesis (Fig. 7-27).

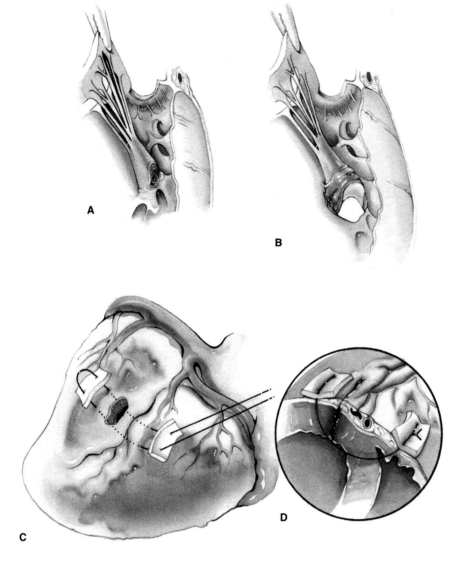

FIG. 7-26. A–D: Mechanism of a buttonhole defect through the left ventricular wall and its surgical repair.

🚫 *ANNULAR CALCIFICATION*
The mural annulus of the mitral valve may become infiltrated with heavily calcified tissue that may extend into and involve the full thickness of the atrioventricular groove and wall. Overzealous removal of this excessive calcium may result in a defect in the atrioventricular groove. Consistency of the surrounding tissues and the location of the circumflex coronary artery in the atrioventricular groove make any attempt to repair this defect most hazardous.

🚫 *ATRIOVENTRICULAR GROOVE DISRUPTION*
Overzealous removal of calcium from the posterior annulus of the mitral valve or forcibly implanting too large a prosthesis may result in disruption of the atrioventricular groove. This catastrophe is often noted as the patient is being weaned off cardiopul-

monary bypass when the operative field is flooded with bright red blood.

NB It is dangerous to attempt to repair this injury from outside the heart.

Cardiopulmonary bypass is resumed, cardioplegic arrest of the heart is once again accomplished. The left atrium is opened and the mitral prosthesis is removed. The extent of the defect is fully evaluated. A large patch of autologous pericardium treated with glutaraldehyde or bovine pericardium is cut to the appropriate size and shape. It is sewn in place, well away from the margin of the defect, to the left ventricular wall, left atrial wall, and left atrioventricular junction. The suture line is reinforced with multiple interrupted sutures buttressed with Teflon felt. A smaller mitral prosthesis is reimplanted in the usual fashion except that it is attached to the pericardium

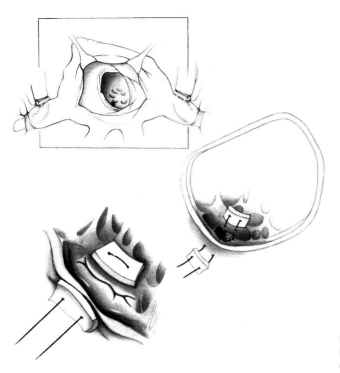

FIG. 7-27. Removal of degenerative calcific material. The hollow cavity in the annulus formed during removal should be irrigated and closed with pledgeted sutures.

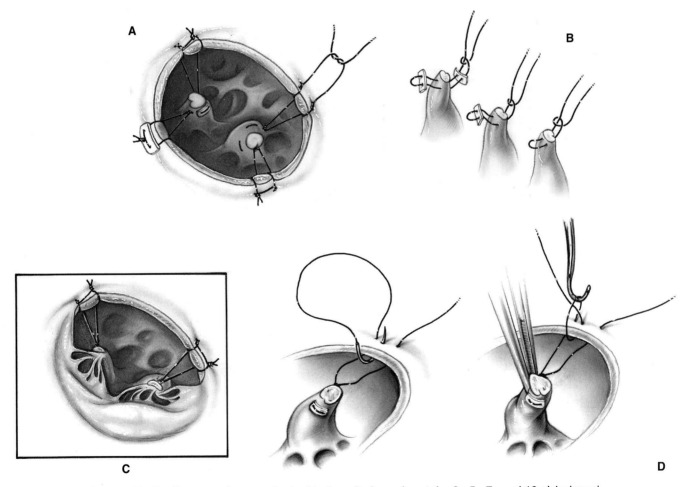

FIG. 7-28. A: Papillary muscles are attached to the mitral annulus at the 2-, 5-, 7-, and 10-o'clock positions with GORE-TEX chorda substitutes. **B:** GORE-TEX sutures are attached to the papillary muscles. Teflon felt pledgets may be used to buttress the sutures. **C:** Anterior chordal replacement with retention of the posterior native chordal attachments. **D:** Locking the GORE-TEX suture at the level of the annulus.

instead of the posterior annulus. The operation is then continued to its completion.

Technique for Chord Replacement

All the native chordal structures are resected if the subvalvular apparatus is markedly diseased, as in patients with rheumatic disease in whom there are fusion of the chordae tendineae, foreshortening of the chordal apparatus, and papillary muscle thickening. Continuity between the mitral annulus and the papillary muscle then is recreated with 4-0 GORE-TEX sutures to produce artificial chordae tendineae that extend from the heads of the papillary muscle to the annulus (Fig. 7-28).

A suture of 4-0 GORE-TEX on a double-armed needle is sutured to the fibrous tip of the papillary muscle. If there is no fibrous tissue, the suture is buttressed with a small, soft felt or pericardial pledget and the suture is tied snugly or locked on itself (Fig. 7-28B). Both needles of each suture are passed through the annulus of the mitral valve at approximately the 2-, 5-, 7-, and 10-o'clock positions (Fig. 7-28A). The precise length of the GORE-TEX artificial chord is determined, and each suture is locked on itself and then tied. Locking the stitch prevents any pulling on the GORE-TEX, resulting in shortening of its length. The correct length of the artificial chords allows both the papillary muscle and the GORE-TEX suture to be barely taut, not tight and certainly not too loose. There should be no "bowing" of the GORE-TEX chord. Often

it is possible to retain the native posterior chordal attachments and replace only the anterior chords with GORE-TEX suture (Fig. 7-28C).

Sizing the Mitral Orifice

The largest possible prosthesis should be chosen for mitral valve replacement. Sizers are introduced sequentially into the annulus until the correct size can be selected. The sizer should fit loosely.

INJURY FROM THE SIZER
It is important not to push the sizer forcefully into the annulus.

COMBINED MITRAL AND AORTIC VALVE REPLACEMENT
When a double valve replacement is performed, both prostheses should be undersized to ensure proper seating of both valves.

VALVE CHOICES

Although many prostheses have been successfully used in the past, we believe that technical complications are markedly reduced when a bileaflet mechanical or a low-profile tissue valve is implanted in the mitral position, especially when the subvalvular apparatus is retained.

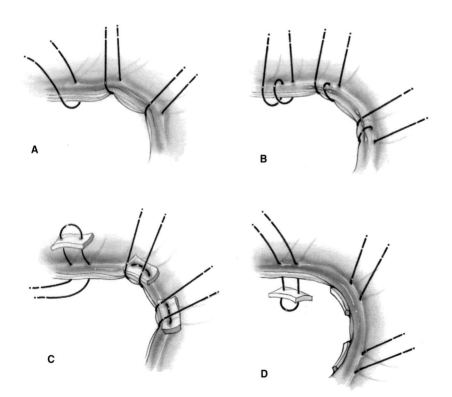

FIG. 7-29. Sutures to anchor the mitral prosthesis. **A:** Simple sutures. **B:** Figure-of-eight sutures. **C:** Everting pledgeted mattress sutures. **D:** Ventricular pledgeted mattress sutures.

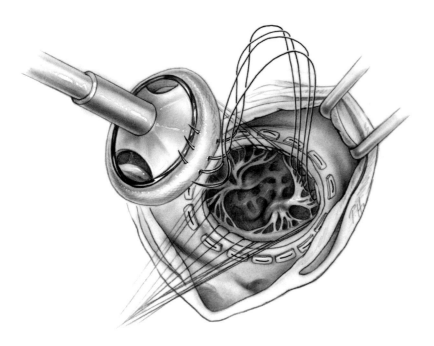

FIG. 7-30. Placement of sutures into the sewing ring of the bileaflet prosthesis (St. Jude Medical, Minneapolis, MN).

Technique for Suture Insertion

Simple, figure-of-eight, everting pledgeted mattress, and ventricular pledgeted mattress sutures are commonly used in anchoring the mitral prosthesis. If the annulus is well defined and strong, simple or figure-of-eight sutures of 2-0 Tevdek will be adequate. Conversely, if the annulus is degenerative, pledgeted, horizontal mattress sutures provide added security (Fig. 7-29). Occasionally, a continuous 2-0 Prolene suture may be preferred. The use of everting, pledgeted mattress sutures (Fig. 7-29C) is

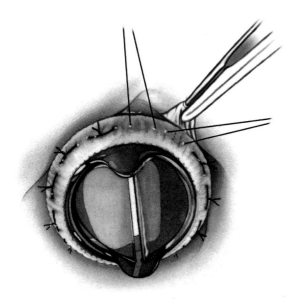

FIG. 7-31. Pulling retained chordal button tissue above the mitral annular plane as valve sutures are tied.

favored by most surgeons and is the preferred technique in our unit.

Simple sutures can be inserted in the sewing ring of the prosthesis, either singly or in vertical mattress fashion. Figure-of-eight sutures and mattress sutures are placed into the sewing ring in horizontal mattress fashion (Fig. 7-30). When all the sutures have been passed through both the annulus and the valve sewing ring, the prosthesis is gently lowered into position and the sutures are tied snugly. Any retained redundant subvalvular apparatus must be pulled above the mitral annular plane when the sutures are tied to prevent interference with the mechanism of the mechanical prostheses or left ventricular outflow tract obstruction (Fig. 7-31). If extensive retained leaflet tissue is present in the left atrium, it may be secured away from the prosthetic sewing ring with a 4-0 Prolene suture attaching the leaflet tissue to the left atrial wall.

 SITES OF SUTURE INJURY
There are important anatomic structures in the immediate vicinity of the mitral annulus (Fig. 7-32). The left circumflex coronary artery courses through the atrioventricular groove just outside the posterior mitral annulus. The coronary sinus also traverses around the annulus and is likely to be encountered in the region of the posteromedial commissure. The artery to the atrioventricular node sometimes runs parallel to the annulus just above the posteromedial commissure. The aortic leaflets, being continuous with the aortic (anterior) leaflet of the mitral valve, can also be occasionally incorporated in a stitch.

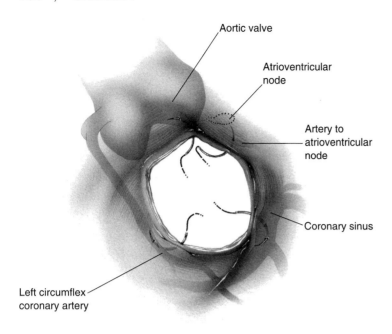

Aortic valve

Atrioventricular node

Artery to atrioventricular node

Coronary sinus

Left circumflex coronary artery

FIG. 7-32. Possible sites of suture injuries.

⊘ ***DEGENERATIVE OR DELICATE ANNULAR TISSUE***
Degenerative or otherwise delicate annular tissue will not hold sutures securely enough to support a valve prosthesis. Pledgets should always cushion the sutures so that they will not cut through the friable annulus and allow paravalvular leaks. Sutures that are not adequately tightened will also result in leaks.

⊘ ***HANDLING OF TISSUE VALVES***
Tissue valves must be kept moist by intermittently rinsing them with room temperature physiologic saline solution. If this vital precaution is not taken, the heat of the operating room lights will soon dry and permanently damage the valve tissue.

⊘ ***ANTIBIOTICS AND TISSUE PROSTHESIS***
Tissue prostheses should never be exposed to antibiotic solutions because of possible tissue-chemical interaction that may result in premature fibrosis and calcification.

⊘ ***INTERFERENCE WITH THE OCCLUDING MECHANISM OF MECHANICAL PROSTHESES***
Pledgets on the ventricular aspect may occasionally interfere with the normal function of disc prostheses.

⊘ ***EXCESS SUTURE MATERIAL***
The sutures, when tied, should be cut short. Excessive suture material will interfere with the normal occluding mechanism of some prostheses.

⊘ ***EXCESS RETAINED CHORDAL BUTTON TISSUE***
Excess retained chordal and leaflet tissue above the mitral annular plane should be sutured to the atrial wall away from the sewing ring to prevent interference with the prosthetic mechanism.

⊘ ***DETACHED CHORDAE***
Unattached chordae hanging loose can be drawn into the prosthesis and prevent its normal closure, resulting in incompetence of the prosthesis (Fig. 7-33).

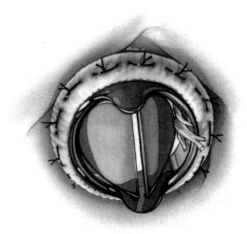

FIG. 7-33. Calcium or loose chordae impairing the movement of prosthetic disc mechanisms.

OBSTRUCTIVE CALCIUM DEPOSITS
Calcium in the ventricular wall that protrudes into the ventricular cavity near the annulus can seriously impair normal excursion of the mechanical leaflet mechanism.

 STRUT PROJECTION
The struts of the prosthesis must project freely into the left ventricular cavity. Every precaution must be taken to prevent these struts from coming into contact with or becoming embedded in the left ventricular wall. This can result in intractable dysrhythmia and can also interfere with normal prosthetic function (Fig. 7-34).

 PROSTHETIC OBSTRUCTION OF THE LEFT VENTRICULAR OUTFLOW TRACT
The prosthesis must be placed in such a way that the struts of tissue valves or the cage of ball valves do not obstruct the adjacent left ventricular outflow tract (Fig. 7-35).

The stented porcine aortic valve is, at this time, the standard tissue prosthesis for the mitral position. One of the three leaflets of the porcine aortic valve is usually larger than the other two, and a correspondingly larger third of the sewing ring is aligned with it. Therefore, just a little more than one-third of the sewing ring of these prostheses, from one strut to another, should be reserved for alignment with the anterior mitral annulus and the remaining two-thirds of the sewing ring for the posterior mitral annulus. In this position, the struts of the prosthe-

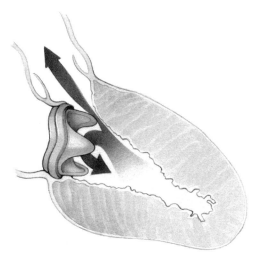

FIG. 7-35. Prosthetic obstruction of the left ventricular outflow tract.

sis are unlikely to obstruct the left ventricular outflow tract.

 STRUT ENTANGLEMENT
The struts of the prosthesis can become encircled by the sutures, which causes distortion of the leaflets and prevents valve function. All tissue prostheses come with the tips of the struts already temporarily held together with sutures, which are easily removed after the prosthesis is properly seated.

 SUTURE PLACEMENT
Sutures must always incorporate annular and leaflet tissues. Inadvertent placement of sutures into left ventricular musculature will cut through the left ventricular wall (Fig. 7-36). This can cause a hematoma of the left ventricle, which may enlarge and rupture outside the heart after ventricular contraction resumes.

 PARAVALVULAR LEAK
Weakness or tearing of the posterior annulus may result in disruption of the prosthetic attachment during the operation as well as postoperatively; consequent paravalvular leak may ensue. Such a complication must be noted and corrected by reinserting the sutures, now reinforced with pledgets, into a stronger part of the posterior annulus. This should allow the prosthesis to be securely reseated.

NB *EXCLUSION OF THE LEFT ATRIAL APPENDAGE*
The left atrial appendage can be closed to prevent blood stasis and subsequent possible thromboem-

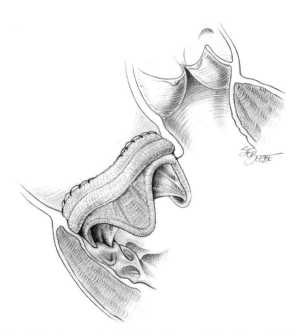

FIG. 7-34. Strut embedded in the posterior left ventricular wall.

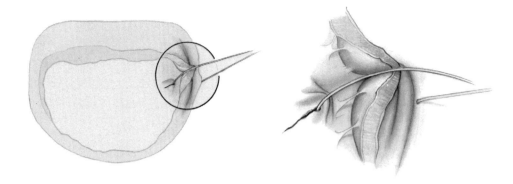

FIG. 7-36. Deeply placed sutures cutting through the left ventricular wall.

bolism. This is especially important when the patient is in atrial fibrillation. Exclusion is accomplished by tying off the auricle from the outside or by occluding its orifice from the inside of the left atrium with a purse-string suture (Fig. 7-37).

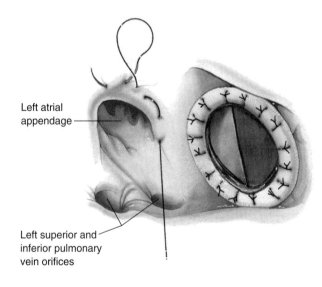

Left atrial appendage

Left superior and inferior pulmonary vein orifices

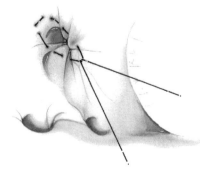

FIG. 7-37. Exclusion of the left atrial appendage.

Mitral Valve Replacement in Children

Selection of an appropriately sized mitral prosthesis in the very young can be challenging. We have found aortic bileaflet mechanical prostheses satisfactory when implanted upside down in the mitral position. In this fashion, the leaflets and occluding mechanism will be well above the mitral annulus, sitting entirely in the left atrium, thus allowing a larger prosthesis to be implanted safely.

This concept can also be used in reoperation for mitral prosthetic malfunction when there has been prosthetic patient mismatch and the mitral annulus is fibrotic or too small for the patient's body surface area.

🚫 **SUPRAANNULAR BILEAFLET AORTIC PROSTHESIS**
This modification of the bileaflet aortic prosthesis must never be used in an upside-down fashion in the mitral position because this would result in the entire valve housing and leaflets residing in the left ventricle itself.

🚫 **REGURGITANT FRACTION OF THE BILEAFLET VALVE**
There is an 8% to 10% regurgitant flow across the bileaflet prosthesis. In young hearts with a small left ventricle, the regurgitant fraction may be significant compared with the stroke volume, and the prosthesis may not therefore provide optimal hemodynamics.

An alternative technique is to implant a tissue prosthesis. The struts are first introduced through the mitral annulus. The sewing ring is then sewn to the atrial wall. Of course, this is a temporary measure because the prosthesis calcifies in children rather rapidly. The prosthesis perhaps can be replaced with a larger one at reoperation when the child is older and much bigger.

 OBSTRUCTION TO PULMONARY VEINS
The sewing ring must be sewn to the atrial wall well away from the orifices of the pulmonary veins to prevent pulmonary venous obstruction.

LATE ANNULAR COMPLICATIONS

Posterior Subannular Aneurysm

Inadvertent injury to the subvalvular membrane of the mural (posterior) mitral annulus (see Surgical Anatomy of the Mitral Valve section) during mitral valve replacement predisposes to the development of a subannular aneurysm. This kind of injury commonly occurs during leaflet excision or an aggressive removal of annular calcific deposits. Patients with this condition require reoperation. The prosthesis is removed so that the edges of the aneurysm can be identified and closed either with horizontal pledgeted mattress sutures or with a Dacron patch (Fig. 7-38). The valve can then be reinserted placing the posterior annular sutures through the reinforced aneurysm suture closure or the upper edge of the Dacron patch.

Paravalvular Leaks

In most patients, paravalvular dehiscence resulting in leaks around the mitral prosthesis is owing to imperfect surgical technique. Some of the predisposing factors, such as calcified or degenerative annulus (which allows the sutures to cut through the tissues), have been referred to previously. Paravalvular leaks tend to occur commonly along the mural (posterior) annulus. Massive calcification affecting the aortomitral leaflet continuity may obscure the annulus and interfere with correct placement of anchoring stitches. In addition, exposure of the annulus in the vicinity of the aortic valve may not be ideal. The annulus stitches may be inadvertently placed in the atrial wall or fleshy muscular ventricular wall instead of the annulus. In time, these sutures may cut through the muscular walls and produce paravalvular leaks. It is therefore important for surgeons to be aware of these fine details so that necessary precautions can be taken.

The paravalvular defect is identified under direct vision. The tissue margin of the defect has commonly become fibrous since the time of operation. Pledgeted sutures are passed deeply through the tissue margin of the defect and then through the sewing ring of the prosthesis before tying.

When the tissue margin of the defect is not satisfactory, sutures are first passed through the sewing ring of

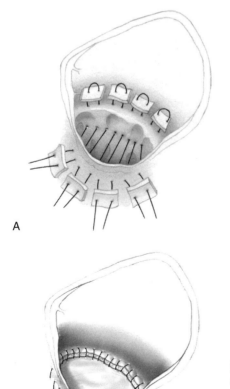

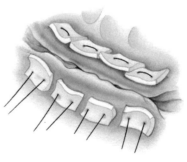

FIG. 7-38. **A and B:** Primary suture closure of a mitral subannular aneurysm. **C:** Closure of a mitral subannular aneurysm with a Dacron patch.

the prosthesis before taking a deep bite in the vicinity of the annulus through the full thickness of the atrial wall. The sutures are then tied over a strip of Teflon felt. If dehiscence of the annulus suture line is extensive, the prosthesis may need to be removed. Taking all the aforementioned precautions into consideration, the surgeon must implant a new prosthesis into position.

 INJURY TO THE CIRCUMFLEX ARTERY
Deep sutures may cause injury to the circumflex artery. This will result in myocardial injury, bleeding, and inability to wean the patient from bypass.

ATRIAL CLOSURE

Interatrial Groove Approach

A double-armed suture of 4-0 Prolene with large half-circle needles is used, starting at each end of the left atriotomy. For a secure closure, the interatrial groove tissue should be included for its buttressing effect (Fig. 7-39). To lessen the tendency to bleed from the ends of the atriotomy, the suture line should also include tissue beyond the ends of the incisions before continuing the closure (Fig. 7-39, inset). Suturing is continued in both directions. The suture line on each side is then oversewn with the other arm of the suture. Whenever the left atriotomy is extended inferiorly

behind the heart, the closure is facilitated if the sewing is started from the inside of the atrium under direct vision (Fig. 7-39).

 ATRIOTOMY CLOSURE
Although a single-layer closure is adequate, a second over-and-over suture provides a more secure atriotomy closure.

Transatrial Oblique Approach

The divided interatrial septum is approximated with a continuous suture of 4-0 Prolene, starting at the far end (anterior) end of the incision and progressing toward the right superior pulmonary vein. Another suture is used to close the right atriotomy. The edges of the right superior pulmonary vein are then approximated with a third suture (Fig. 7-40).

 INJURY TO THE RIGHT PHRENIC NERVE
Caution must be exercised in closing the right superior pulmonary vein to avoid incorporating the phrenic nerve in the suture line.

 DEPTH OF SUTURES IN THE SEPTUM
The septum is quite thick at times; the sutures should incorporate the whole thickness, including the endocardium on both sides of the septum. Oth-

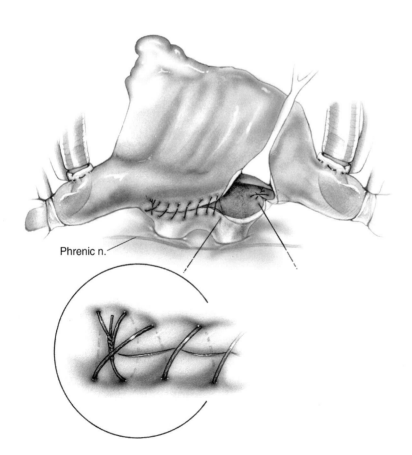

FIG. 7-39. Closure of the posterior interatrial groove. **Inset:** Inclusion of tissue beyond the ends of the incision.

Phrenic n.

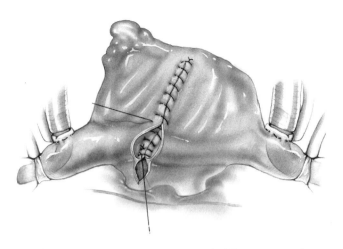

FIG. 7-40. Closure in the transatrial oblique approach.

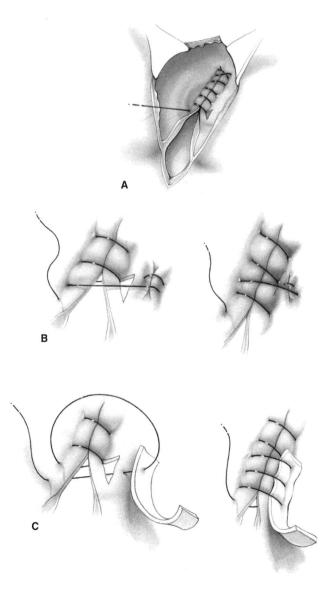

FIG. 7-41. A: Closing tears in the fossa ovalis. **B:** Buttressing with adjacent fossa tissue. **C:** Buttressing with Teflon felt.

erwise, the suture may tear through the muscular septum , resulting in a septal defect.

 BUTTRESSING THE SUTURES
Fossa ovalis tissue can be friable and may not hold sutures well (Fig. 7-41A). The adjacent fossa tissue may be used to buttress the sutures (Fig. 7-41B). Alternatively, Teflon felt or pericardial strips may be used (Fig. 7-41C).

 TRANSATRIAL LONGITUDINAL SEPTAL APPROACH
After completion of the procedure, the septum is reapproximated with continuous a 4-0 Prolene suture. The right atrial wall is closed with a second 4-0 Prolene suture line.

CLOSED MITRAL COMMISSUROTOMY

Closed mitral commissurotomy is now rarely performed in most Western countries. Consequently, only a few of the current generation of cardiac surgeons have had adequate experience with this technique. In Third World countries, where mitral valve disease continues to be the dominant form of cardiac lesion, closed valvotomy continues to be the preferred form of therapy because of its simplicity and low cost compared with open heart procedures. Nevertheless, closed mitral valvotomy remains a good operation in selected subgroups of patients, and the long-term results have been consistently satisfactory.

Technique

A left posterolateral or anterolateral thoracotomy is made through the bed of the fifth rib. The lung is retracted posteroinferiorly, and a long incision is made anterior and parallel to the left phrenic nerve. The pericardium is then suspended with traction sutures. The left atrial appendage is identified and excluded with a side-biting clamp. A purse-string suture of 2-0 Prolene is placed around the left appendage. Another purse-string suture, reinforced with pledgets, is then placed into the apex of the left ventricle. The left atrial appendage is incised within the purse-string suture, and the surgeon's right index finger is introduced into the left atrium. The mitral valve is palpated to detect calcification, the degree of mitral stenosis, or the presence of insufficiency (Fig. 7-42).

 TEAR IN THE ATRIAL APPENDAGE
The index finger should be introduced gently, without undue pressure. If the atrial appendage tears, it will result in brisk bleeding.

 BLOOD CLOT
Preoperative echocardiography is always performed to study the mitral valve pathology and to

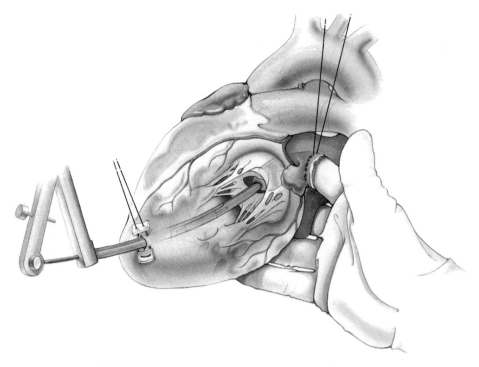

FIG. 7-42. Technique for a closed mitral commissurotomy.

detect the presence of a blood clot in the left atrial appendage. Nevertheless, before applying clamps to the appendage or introducing a finger into the atrial cavity, the left atrial appendage should be palpated carefully to detect a blood clot. If thrombus is suspected, it should be excluded through an atriotomy. If this is not possible, the closed procedure should be abandoned, and the operation converted to an open valvotomy with the use of extracorporeal circulation.

 MITRAL ORIFICE OCCLUSION
The index finger should not occlude the mitral orifice for more than two or three cardiac cycles to avoid precipitating dysrhythmia and possible cardiac arrest.

When the right index finger is in the left atrium, the heart is elevated with the remaining three fingers and palm of the right hand to bring the left ventricular apex into view. With a no. 11 blade held in the left hand, the surgeon makes a small ventriculotomy within the apical purse-string suture. This can also be performed by the surgeon's assistant if desired. This opening is now enlarged with a series of Hegar's dilators until it accommodates the diameter of the Tubb's valvulotome. The Tubb's dilator is then introduced into the left ventricle with the surgeon's left hand and advanced through the mitral valve into the left atrium. It is then opened quickly to the preset limiting extent of 3.5 to 4.5 cm, closed, and

removed. The surgeon's finger is then removed, and the purse-string suture on the left ventricular apex is then snugged down and tied over pledgets.

 PREMATURE OPENING OF THE DILATOR
It is most important not to open the dilator until the surgeon can feel its tip with the right index finger in the left atrial cavity. Premature opening of the dilator may injure or tear the subvalvular structures and result in mitral insufficiency (Fig. 7-43).

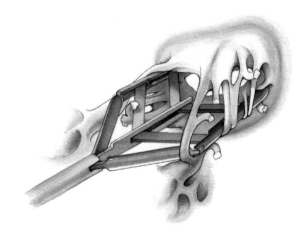

FIG. 7-43. Premature opening of the dilator, which may injure or tear the subvalvular structures and result in mitral insufficiency.

INADEQUATE DILATOR CLOSURE
After completion of the dilation, the dilator must be closed completely before removal. Inadequate closure of the dilator will cause tearing of the left ventricular opening during withdrawal.

 VALVOTOMY ADEQUACY
Adequacy of the valvotomy and any evidence of a mitral insufficiency jet must be ascertained with the surgeon's index finger while it is still in the left atrium.

 AIR EMBOLISM
Every precaution should be taken to prevent air from entering the left atrium or left ventricle during the procedure.

Conversion of a Closed Mitral Valvotomy to the Open Technique

In young adults, the mitral lesion may be fibrotic but elastic and without calcification. The surgeon may find it possible to stretch the orifice maximally with a Tubb's dilator only to note that the orifice resumes its previous stenotic size on removal of the dilator. Such patients must be treated with open mitral commissurotomy.

NB *STANDBY CARDIOPULMONARY BYPASS*
It is always a prudent precaution to perform this procedure with a heart-lung machine available on

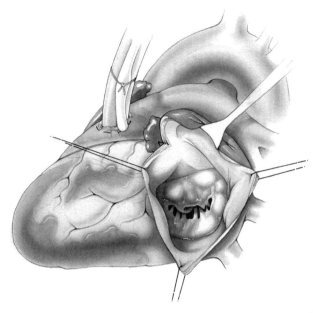

FIG. 7-44. Left atriotomy for exposure of the mitral valve if cardiopulmonary bypass becomes necessary.

standby so that the surgeon will have the option of using cardiopulmonary bypass if it becomes necessary. Venous drainage can be accomplished through a cannula placed in the main pulmonary artery. Arterial return may be through a cannula either in the descending aorta or femoral artery. A left atriotomy will give excellent exposure of the mitral valve (Fig. 7-44).

CHAPTER 8

Surgery of the Tricuspid Valve

Rheumatic fever continues to be the most common cause of organic tricuspid valve disease. With rare exceptions, it is associated with mitral and, in most patients, aortic valve disease as well. Usually both stenosis and insufficiency coexist because pure tricuspid stenosis of rheumatic origin as an isolated entity is rarely seen. Functional tricuspid insufficiency occurs frequently in patients with advanced mitral valve disease and often disappears or improves greatly when successful mitral valve repair or replacement is accomplished. Not infrequently, however, some form of reparative procedure is indicated when the tricuspid valve incompetence is severe.

The tricuspid valve may be affected by itself or as part of a general picture of infective endocarditis. Isolated, tricuspid valve bacterial endocarditis is seen in intravenous drug abusers and occasionally in patients with long-standing central venous catheters.

TECHNICAL CONSIDERATIONS

Surgical Anatomy of the Tricuspid Valve and the Right Ventricle

The tricuspid valve guards the right ventricular orifice. It consists of a septal leaflet, a large anterior leaflet, and a small posterior leaflet, all three of which are attached to and continuous with the tricuspid ring. These valve leaflets are folds of endocardium strengthened by fibrous tissue. Small accessory leaflets are often present in the angles between the major leaflets. The atrioventricular node lies in the atrial septum adjacent to the septal leaflet, just anterior to the coronary sinus. Its location can be pinpointed at the apex of the triangle of Koch (which is bordered by the septal leaflet, the tendon of Todaro, and the orifice of the coronary sinus). The atrioventricular conduction bundle (His's bundle) extends from the atrioventricular node through the central fibrous body into the ventricles under the membranous part of the interventricular septum. It is approximately 2 mm thick and consists of bundles of fine muscular fibers. There is normally no muscular continuity between the atria and the ventricles except through the conducting tissue of the atrioventricular bundle, but aberrations may exist that can give rise to rhythm disturbances (Fig. 8-1) (see also Surgical Anatomy of the Right Atrium section in Chapter 17).

The right ventricular cavity is tubular and triangular in contrast to that of the left ventricle, which is conical. It is bounded by concave anterior and posterior walls and a convex septal wall. There are at least three groups of papillary muscles that stem from the inner aspect of the right ventricular cavity. Chordae tendineae, which are nonelastic chords of tissue, arise from the papillary muscles and fuse to the free edges and the ventricular surfaces of the leaflets of the tricuspid valve. The chordae of each papillary muscle control the contiguous margins of two cusps. Hence, chordae pass from a large anterior papillary muscle to the anterior and posterior leaflets; from a posterior papillary muscle, often represented by two or more components, chordae attach to the posterior and septal leaflets; finally, from a variable group of small septal papillary muscles, chordae fan out and fasten to the anterior and septal leaflets of the tricuspid valve. A bridge of muscle, the moderator band, stems from the septum, crosses the cavity of the right ventricle to the free wall, and contributes to the origin of the anterior papillary muscle. A tract of specialized tissue associated with the conduction system runs through the moderator band (Fig. 8-2).

Incision

A median sternotomy is the preferred approach for acquired valvular disease because it offers complete exposure for exploration of the mitral, aortic, and tricuspid valves.

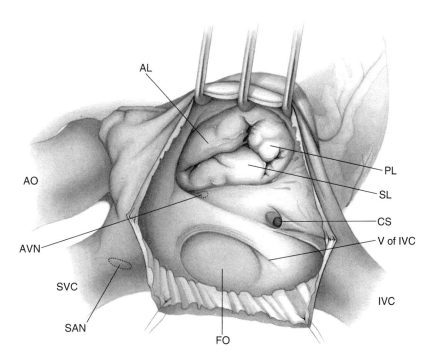

FIG. 8-1. Surgical anatomy of the right atrium and tricuspid valve. *AL*, anterior leaflet; *PL*, posterior leaflet; *AO*, aorta; *SL*, septal leaflet; *AVN*, atrioventricular node; *SVC*, superior vena cava; *FO*, fossa ovalis; *CS*, coronary sinus; *V of IVC*, valve of inferior vena cava; *SAN*, sinoatrial node; *IVC*, inferior vena cava.

Myocardial Preservation

When satisfactory cardiopulmonary bypass has been established, the aorta is cross-clamped and cold blood cardioplegic solution is administered into the aortic root to bring about prompt diastolic cardiac arrest. This is usu-ally complemented by the retrograde technique (see Chapter 3). If isolated tricuspid valve surgery is indi-cated, it can be performed on cardiopulmonary bypass with a warm, beating heart.

Cannulation

Any procedure that entails internal exposure of the right side of the heart requires bicaval cannulation. There-fore, whenever surgery on the tricuspid valve is contem-plated, both vena cava are cannulated (Fig. 8-3). The ascending aorta is cannulated for arterial return, and car-diopulmonary bypass is initiated.

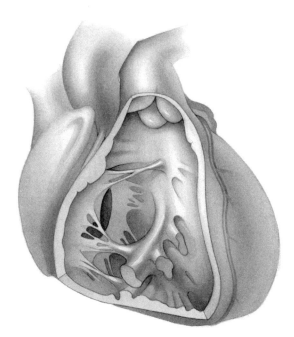

FIG. 8-2. Surgical anatomy of the tricuspid valve as seen from the right ventricle. The free wall of the ventricle has been removed to show the tricuspid subvalvular apparatus and the convex septal wall.

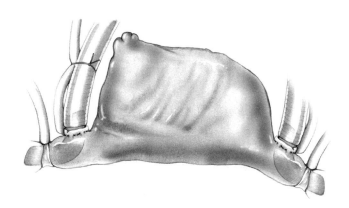

FIG. 8-3. Direct caval cannulation.

Exposure of the Tricuspid Valve

A longitudinal or oblique atriotomy is made approximately 1 cm posterior to and parallel with the atrioventricular groove. The atriotomy edges are retracted with sutures, and exposure of the tricuspid valve is further facilitated by means of appropriately sized retractors.

 INJURY TO THE SINOATRIAL NODE
The sinoatrial node is always prone to injury, either during cannulation, during passage of tapes around the superior vena cava, or by atriotomy. The incision should be well away from the sinoatrial node, and its superior extension should be limited to approximately 1 cm from the superior margin of the right atrium.

It has always been the rule to digitally palpate and evaluate tricuspid insufficiency before the initiation of cardiopulmonary bypass through a purse-string suture in the right atrial appendage. With the use of intraoperative transesophageal echocardiography, digital palpation of the tricuspid valve has gone out of vogue. However, clinical history, preoperative echocardiography, right heart catheterization data, and intraoperative transesophageal echocardiography confirming the diagnosis of tricuspid insufficiency are definite indications to explore and evaluate the tricuspid valve. Isolated tricuspid valve surgery is not frequently performed; it is usually part of a complex procedure that includes mitral valve surgery or aortic valve surgery, with or without concomitant coronary artery bypass grafting. Surgery on the tricuspid valve is the last step of the operation and is carried out when other procedures have been completed and the patient is being rewarmed.

Annuloplasty of the Tricuspid Valve

Irreversible functional tricuspid insufficiency is the outcome of chronic right ventricular dilation, with permanent increase in right ventricular volume and loss of its bellows shape. After satisfactory relief of associated valvular disease, the regurgitant jets will remain and may even progress, resulting in increased postoperative mortality and morbidity. The controversy regarding the management of functional tricuspid insufficiency reflects the difficulty of precisely distinguishing the two stages of the same disease process, i.e., irreversible and reversible tricuspid valve insufficiency. Both the DeVega and ring annuloplasty techniques are satisfactory procedures for the repair of the tricuspid valve. Neither technique incorporates the margin of the septal leaflet that is usually minimally involved in functional dilation of the tricuspid valve.

DeVega Annuloplasty

This procedure is an effective method in the management of *functional* tricuspid insufficiency and is recommended even for patients in whom the only indication may be a history of tricuspid insufficiency. Because of its simplicity, it requires little additional time and can be performed concomitantly with the mitral or aortic valve surgery.

The right atrium is opened obliquely or longitudinally, and the tricuspid valve is inspected. A double-armed suture, usually 2-0 Ticron or Prolene, is started on the annulus at the posterior septal commissure. It is then extended around the circumference of the valve in a counterclockwise direction, taking deep bites (every 5–6 mm) into the endocardium (Fig. 8-4) and into the fibrous ring of the posterior septal commissure, posterior leaflet, anteroposterior commissure, anterior leaflet, and anterior septal commissure. The second needle of the suture traverses the same route 1 to 2 mm outside the previous suture. At each end of the course of suturing, a small pledget of Teflon is used for a buttress, and the suture is then tied securely around an appropriately sized Starr-Edwards mitral prosthesis obturator to ensure a predictable annuloplasty. A strip of autologous pericardium previously treated with glutaraldehyde or a strip of Teflon felt can be incorporated in the suturing process to add durability and contour to the reparative process (Fig. 8-5).

Ring Annuloplasty

The DeVega annuloplasty has been criticized for its inability to adequately plicate commissures where dilation is predominant. At times, infolding of the leaflet as a

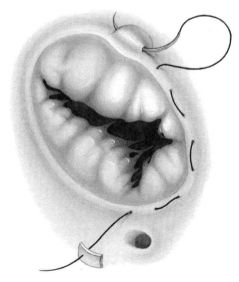

FIG. 8-4. Suturing technique in DeVega annuloplasty.

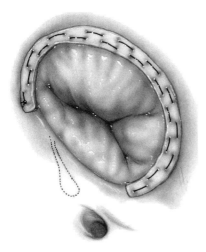

FIG. 8-5. Annuloplasty reinforced with a Teflon felt strip.

consequence of annular plication may defeat the normal function of the valve. It may therefore be preferable to choose a flexible annuloplasty band that conforms to the normal shape of the tricuspid valve and does not include the area of the septal annulus. The sizes vary according to the length of the fibrous septal annulus.

The band is anchored in position by means of multiple simple or mattress sutures of 3-0 Tevdek incorporating the fibrous annulus of the anterior and posterior leaflets and excluding the septal leaflet (Fig. 8-6A). The sutures are then brought up through the annuloplasty band at shorter intervals than in the annulus to reduce the size of the annulus (Fig. 8-6B). They are then individually tied in place. The completed annuloplasty thus not only reduces the size of the tricuspid orifice but also restores the valve to its normal configuration when severe annular dilation or mixed valvular disease is present (Fig. 8-6C).

Tricuspid Annuloplasty system [Baxter Healthcare Corporation Edwards CVS Division, Santa Ana, CA] is the most recent modification of flexible tricuspid annuloplasty bands. It has the distinct advantage of having a template that is left in place while the sutures are tied, resulting in a normally shaped tricuspid orifice that can still flex as ventricular contraction occurs.

⊘ *INADEQUATE DEPTH OF EACH SUTURE BITE*
The depth of the bites at the annulus must be quite substantial; otherwise, the suture will tear through and result in an inadequate annuloplasty.

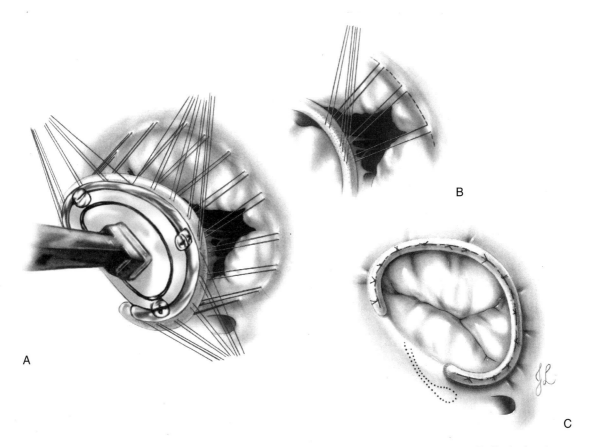

FIG. 8-6. Edwards mc³ Tricuspid Annuloplasty system. **A:** Anchoring mattress sutures. **B:** Reducing the size of the annulus. **C:** Restoring the valve to its normal configuration.

INJURY TO THE ATRIOVENTRICULAR NODE
The suture should exclude the septal segment and be well away from the orifice of the coronary sinus to avoid producing postoperative heart block.

LEAFLET TEAR
Sutures should be limited to the fibrous annulus and must not include the thin and otherwise normal leaflet tissue, which may tear, resulting in valvular insufficiency and an inadequate repair.

NB **INDICATION FOR TRICUSPID RECONSTRUCTION**
When the decompressed heart is opened, the tricuspid valve may look completely normal and competent. The features of ventricular-valvular disproportion are not evident in the decompressed heart, and the slight thickening of the subvalvular mechanism is not easily detected from the atrial view. The decision to attempt to repair the valve must be made preoperatively based on the clinical history, cardiac catheterization, and echocardiographic data.

Bicuspidization of the Tricuspid Valve

Annuloplasty at the anteroposterior and posterior septal commissures may also be employed in the repair of tricuspid valve insufficiency. Often, however, the whole posterior annulus is excluded, converting the tricuspid valve to a bicuspid valve. This is achieved by multiple figure-of-eight sutures of 2-0 Ticron (Fig. 8-7) placed well away from the orifice of the coronary sinus to avoid producing postoperative heart block.

TRICUSPID COMMISSUROTOMY

Pure tricuspid stenosis is rare. When it occurs, it is usually of rheumatic origin and thus manifests typical fibrotic changes, that is, commissural fusion, thickening of the leaflets, and variable fibrosis and shortening of the chordae tendineae.

Commissurotomy is carried out meticulously with a no. 11 knife blade along the commissures up to 1 to 2 mm from the annulus. Because of the tricuspid nature of the valve, commissurotomy is limited to one or two commissures to avoid producing insufficiency (Fig. 8-8).

 ANTERIOR SEPTAL COMMISSURE
The anterior septal commissure is rarely incised because it is prone to produce insufficiency.

 REMODELING THE TRICUSPID VALVE
If insufficiency occurs, the valve must be remodeled with an annuloplasty band (see techniques for tricuspid valve annuloplasty previously described). Often bicuspidization of the tricuspid valve is indicated to ensure a competent valve.

TRICUSPID VALVE REPLACEMENT

Because it is usually possible to repair the tricuspid valve, its replacement is rarely necessary. Nevertheless, when the severity of the valvular distortion prevents a satisfactory reconstructive procedure, valve replacement becomes mandatory. If possible, the subvalvular apparatus is retained and the leaflet tissues are incorporated in suturing the prosthesis to the annulus (see discussion on mitral valve replacement with retaining the subvalvular apparatus in Chapter 7). Often, however, when tricuspid valve replacement becomes necessary, all the subvalvular apparatus and the leaflet tissues are diseased to a degree that precludes their use. Therefore, resection of the tricuspid valve is started by incising the anterior and poste-

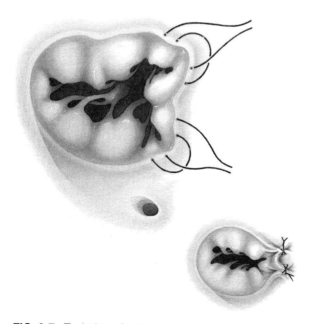

FIG. 8-7. Technique for bicuspidizing the tricuspid valve.

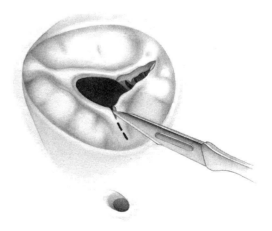

FIG. 8-8. Tricuspid valve commissurotomy.

rior leaflets and dividing the chordal attachments deep in the right ventricle. The mobilized valve may now be inverted up into the right atrium, and with visual control from both the atrial and ventricular sides, the septal leaflet is dissected. A broad zone of the attached margin of the septal leaflet and its chordal attachments is left in place, if possible. Preferably, the septal leaflet or all the leaflets are left intact and used to anchor the appropriate prosthesis. The normal tubular and triangular configuration of the right ventricle is often lost in patients with chronic tricuspid valve disease. The dilated right ventricle can easily accommodate the struts of a tissue prosthesis or even the cage of a ball valve prosthesis.

Size 3-0 Teflon pledgeted sutures are passed through the annulus, except in the region of the septal leaflet. In this area, sutures are placed only through the leaflet tissue and its attached structures to avoid producing heart block. The sutures are then passed through the sewing ring of the prosthesis exactly as in mitral valve replacement (Fig. 8-9). The prosthesis is slipped down into its bed, and the sutures are tied and cut. Care is taken to avoid injury to the right ventricular endocardium by pressing the prosthesis into the decompressed cardiopleged ventricle. As in mitral valve replacement, size selection is based not only on the diameter of the atrioventricular ring but also on the size of the ventricular cavity. No problems have been encountered in reducing the annulus by placing sutures close together in the prosthesis. Serious injury to

the interventricular septum may occur, however, if the prosthesis selected is too large.

 DISC VALVE DYSFUNCTION CAUSED BY LEAFLET TISSUE
When the leaflets with their subvalvular attachments are left intact to preserve right ventricular function, disc prostheses should not be used. Bileaflet prostheses and bioprostheses are the valves of choice in the tricuspid position.

 INJURY TO THE ATRIOVENTRICULAR NODE AND CONDUCTION TISSUE
The anchoring of sutures for the prosthesis must be well away from the conduction tissue to avoid producing heart block.

SEPTAL INJURY
A ball valve or a large bioprosthesis protruding into a very small right ventricular cavity can produce a septal injury. Therefore, under these circumstances, an appropriately sized bileaflet mechanical prosthesis or a very low profile bioprosthesis should be used.

NB Consideration should be given to placing permanent epicardial ventricular pacing leads in patients undergoing tricuspid valve replacement. These leads can be buried in a pocket anterior to the posterior rectus sheath in the left upper quadrant for later permanent pacemaker implantation if required.

TRICUSPID VALVE ENDOCARDITIS

Tricuspid valve endocarditis is seen with increasing frequency, especially in patients who are intravenous drug abusers. When tricuspid valve endocarditis has not responded to antibiotic therapy, valve excision and its removal may be recommended. Valve replacement is then indicated approximately 3 months after all evidence of residual infection has disappeared. In addition, intravenous drug abusers should be completely free of their addiction before being subjected to further valve surgery to lessen the risk of subsequent prosthetic valve endocarditis. This can be difficult to establish with certainty, and there is an inherent risk involved with valve replacement in these patients owing to the high incidence of their recurring addiction.

NB *HEMODYNAMIC CONSEQUENCES*
Removal of the tricuspid valve necessarily results in the right atrium and the right ventricle becoming a single chamber. The hemodynamic consequences may not be revealed in the immediate postoperative period, partly because of the otherwise healthy myocardium in these patients. Nevertheless, right-sided heart failure ensues in due course. Conse-

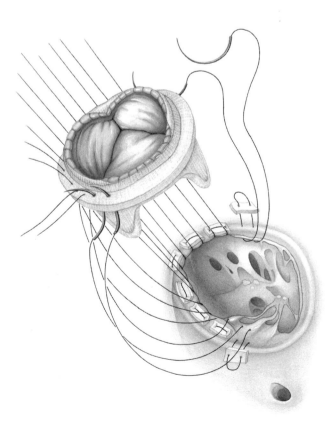

FIG. 8-9. Technique for tricuspid valve replacement.

quently, valve replacement in the not too distant future will become necessary.

Interest in tricuspid valve repair has led to an attempt to resect diseased leaflet tissue and to remodel the valve in patients affected with endocarditis of the tricuspid valve. Vegetations are usually found to be large and adherent to the leaflet tissue. Often the infection destroys the leaflet and its attachments. If the posterior leaflet is involved, the necrotic area with a good margin of healthy tissue is removed. Posterior annuloplasty with 2-0 Ticron sutures buttressed with autologous pericardial pledgets is carried out, and bicuspidization of the tricuspid valve results in a competent valve (Fig. 8-10). When the septal or anterior leaflets are involved, the affected portion is excised in a trapezoidal fashion. A limited annuloplasty with figure-of-eight sutures of 2-0 Ticron is then performed, and the resected leaflet edges are reapproximated with interrupted 6-0 or 7-0 Prolene sutures (Fig. 8-11). Because septal leaflet resection and repair may at times result in complete heart block, permanent pacemakers may be necessary in this subgroup of patients.

In patients with ventriculoseptal defects associated with bacterial endocarditis affecting the tricuspid valve, the septal defect is repaired through the tricuspid valve using a double velour Dacron patch (Fig. 8-12). The edges of the ventriculoseptal defect are first debrided, and the necrotic tissue and vegetations are removed meticulously. A patch of double velour Dacron is then cut to match the size and shape of the resultant defect. This is secured to the edges of the septal defect with running 4-0 Prolene or interrupted horizontal mattress sutures of 4-0 Ticron. At the superior aspect of the ventriculoseptal defect located under the septal leaflet of the tricuspid valve, the patch is secured to leaflet tissue adjacent to the annulus. If possible, sutures should not be passed through the annulus in this area because the atrioventricular node is likely to be injured. If this portion of the septal leaflet is involved with vegetation and requires excision, an attempt is made to preserve a rim of leaflet tissue next to the annulus. After the ventriculoseptal defect patch is secured in place, the septal annulus is reapproximated with figure-of-eight sutures of 2-0 Ticron and the leaflet tissue is brought together with interrupted 6-0 Prolene sutures (Fig. 8-12). Results of tricuspid valve repair in patients with endocarditis have been very gratifying.

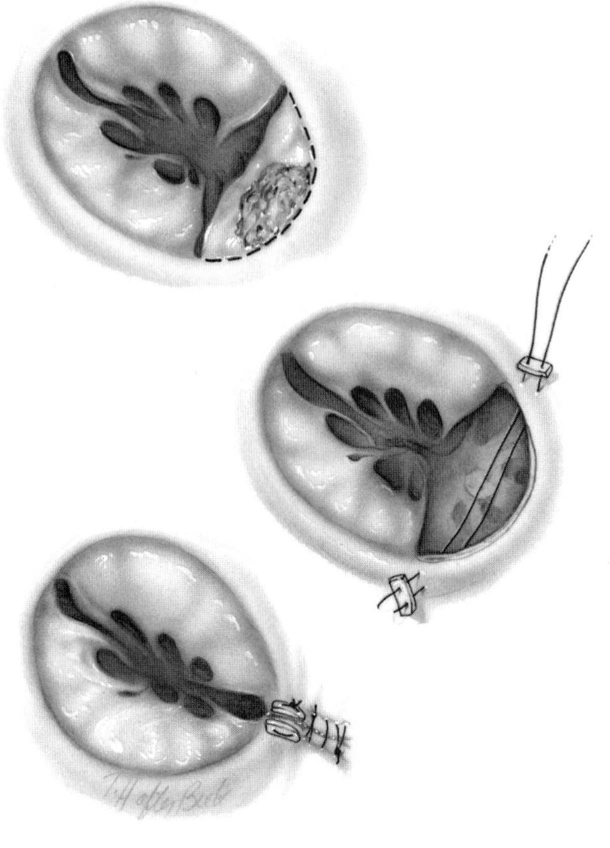

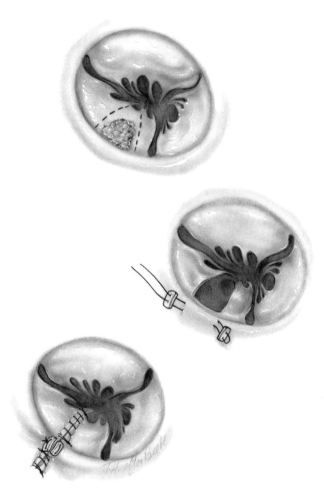

FIG. 8-10. Technique for posterior leaflet resection and bicuspidization of the tricuspid valve.

FIG. 8-11. Technique for resection of a portion of tricuspid septal valve leaflet with subsequent annuloplasty and leaflet reapproximation.

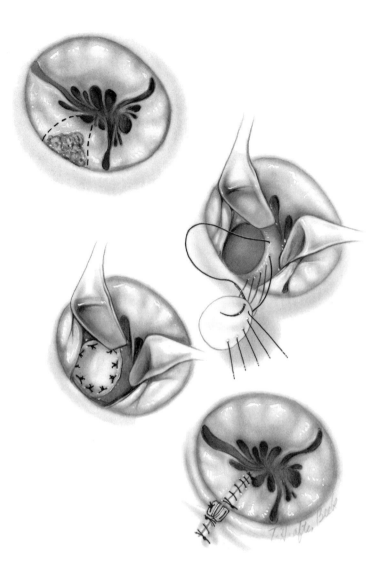

FIG. 8-12. Technique for patch closure of a ventricular septal defect combined with partial septal leaflet resection and reconstruction.

CHAPTER 9

Surgery of the Aorta

ACUTE AORTIC DISSECTION

Acute aortic dissection has a sudden onset and is a true surgical emergency. It is usually initiated by a transverse tear in the intima or the intima and media. This disruptive injury gives rise to a hematoma within the media. The pulsatile force of ejection of the left ventricle causes a longitudinal separation of the aortic wall, mainly along and within the media. This dissection can progress both distally and proximally. Distal progression beyond the aortic arch can continue along the course of the descending thoracic and abdominal aorta to a variable extent and can involve its branches. Proximal extension of the dissecting hematoma may infiltrate the aortic root, distorting the aortic valve leaflets or compressing the ostia of the coronary arteries. This can produce aortic valve insufficiency and acute myocardial ischemia, respectively, both of which can cause death. In addition, acute dissection can cause rupture of the aorta into the pericardium. Thus, the symptomatology of aortic dissection varies depending on its effect on the aortic valve, aortic wall, or aortic branches.

The underlying cause for the development of acute aortic dissection is associated with many factors. Of great significance is medial degeneration or cystic medial necrosis of the aortic wall. Marfan's syndrome, an autosomal dominant disorder, is commonly associated with acute aortic dissection. However, annuloectasia can occur in patients without Marfan's syndrome and result in acute aortic dissection. Of significant clinical importance is the association of hypertension, the presence of a bicuspid aortic valve, and coarctation of the aorta with acute aortic dissection.

The current classification (Stanford) distinguishes two types of aortic dissection based on the involvement of the descending aorta. Type A, or anterior, dissection commonly starts in the ascending aorta, usually 1 to 2 cm above the aortic annulus, and may progress along the course of the aorta for a variable distance. Type B, or posterior, dissection typically starts in the descending aorta distal to the origin of the subclavian artery. The dissection can progress dis-

tally to a variable distance; less commonly, it may extend proximally thereby resulting in a type A dissection.

DeBakey's classification is based on the anatomic location of the dissection. Therefore, type A Stanford classification conforms to DeBakey types I and II, whereas type B Stanford classification includes DeBakey types IIIA and IIIB (Fig. 9-1). From the practical point of view, the Stanford classification is simple and provides guidance as to the initial method of management (surgical versus medical) as well as surgical approaches (median sternotomy versus left lateral thoracotomy).

The immediate management of all acute aortic dissections is to reduce and maintain the patient's systolic blood pressure at a level that still ensures satisfactory cerebral and renal perfusion. All patients suspected of acute aortic dissection should undergo transesophageal echocardiography immediately. This can usually be performed in the intensive care unit, in the emergency department, or even in the operating room. There are occasions when diagnosis of acute aortic dissection cannot be made with transesophageal echocardiography. In these cases, if the patient's condition permits, computed tomography with contrast, magnetic resonance imaging, or aortography should be performed to establish the precise entry site and extent of dissection. Acute ascending aortic dissection is a surgical emergency because conservative therapy is not effective in most instances. Antihypertensive therapy plays an important role, at least in the initial management of patients with acute dissection of the descending thoracic aorta.

AORTIC ANEURYSMS

Aortic aneurysm is a localized enlargement and dilation of the arterial wall. It can affect any segment of the aorta. The ascending aorta is most commonly affected (45%), followed by the descending aorta (35%). The aortic arch (10%) is involved either as an isolated lesion or as an extension of the ascending or, less commonly, descending thoracic aorta. Progressive enlargement of the aneurysm is an indication for resection and replace-

116

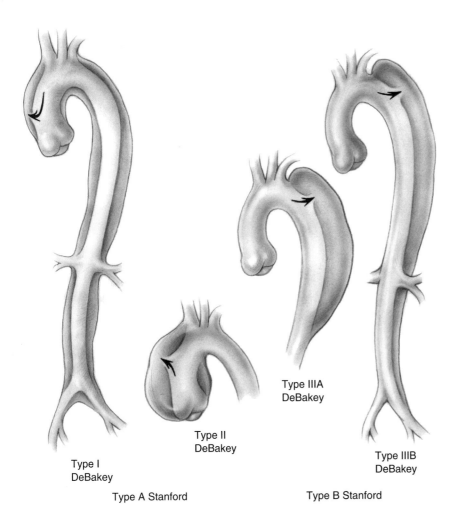

Type IIIA
DeBakey

Type II
DeBakey

Type IIIB
DeBakey

Type I
DeBakey

Type A Stanford

Type B Stanford

FIG. 9-1. Classification of aortic dissection.

ment with a tube graft because it will eventually rupture, culminating in the death of the patient.

The techniques for excision and graft replacement for aneurysms of the ascending and descending thoracic aorta are similar to those described for surgical management of types A and B aortic dissections.

Replacement of the Ascending Aorta

The ascending aorta is approached by median sternotomy. Both groins should be in the operative field, and the arterial return is accomplished by cannulating either femoral or external iliac arteries. In patients with ascending aneurysms, direct aortic cannulation may be feasible. In many centers, right axillary artery is used.

NB The right femoral artery is less commonly involved in aortic dissection and therefore should be the cannulation site of choice.

 RETROGRADE PERFUSION THROUGH FALSE LUMEN
In patients with aortic dissection, the disease often extends distally, sometimes down to the femoral vessels; therefore, care must be exercised not to cannulate and perfuse through the false lumen of the femoral artery in a retrograde fashion.

 OCCLUSIVE DISEASE OF THE EXTERNAL ILIAC AND FEMORAL VESSELS
In elderly patients with severe atherosclerosis, the femoral and iliac arteries are markedly diseased and cannulation may be hazardous. Cannulae are available that can be introduced into these vessels percutaneously or under direct vision with a needle and wire technique (Fig. 9-2). The flow through a size 20 cannula is adequate for all but very large patients. Alternatively, the axillary artery may be used.

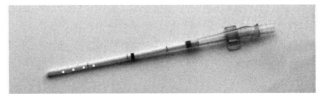

FIG. 9-2. Multiple side hole femoral cannula that can be introduced over a guidewire.

A dual-stage atriocaval cannula is usually used for venous drainage.

NB If the ascending aorta is too large, preventing adequate exposure of the right atrium for venous cannulation, femoral vein cannulation is performed.

 REPEAT STERNOTOMY
If the procedure is a reoperation, it is preferable to achieve cardiopulmonary bypass through a femoral artery and femoral vein before opening the sternum (see discussion in Chapter 2).

 HEMODYNAMIC INSTABILITY
It is prudent to initiate cardiopulmonary bypass promptly by means of the groin vessels before the administration of general anesthesia in patients with unstable hemodynamics to prevent circulatory collapse. This is especially important if pericardial tamponade is apparent or suspected.

Femoral vein cannulation can be achieved by introducing a long, hydraulically superior cannula with multiple side holes for excellent venous return. The important characteristic of this device is that it comes with a guidewire and contains a tapered, dilated sheath inside the cannula. The guidewire allows easy, comfortable, and safe passage of the cannula over the pelvic rim. The cannula has multiple side holes and may be advanced into the right atrium, providing superior drainage.

 ILIAC VEIN INJURY
Venous cannulae that lack guidewires often hang up at the pelvic rim, resulting in inadequate venous return. If an attempt is made to push the cannula farther into the inferior vena cava, perforation of the iliac vein with catastrophic consequences may ensue. It is usually easier to pass the cannula via the right femoral vein because of its straighter course compared with the left femoral vein.

After completion of a median sternotomy, an additional venous cannula is placed in the right atrium if required. A left ventricular vent through the right superior pulmonary vein (see Chapter 4) decompresses the heart and expedites the procedure. Venting is especially important if aortic valve insufficiency is present.

Retrograde Cerebral Perfusion

Whenever deep circulatory arrest is contemplated, the patient is generally cooled down to bladder temperature of 18° to 24°C. Ice is packed around the patient's head. A tape is passed around the superior vena cava (see Chapter 2). A purse-string suture of 4-0 Prolene is applied to the adventitia of the superior vena cava at its junction with the pericardium. The adventitial tissue within the purse-string suture is cleaned off the superior vena cava, and an incision is made on the vein. The opening is enlarged with the tip of a clamp or scissors, and a long, metal-tipped, right-angled cannula is introduced into the superior vena cava and guided upward past the innominate vein (Fig. 9-3). This cannula is then connected to an arm of the cardioplegia delivery system or the arterial line to perfuse cold blood into the superior vena cava whenever circulatory arrest is initiated. The tape around the superior vena cava is snugged down on the cannula to prevent perfusate from flowing back into the right atrium.

 EXCLUSION OF THE AZYGOS VEIN
Tape is snugged down on the superior vena cava above the azygos vein to prevent runoff of cold blood into the azygos system (Fig. 9-3).

NB Some thought has to be given to extending the concept of retrograde cerebral perfusion with cold blood to retrograde perfusion of the gastrointestinal tract and even the rest of the body! Consequently, at times, perfusion of cold blood through the azygos vein may be advantageous.

The central venous pressure should not exceed 30 to 40 mm Hg as measured by the side arm of the Swan-Ganz introducer in the internal jugular or subclavian vein. The perfusion flow should be approximately 400 to 800 mL per minute. It is not quite evident that the retrograde cerebral perfusion provides any nutritive support to the brain. However, it is clear that it does provide a uniform cooling of the brain. Its most important benefit is prevention of air or debris from flowing upward into the arch vessels, which would cause cerebral emboli. This is very evident when much debris is seen floating on the very dark desat-

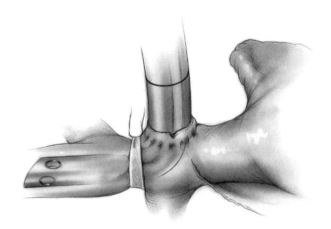

FIG. 9-3. Direct cannulation of the superior vena cava for retrograde cerebral perfusion.

urated blood flowing out of the arch vessels into the operative field.

At the end of circulatory arrest, retrograde cerebral perfusion is discontinued and the cannula is removed and the purse-string suture on the superior vena cava is tied down. If retrograde cerebral perfusion has been accomplished using an arm of the cardioplegia system, retrograde flow is continued for the first 1 to 2 minutes after resuming cardiopulmonary bypass to help to prevent air embolism to the arch vessels.

Technique

On cardiopulmonary bypass with the heart decompressed, preliminary evaluation is made. Any concomitant additional procedures, such as the need for coronary artery bypass grafting, must be noted. The conduct of the operation should be choreographed precisely at this time.

When the nasopharyngeal temperature reaches 18° to 24°C, the patient is placed in the Trendelenburg position. The heart-lung machine is halted, and retrograde cerebral perfusion is started. A transverse or longitudinal aortotomy is made on the anterior aspect of the aortic wall (Fig. 9-4). When dissection is present, the false lumen may be entered first. This necessitates opening of the true lumen.

Clamping of the Aorta

The aorta should only be clamped if there is a localized aneurysm of the ascending aorta with a generous normal distal segment. Only under this very precise condition should the aorta be cross-clamped. Deep circulatory arrest with retrograde cerebral perfusion is used when the ascending aortic aneurysm fades away into the arch or involves the arch as well as in all patients with aortic dissection.

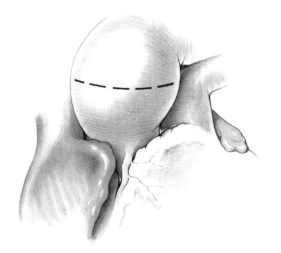

FIG. 9-4. The aortic aneurysm is opened transversely.

 AORTIC CROSS-CLAMP INJURY
Application of a clamp to the aorta in the presence of acute aortic dissection further traumatizes the aortic wall. In addition, it may pressurize the false lumen and result in progression of the dissection and possible obstruction of some aortic branches or even aortic rupture.

 BLOOD CLOTS IN THE AORTIC WALL
Blood clots are often evident within the aortic wall. In patients with aneurysms, the clots may be old and organized. They must be carefully removed along with atherosclerotic debris to prevent possible subsequent embolization.

Myocardial Protection

Cold blood cardioplegic solution may be administered antegrade into each coronary artery if deemed necessary. This is especially important if the dissection has involved one of the coronary ostia because the myocardium fed by this vessel may not have cooled sufficiently owing to obstructed flow. Retrograde infusion of cardioplegia into the coronary sinus should also be performed.

NB If the cardioplegic line is used for the retrograde cerebral perfusion of cold blood, this will have to be delayed until the cardioplegic infusion is completed and the line purged of cardioplegic solution.

The entry site of the aortic dissection is identified. The dissection may have extended into the aortic arch and the aortic root involving a coronary ostium, most commonly that of the right coronary artery. The aorta is resected from just above the sinotubular ridge to the level of the innominate artery.

NB The divided aortic wall may at times be left in situ to be reapproximated loosely over the tube graft at the completion of the procedure. This technique may provide added protection from possible mediastinal infection.

Typically, the lesser curvature of the aortic arch is resected to remove as much diseased aorta as possible, A 1-cm cuff of relatively normal aorta is dissected with as much adventitial tissue as possible left intact for the distal anastomosis.

 REINFORCEMENT OF THE AORTIC WALL
If the distal aortic wall is dissected, BioGlue Surgical Adhesive (CryoLife, Inc., Kennesaw, GA) is injected into the false lumen to bond and strengthen the aortic wall (Fig. 9-5). A sponge is placed in the true lumen to prevent spillage.

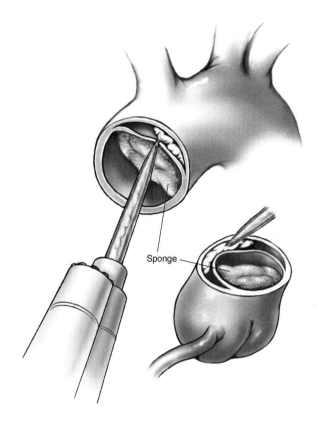

Sponge

FIG. 9-5. Injection of glue into the false lumen to bond and strengthen the aortic wall.

 NB The sponge within the lumen of the aorta is gently pressed against the aortic wall in close proximity to the coronary ostia to prevent the glue material from reaching too far down to occlude the coronary arteries.

🚫 ***GLUE EMBOLIZATION***
Glue material is not introduced within the dissected distal wall of the aorta if there appears to be reentry sites within the aortic arch. The possibility of glue material becoming detached and embolized through the distal reentry site is a grave complication of this procedure.

Further reinforcement can be obtained with Teflon felt strips attached to both the inside and/or outside of the aortic wall first with six to 10 interrupted mattress sutures or a continuous mattress suture of 3-0 Prolene (Fig. 9-6). Teflon felt strips may not be required if the integrity of the aortic wall appears to be satisfactory with the glue.

An appropriately sized Hemashield tube graft (Medox Medical, Oakland, NJ) is cut and tailored obliquely to be attached to the undersurface of the arch or cut straight to be attached to the aorta at the level of the innominate

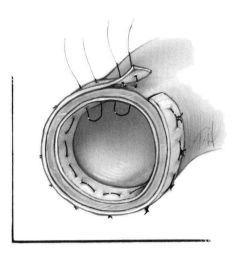

FIG. 9-6. Reinforcement of the distal aorta with double layers of Teflon felt.

artery. The tube graft is then anastomosed to the reinforced aortic cuff with a continuous suture of 3-0 Prolene.

NB ***TENSION ON THE SUTURE LINE***
It is important for the assistant surgeon to follow the suture meticulously to provide appropriate tension on the suture line. Otherwise, multiple reinforcing interrupted sutures may be required to ensure a watertight anastomosis.

With the patient in the Trendelenburg position, the perfusion of retrograde cerebral blood is allowed to accumulate and fill the aortic arch. All air and debris are allowed to flow out through the graft. At this time, another arterial cannula is introduced through the tube graft, and the perfusionist is asked to initiate arterial perfusion through this cannula in an antegrade fashion with extremely low flow. A clamp is now applied to the tube graft well away from the anastomosis and proximal to the cannula, and the retrograde cerebral perfusion is gradually discontinued and venous drainage is reinstituted (Fig. 9-7). Normal perfusion flow and pressure are gradually restored, and the patient is rewarmed. The posterior distal suture line is now examined, and additional stitches are placed for control of hemostasis if required.

NB In patients with aortic aneurysm, the femoral arterial cannula may be used to reinstate cardiopulmonary bypass. This retrograde arterial perfusion is gradually increased to normal flow, and rewarming is started. Antegrade perfusion is not essential. However, antegrade perfusion with a separate cannula through the tube graft allows earlier removal of the femoral arterial cannula and repair of the femoral artery while the remainder of the operation is being completed.

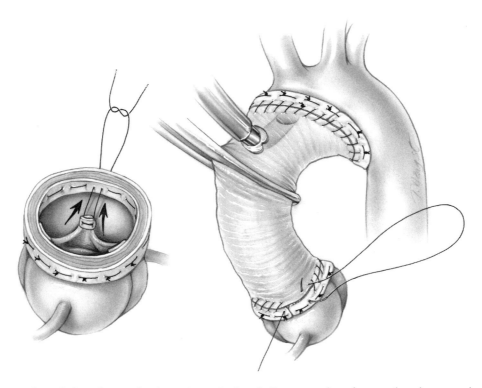

FIG. 9-7. Completion of a proximal anastomosis. **Inset:** Resuspension of an aortic valve commissure.

🚫 ***RETROGRADE ARTERIAL PERFUSION AND***
AORTIC DISSECTION
In patients with aortic dissection, blood gains access through the entry site into the aortic wall. This dissection may result in a reentry site by tearing the intima distally along the course of the aorta. When cardiopulmonary bypass is reinitiated, the retrograde flow may enter the false lumen through this distal intimal tear and reenter the lumen at the entry site. However, when the aorta has been repaired and the entry site is excluded by tube graft interposition, the retrograde flow of blood cannot escape and may cause further dissection of the aorta. *Therefore, it is important to establish antegrade flow when restarting cardiopulmonary bypass.*

NB After cardiopulmonary bypass is reestablished, additional doses of blood cardioplegic solution are administered by the retrograde technique and antegrade into the coronary ostia at 10- to 20-minute intervals (see Chapters 3 and 5).

When the aorta is otherwise normal and there is no aortic valve insufficiency, the proximal aorta that has been transected at approximately 1 cm above the level of aortic commissures is reinforced with glue and a single or double layer of Teflon felt, as described for the distal anastomosis. The tube graft is tailored to an appropriate length and anastomosed to the proximal aorta with 3-0 Prolene continuous suture (Fig. 9-7).

Often, however, there may be associated aortic insufficiency from aortic root dissection or dilation. When the valve leaflets are not diseased and the remainder of the aortic root is normal, every attempt is made to retain the aortic valve. Any incompetent commissure is resuspended by curing the dissected root with BioGlue and reinforced with an external felt strip. This tailored proximal anastomosis reestablishes a new *sinotubular junction*, incorporating the resuspended commissures to ensure a competent aortic valve (Fig. 9-7).

Aortic Root Replacement

When the aortic valve is so diseased that its repair is not feasible or the dissection extends proximally into the sinuses, complete aortic root replacement with an aortic valve conduit and reimplantation of the coronary arteries become necessary.

Aortic root replacement as originally described by Bentall consisted of replacement of the aortic valve and the ascending aorta including the aortic root and of reimplantation of the coronary arteries into the tube graft all within the native aorta and then wrapping the tube graft with redundant aortic wall. There appears to be an increased incidence of pseudoaneurysm formation, probably because of insecure hemostasis at the anastomotic suture lines masked by the wrapping of the aorta. With the introduction of improved tube grafts and aortic root conduits and better surgical techniques for anastomosis and hemostasis, simple interposition of a valve conduit is now the method of choice.

The Interposition Technique

The aorta is divided approximately 15 mm above the commissures, followed by excision of all the diseased aortic wall up to the lesser curvature of the aortic arch. Buttons of aortic wall, approximately 1.5 to 2 cm wide, containing the coronary artery ostia are detached from the aortic root with an electrocautery blade. The aortic valve leaflets are excised and an appropriately sized composite tube graft is selected. St. Jude Medical (Minneapolis, MN) provides a collagen-impregnated tube graft (Hemashield) attached to a bileaflet valve with a tall sewing cuff. Interrupted pledgeted sutures of 2-0 Ticron are placed close together in the aortic annulus (Fig. 9-8). Subsequently, they are passed through the lower portion of the sewing ring of the composite valve graft, leaving 2 to 3 mm of the upper sewing cuff free. The prosthesis is lowered into position, and the sutures are tied, taking all the same precautions as in aortic valve replacement (see Chapter 5).

NB Six to 8 mm of the aortic wall should be left attached to the annulus. This remaining aortic wall with its adventitial tissue is now brought forward and sewn to the upper portion of the sewing ring of

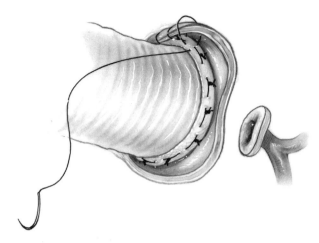

FIG. 9-9. Technique (Copeland) for reinforcing the proximal suture line.

the prosthesis with a continuous suture of 3-0 Prolene (Fig. 9-9). In addition, a Teflon strip can be used to buttress the proximal suture line (Fig. 9-10). This reduces the possibility of leaks at the aortic root.

Circular holes are made in the tube graft with an ophthalmologic cautery device for reimplantation of the coronary artery buttons. These openings should preferably be some distance above the sewing ring for ease of suturing. The coronary artery buttons are now attached to these openings with continuous 5-0 Prolene sutures (Fig. 9-11).

NB Often this suture line is buttressed and reinforced with a strip of autologous pericardium on the coronary button for a more secure anastomosis.

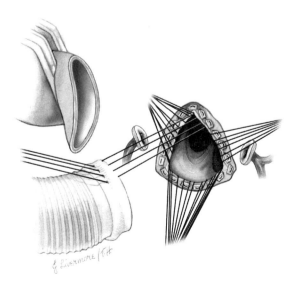

FIG. 9-8. Technique for aortic root replacement: placement of annular sutures in valve conduit.

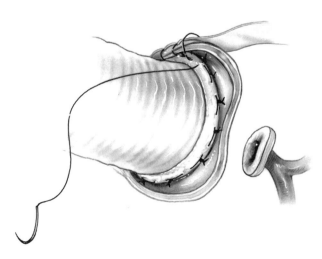

FIG. 9-10. Copeland technique reinforced with a felt strip.

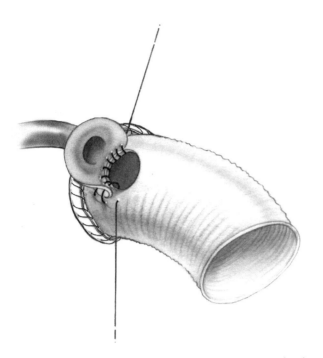

FIG. 9-11. Technique for aortic root replacement: reimplantation of coronary ostial buttons.

NB It is often advisable to delay reimplantation of the right coronary button until the distal aortic anastomosis in completed. The cross-clamp is briefly removed, and the heart is allowed to fill so that the correct site for reimplantation of the right coronary can be marked.

⊘ BLEEDING FROM THE CORONARY ARTERY SUTURE LINE

Implantation of the coronary artery buttons to the graft must be performed meticulously. The suture bites must be very close together and preferably buttressed with a pericardial strip. Control of bleeding from these sites, particularly the left coronary artery anastomosis, at a subsequent stage is challenging.

The tube graft is now cut appropriately and attached to the distal aorta as described earlier. If a tube graft is already attached to the distal aorta, the proximal and distal tube grafts are now tailor cut and anastomosed to each other with a continuous suture of 3-0 or 4-0 Prolene.

NB *COMPOSITE VALVE–TUBE GRAFT INTERPOSITION*
Many of these patients have diffuse aortic wall disease. Use of the composite valvular conduit should be preferred to isolated aortic valve replacement followed by tube graft replacement of the aorta above the sinotubular junction. This latter tech-

nique may leave behind diseased sinus of Valsalva and put the patient at risk of later development of aortic sinus aneurysms.

⊘ INABILITY TO DIRECTLY CONNECT THE CORONARY ARTERIES TO THE TUBE GRAFT

Composite valvular tube graft replacement entails reimplantation of the coronary arteries into the graft. Use of saphenous vein grafts to bypass the major branches of the coronary arteries can be an alternate technique and is implemented whenever direct coronary artery to graft continuity cannot be safely accomplished. This entails the oversewing of the coronary ostia. An alternative technique uses an 8-mm GORE-TEX tube graft interposition between the coronary ostia and the tube graft. This modification introduced by Cabrol has been found to be useful in some patients.

⊘ CORONARY ARTERY IMPLANTATION

A kink or twist of the coronary arteries at the implantation site interferes with normal coronary perfusion and can give rise to myocardial ischemia. The surgeon must be aware of this possibility during anastomosis of the coronary ostia to the graft to prevent misalignment.

⊘ STENOSIS OF THE CORONARY ARTERY OSTIA

To minimize the possibility of ostial stenosis, the anastomosis should incorporate a wide margin of the aortic wall around each coronary ostium. The window cut in the graft wall must be correspondingly generous (Fig. 9-11).

⊘ SAPHENOUS VEIN BYPASS GRAFTS

When the patient has associated coronary artery disease, it may be necessary to use saphenous vein grafts or appropriate arterial grafts to bypass the occluded branches of the coronary arteries concomitantly with the aortic surgery.

When the patient is rewarmed and all suture lines are secure, deairing is carried out and the patient is gradually weaned from cardiopulmonary bypass.

NB Aortic root venting is performed with an air vent needle through the graft before removing the clamp across the tube graft. The clamp is then reapplied partially across the anterior portion of the graft distal to the needle vent (see Chapter 4, Deairing of the Heart section).

⊘ AIR REMOVAL

The vent needle for air removal should *not* be inserted in the aorta distal to the graft to avoid starting a new site of dissection.

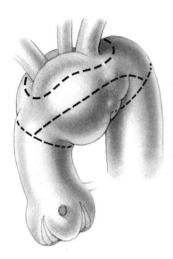

FIG. 9-12. Technique for the repair of an aortic arch aneurysm: initial incision to open the arch and lines of resection.

Technique for Replacement of an Aortic Arch Aneurysm

The aortic arch may have to be replaced if there is an enlarging aneurysm affecting the arch or there is extension of the disease process from the ascending or descending aorta into the arch. The technique involves the use of deep hypothermic arrest and retrograde cerebral protection.

Ice packs are placed around patient's head, and core cooling is continued to a temperature of 18°C. Circulatory arrest is then commenced, and retrograde cerebral perfusion is started. An aortotomy is made across the arch (Fig. 9-12). Blood clots and debris are carefully removed.

An island containing all the three arch vessels is detached from aortic arch with 8- to 10-mm rim of aortic tissue. An 18- to 20-mm Hemashield tube graft is care-

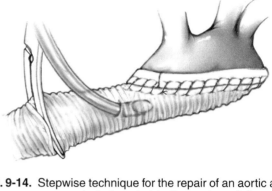

FIG. 9-14. Stepwise technique for the repair of an aortic arch aneurysm: a cannula is inserted in the arch graft for antegrade cerebral perfusion.

fully beveled and tailored to approximate the concavity of the arch vessels. The tube graft is anastomosed to the island. A Teflon felt strip is used to reinforce the suture line (Fig. 9-13). Use of BioGlue along the suture line can provide further reinforcement.

The tube graft is allowed to fill with the retrograde cerebral blood perfusion return from the arch vessels. A separate arterial cannula is introduced into the graft allowed to fill, and its free end is clamped (Fig. 9-14).

Retrograde cerebral perfusion through the superior vena cava is discontinued. Antegrade cerebral perfusion is commenced to maintain a radial artery pressure of 50 mm Hg. This technique minimizes the total circulatory arrest time to the brain while the arch reconstruction is in progress.

The redundant arch tissue with debris and blood clots is removed, and ascending and descending aortic segments are completely divided. A Hemashield tube graft of appropriate size is introduced into the lumen of the descending aorta (Fig. 9-15). It is sewn to the normal aor-

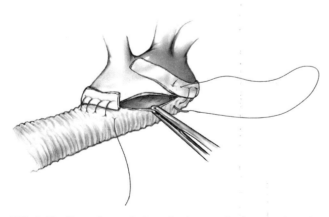

FIG. 9-13. Stepwise technique for the repair of an aortic arch aneurysm: anastomosis of 18-mm tube graft to the island with arch vessels.

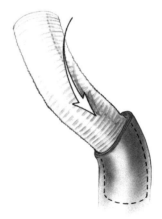

FIG. 9-15. Stepwise technique for the repair of an aortic arch aneurysm: insertion of a tube graft into the descending aorta and performance of a distal suture line.

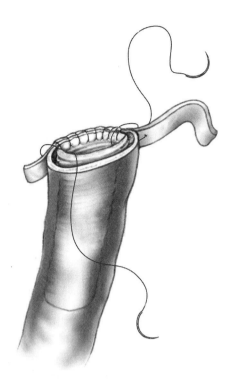

FIG. 9-16. Stepwise technique for the repair of an aortic arch aneurysm: sewing a graft to the aortic wall.

tic wall with a continuous suture of 3-0 Prolene. Sometimes it is buttressed with a Teflon felt strip on the outside of the descending aorta (Fig. 9-16). The suture line may further be secured with BioGlue. The tube graft is then pulled out of descending aorta (Fig. 9-17).

ELEPHANT-TRUNK TECHNIQUE

When the descending aorta is also diseased and requires subsequent excision and replacement, an elephant-trunk technique is used. This entails inverting approximately 3 cm of Hemashield tube graft on itself.

 TUBE GRAFT INVERSION
The short segment is on the outside of the larger segment of the tube graft.

The double-layer tube graft is introduced into the lumen of the descending aorta as before (Fig. 9-18). The double-layer tube graft edge is then sewn to the descending aorta, buttressed with a Teflon felt strip on the outside with a continuous suture of 3-0 Prolene. Again, the use of BioGlue may reinforce the anastomosis.

NB The needle bite includes the two layers of tube graft, aortic wall, and a Teflon felt strip.

At the completion of the anastomosis, the longer segment of the graft is pulled out of the lumen of tube graft, leaving a "trunk" of approximately 3 cm behind within the lumen of the descending aorta.

NB The trunk is anastomosed to another tube graft when excision of descending thoracic aorta is undertaken weeks to months subsequently.

A separate perfusion cannula is introduced into this graft just proximal to the descending aorta suture line. The graft is clamped close to the perfusion cannula, and circulation to the lower body is restored while the antegrade cerebral perfusion is maintained (Fig. 9-19). The proximal segment of this tube graft is now tailor cut to the appropriate length and shape. It is then anastomosed to the ascending aortic wall or composite tube graft with

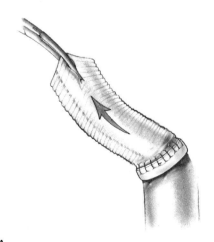

A

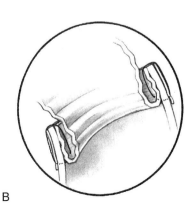

B

FIG. 9-17. Stepwise technique for the repair of an aortic arch aneurysm. **A:** Tube graft is withdrawn from the distal aorta. **B:** Close-up of an inverted distal suture line.

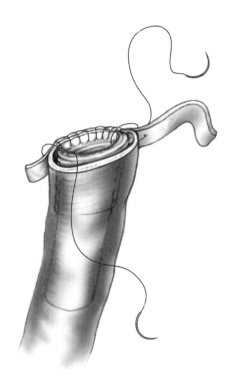

FIG. 9-18. Elephant-trunk technique. A double-layer graft is sewn to the aortic wall.

continuous 3-0 or 4-0 Prolene suture. The anastomosis can be reinforced with a Teflon felt strip and BioGlue.

Complete circulatory arrest is again reinstituted. Retrograde cerebral perfusion is restarted. Both cross-clamps on the tube grafts are removed. The cannula for antegrade cerebral perfusion is removed, and the tube graft is beveled and tailored to match an oval window in the main tube graft. The tube graft openings are then anastomosed to each other with 4-0 Prolene sutures (Fig. 9-20). Cardiopulmonary bypass is reinstituted using the descending aortic arterial cannula. The patient is rewarmed, and the procedure completed. The process of deairing is carried out meticulously.

KINKING OF THE GRAFTS
It is important to correctly trim the arch graft for its anastomosis to the descending aortic graft. Similarly, the oval opening in the main graft should match the beveled opening of the arch graft. Any discrepancy may result in kinking of the graft anastomosis on the convexity or concavity or both aspects of the reconstructed arch (Fig. 9-21).

Management of Type B Aortic Dissection

Initial management of patients with type B dissection affecting the descending aorta is to control the high blood

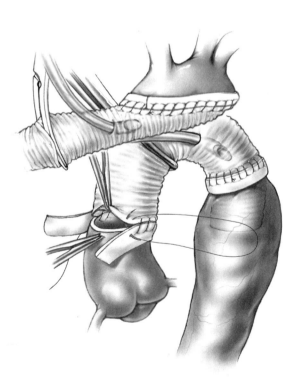

FIG. 9-19. Stepwise technique for the repair of an aortic arch aneurysm: a longer segment of tube graft has been pulled out of the descending aorta. Perfusion of the lower body through a cannula in the aortic graft while performing a proximal aortic suture line.

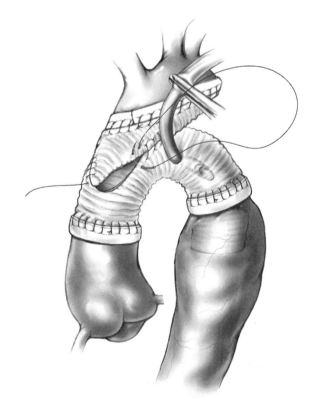

FIG. 9-20. Stepwise technique for the repair of an aortic arch aneurysm. Anastomosing the arch graft to the aortic graft under hypothermic arrest.

after ascending aortic replacement. These patients may also be successfully treated by the interventional radiologist.

Technique for Replacement of the Descending Thoracic Aorta

A posterolateral thoracotomy through the fifth intercostal space provides ample exposure of the descending thoracic aorta. At times, a second lower incision may facilitate the distal anastomosis. Adhesions must be taken down with utmost care to prevent injury to the lung or the diseased aorta. A plane of dissection is identified, and vascular loops or umbilical tapes are passed around the transverse arch between the left carotid and the left subclavian arteries, the left subclavian artery, and the descending aorta distally. The left groin area is always prepared and should be within the operative field in all cases.

We routinely use partial left-sided heart bypass for nearly all surgery on the descending thoracic aorta. The femoral artery is cannulated for arterial return, and either the femoral vein, pulmonary artery, or pulmonary vein is selected for venous drainage (see Replacement of the Ascending Aorta section). The use of partial bypass allows control of the patient's blood pressure. It also provides perfusion of lower body and may protect the spinal cord.

Initially, the transverse arch and the left subclavian artery are clamped. The distal aorta is clamped a short distance below the proximal clamp, even though the distal extent of aortic dissection may have progressed well below the diaphragm. A short aortotomy is made; it is then extended to provide adequate exposure (Fig. 9-22A). When the aorta is opened and decompressed, it is often possible and preferable to reapply a single clamp below the origin of the subclavian artery above the site of dissection to ensure perfusion through the left subclavian artery because this may decrease the incidence of paraplegia. The ostia of the intercostal arteries are oversewn with 3-0 Prolene sutures.

An appropriately sized Hemashield tube graft is sewn into the proximal aortic lumen with continuous sutures of 3-0 Prolene suture (Fig. 9-22B). The suture line is always buttressed and reinforced with strips of Teflon felt, which may be outside and around the aorta or within its lumen or both. A clamp is then applied to the tube graft, and the proximal clamp placed on the aorta is removed. The suture line is checked for bleeding, and additional sutures are placed if deemed necessary. Use of BioGlue on the outside of the anastomosis will provide additional reinforcement of the suture line. The tube graft is cut to the precise length and sewn to the distal aortic wall with continuous 3-0 Prolene suture incorporating a strip of Teflon felt in the suturing to reinforce the anastomotic line (Fig. 9-23A). The remaining aortic wall is then reapproximated

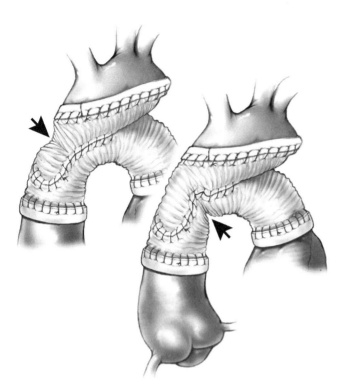

FIG. 9-21. Incorrect length and beveling of an arch graft results in a distorted anastomosis to the aortic graft.

pressure with medical therapy. In contradistinction to type A aortic dissection, which requires urgent surgical intervention, patients with type B dissection have a relatively good prognosis with medical therapy. However, *elective* surgical intervention remains the best form of management and provides superior long-term results in patients who are young and free of other concomitant diseases. Therefore, replacement of the descending thoracic aorta is the treatment of choice in otherwise young, healthy patients with chronic type B dissection and in older patients with expanding descending aortic aneurysms. Nevertheless, patients who continue to have pain despite maximal medical management, have evidence of contained rupture, or have ischemia of a limb or major organ owing to involvement of an arterial branch by the dissection process should undergo urgent surgical intervention.

NB Recently, interventional radiologists have been important participants in the care of patients with aortic dissections. They are often able to reestablish flow to compromised or occluded aortic branches by fenestrating the intimal flap or stenting the true or false lumen. This may allow a patient with a type B dissection to be stabilized and have surgery on an elective basis. Some patients with type A dissections continue to demonstrate clinically significant obstruction to flow in one or more aortic branches

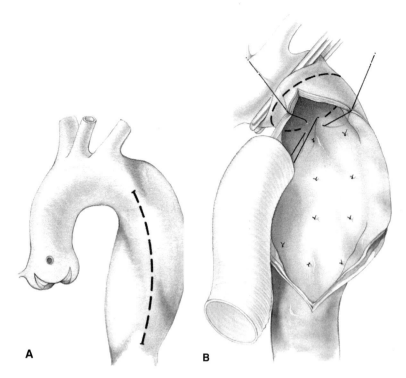

FIG. 9-22. Stepwise technique for the replacement of the descending aorta **(A)**: an aortotomy **(B)** and the proximal suture line.

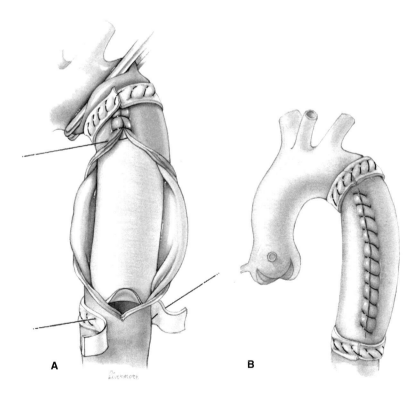

FIG. 9-23. Stepwise technique for the replacement of the descending aorta: the distal suture line **(A)** and wrapping the graft **(B)**.

over the graft (Fig. 9-23B). Alternatively, the aorta may be transected at the proposed site of anastomosis. A generous cuff of aortic wall is dissected free and reinforced with a strip of Teflon felt. The tube graft is then interposed, and both proximal and distal anastomoses are completed with continuous suture of 3-0 Prolene.

NB *REIMPLANTATION OF THE INTERCOSTAL ARTERIES*

The lower thoracic intercostal arteries may on occasion be quite large in patients with chronic dissection or aneurysm. Although oversewing them has been the accepted technique, consideration should be given to their reimplantation to reduce the incidence of paralysis.

Technique

A small, elliptical segment of the tube graft overlying the intercostal arteries is removed. The island of intercostal arteries is then sewn to the tube graft with deep bites of continuous suture of 3-0 Prolene suture (Fig. 9-24). Use of BioGlue may secure the suture line even more.

In patients who have previously undergone ascending aorta and arch replacements with the so-called elephant-trunk technique, the proximal anastomosis is simplified. After the initiation of CPB blood pressure is temporarily lowered to 60. The distal aorta is opened, the graft extension is identified and the clamp is placed on this graft (Fig. 9-25). The proximal descending graft is then anastomosed to the trunk extension with running 3-0 or 4-0 Prolene sutures. The distal anastomosis is completed as described previously.

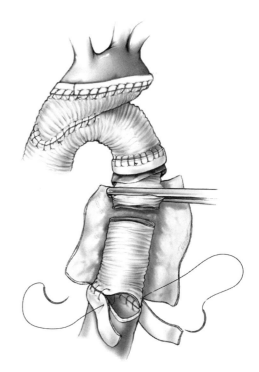

FIG. 9-25. Completing the descending aortic replacement after an elephant-trunk procedure.

The operation can also be performed without the use of left-sided cardiopulmonary bypass. Often the aorta is clamped only proximally. Blood from the distal aorta is removed through a cell saver sucker for reinfusion. The distal anastomosis is carried out by this open technique unimpeded by the distal clamp.

NB *PERFUSION OF UPPER BODY*

Rarely, one may encounter a situation while on left heart bypass in which the descending aortic aneurysm has been opened, only to note that the appropriate proximal margin of resection is indeed beyond the proximal clamp within the arch of the aorta. This necessitates total circulatory arrest. As retrograde perfusion via the femoral artery cannot perfuse the head and the upper part of the body with the thoracic aorta cross-clamped, the ascending aorta needs to be cannulated separately. This can be performed quite easily through the standard left thoracotomy, especially when the heart is decompressed on left heart bypass. Otherwise, the thoracotomy incision is extended medially to provide adequate exposure. It is important for the surgeon and the perfusionist to communicate and choreograph the conduct of the procedure to ensure adequate perfusion of both the lower and upper parts of the body. When the continuity of the aorta has been reestablished, further perfusion and rewarming can be achieved via the femoral or preferably the aortic cannula.

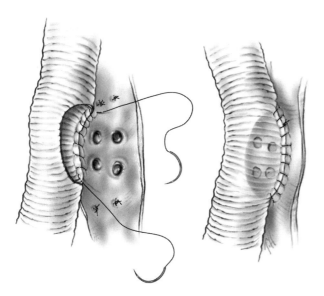

FIG. 9-24. Stepwise technique for the replacement of the descending aorta: reimplantation of the intercostal arteries into the tube graft.

NB *CONNECTION OF THE TRUE WITH THE FALSE DISTAL LUMEN*

It is of utmost importance to maintain a connection between the true and false lumen when chronic the dissection extends distally. This entails removing a short segment of the intima flap wall just distal to the distal anastomosis. In this fashion, all the aortic branches arising from the false as well as true lumen are perfused.

🚫 *ESOPHAGEAL INJURY*

Deep sutures may include the esophagus. Transection and dissection of the posterior aspect of the aorta allow precise placement of the sutures, thus preventing possible esophageal injury.

🚫 *HYPTERTENSION FROM CROSS-CLAMPING*

Aortic cross-clamping often produces proximal hypertension, which must be controlled by hypotensive agents.

🚫 *SPINAL CORD ISCHEMIA*

A significant decrease in distal perfusion pressure can occasionally result in paraplegia. This is a grave complication that should be prevented using all means available. Many techniques, including partial bypass from the left atrium or pulmonary artery to the femoral artery and the femoral vein to the femoral artery necessitating systemic heparinization, have been employed with some success.

Heparin-bonded tubes for left-sided heart bypass have also been used. It seems, however, that keeping the time of aortic cross-clamping short provides the best protection against the development of paralysis.

DRAINAGE OF CEREBROSPINAL FLUID

Cerebrospinal Fluid Pressure

Clamping of the descending aorta causes a significant decrease in distal perfusion pressure, including the spinal arteries. Conversely, there is resultant hypertension proximal to the clamp. This produces engorgement of the intracranial structures and increases in cerebrospinal fluid pressure, which may contribute to spinal cord ischemia. Even though there are no definite data to support the beneficial effect of reducing cerebrospinal fluid pressure, it has been our practice to drain the cerebrospinal fluid in the operating room and continue drainage for the first 1 or 2 days postoperatively, maintaining a pressure of approximately 10 mm Hg.

NB *SPINAL CORD PROTECTION TECHNIQUES*

Spinal cord function can be monitored during the time when the aorta is clamped. Monitoring somatosensory evoked potentials entails stimulating the posterior tibial nerve and recording its response in the cerebral cortex. Although many centers use this monitoring technique, its clinical pertinence has not been totally established.

SECTION III

Surgery for Ischemic Heart Disease

CHAPTER 10

Coronary Artery Surgery

Surgery for revascularization of the myocardium continues to be an effective and lasting means of managing patients with multivessel coronary artery disease. However, the recent evolution of intracoronary stents has enabled interventional cardiologists to treat coronary stenoses percutaneously with early results approaching those of surgical bypass procedures. This has had an impact on the number and types of patients who are referred for coronary artery bypass surgery. Therefore, our surgical patients are now generally older, have more comorbid conditions, and more severe left ventricular dysfunction, and many have had previous catheter-based interventions. These patients are at increased surgical risk and may have poor surgical targets. To handle this group of patients, surgeons need to incorporate newer procedures into their practice, including off-pump surgery and transmyocardial laser revascularization, and pursue such strategies as angiogenic and muscle cell technology.

Ultimately, the goal in the operating room is to provide patients with grafts that have the best long-term patency. The internal thoracic artery has proven to be the gold standard of conduits. Its patency is better than 90% at 15 years, and its use has been proven to prolong patient survival. The *in situ* left internal thoracic artery is the graft of choice to the left anterior descending coronary artery. The *in situ* right internal thoracic artery has slightly lower patency compared with the *in situ* left internal thoracic artery. In younger patients, this is an excellent choice of graft to the ramus intermedius or proximal obtuse marginal coronary artery. Bilateral internal thoracic arteries should be avoided in patients with insulin-dependent diabetes because of increased sternal complications. A free internal thoracic artery graft has a lower patency rate than an *in situ* graft.

Other arterial conduits have been used including the inferior epigastric artery, gastroepiploic artery, and radial artery. The inferior epigastric artery was found to have poor patency rates and is used rarely if at all. The gas-troepiploic artery is still used by some surgeons, but harvesting this conduit requires entry into the peritoneal cavity and its use is therefore limited. The radial artery has recently been reintroduced and is now considered the second arterial conduit of choice. One or both radial arteries can be used along with one or both internal thoracic arteries to provide complete arterial revascularization. The radial artery may be anastomosed proximally to the aorta or sewn in an end-to-side fashion to an internal thoracic artery to create a Y graft.

The greater saphenous vein has been extensively used as a conduit because it can be quickly procured, is easy to handle, and ensures excellent inflow. Renewed enthusiasm for this graft has been generated by the development of less invasive endoscopic vein-harvesting techniques. The 10- year patency of greater saphenous vein grafts is 60% to 70%; however, this may be improved with the routine use of cholesterol-lowering agents and anticholinesterase inhibitors.

TECHNIQUE FOR INTERNAL THORACIC ARTERY HARVEST

The internal thoracic artery is a very delicate vessel that can be injured easily. Consequently, the artery should be dissected as a pedicle with great care.

A median sternotomy is made in the usual fashion. The parietal pleura and pericardium are depressed gently, and the course of the internal thoracic artery is identified from its origin near the first rib to its termination beyond its bifurcation in the rectus sheath. A Favaloro retractor provides excellent exposure. The Rultract System retractor also provides superb exposure and is probably less traumatic. The posterior rectus sheath is freed from the undersurface of the sternum and costal cartilages, allowing more extensive retraction with improved exposure of the internal thoracic artery.

INJURY TO THE RIBS AND COSTOCHONDRAL JUNCTION
Overzealous elevation of the hemisternum by retractors may result in rib fractures or even costo-chondral disruption. This is more apt to occur in patients with pectus deformities or morbid obesity and in elderly patients with osteoporosis.

Although it is possible to dissect the internal thoracic artery without entering the pleural cavity, we prefer to routinely open the left pleura widely to provide excellent exposure and greatly facilitate harvesting of the internal thoracic artery.

NB Opening the pleura allows the left internal thoracic artery pedicle to fall away from midline. This decreases the risk of injury at reoperation.

Alternatively, the left internal thoracic artery can be harvested through a lower ministernotomy, dividing the left half of the sternum (see Chapter 1). A Favaloro retractor allows the left hemisternum to be elevated to provide adequate exposure for mobilizing the internal thoracic artery. This approach allows off-pump bypass grafting of the left internal thoracic artery to the left anterior descending coronary artery (see later).

The internal thoracic artery is usually harvested as a pedicle with extensive use of electrocautery *for chest wall hemostasis but not pedicle hemostasis.* The parietal pleura on the internal intercostal musculofascial layer of the chest wall is incised approximately 7 to 10 mm medial to the internal thoracic artery along its entire course (Fig. 10-1). The blade of the electrocautery is then used to depress and dissect the pedicle from the chest wall. The lowest current is used to coagulate the internal thoracic artery and vein branches, well away from the parent trunks. The side branches on the artery are then occluded with fine metal clips. The pedicle is dissected from the level of the rectus sheath to the level of the sub-clavian vein where the artery passes beneath this vessel. Care is taken to identify and divide two intercostal branches, one passing anterior to the subclavian vein and a high first intercostal branch coursing laterally above the subclavian vein.

 UNSTABLE HEMODYNAMICS
When the patient's condition is unstable, it is preferable to harvest the internal thoracic artery while the patient is on cardiopulmonary bypass.

 INJURY TO THE INTERNAL THORACIC ARTERY
Because the internal thoracic artery is a delicate structure, any undue stretching, clamping, or mis-placed metal clips results in permanent vascular injury and thus unsatisfactory short- and long-term results.

HEAT INJURY
When an electrocautery is used to divide the internal thoracic artery branches after application of metal clips, the heat and the electric current may conduct through the metal clip adjacent to the parent trunk and cause a burn injury. Therefore, branches must be divided with scissors or coagulated well away from the metal clip adjacent to the internal thoracic artery.

 MAXIMAL LENGTH OF THE INTERNAL THORACIC ARTERY
The internal thoracic artery pedicle must be dissected free from the chest wall along its entire course, from near its origin in the first intercostal space to well past its bifurcation into the rectus sheath to provide maximal length.

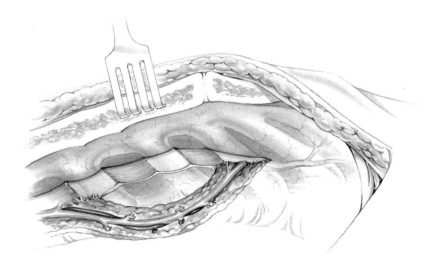

FIG. 10-1. Harvesting an internal thoracic artery.

INTERNAL THORACIC STEAL SYNDROME
The first intercostal branch of the internal thoracic artery must be identified and divided to avoid any possible steal phenomenon from the internal thoracic flow.

Before commencing cardiopulmonary bypass, papaverine is sprayed gently over the pedicle and the adequacy of flow is determined. If there is no flow, a 1-mm vascular probe (Parsonnet) is *cautiously* introduced into the lumen of the vessel for a varying distance. *This should be done with extreme care to avoid intimal injury.* Usually very good flow is noted. Unless traumatized during harvesting, the internal thoracic artery usually provides adequate flow and should not be discarded.

NB In elderly patients, it may be preferable to harvest only the internal thoracic artery rather than a pedicle. This may decrease the incidence of vascular necrosis and infection affecting the sternum.

The pedicle is laid on the heart to judge the appropriate length. The end of the pedicle is then grasped with forceps, allowing the thoracic artery to distend with blood. The artery is then cleaned free of the surrounding tissues, using sharp dissection. The artery is transected obliquely with the heel on the fascial side of the pedicle and prepared as a large hood orifice.

NB The internal thoracic artery can be lengthened considerably with multiple *pedicle fasciotomies.* Maximal length can be obtained by *skeletonizing* the vessel along its course. Division of the internal thoracic veins should be avoided when performing the fasciotomies. If the pedicle remains too short, the artery may be divided proximally and used as a free graft.

 STRING SIGN
Excessive stretch and tension on the internal thoracic artery result in narrowing of the lumen and graft failure. This is seen as a *string sign* on a selective angiogram of the artery.

 OPTIMAL LENGTH OF THE THORACIC PEDICLE
Before the distal end of the thoracic artery is divided, its correct length must be ascertained. The thoracic pedicle should lie very comfortably on the heart when it is full and the lungs are fully inflated; otherwise, the artery will be stretched and could become detached at the anastomotic site.

Similarly, it should not be redundant because too long a pedicle may curl or kink into the substernal area, increasing the risk of injury at reoperation.

NB The caliber of the thoracic artery is smaller and resistance to flow is higher the longer the pedicle is. A tortuous thoracic artery course makes later catheter intervention nearly impossible.

 CLOT FORMATION WITHIN THE INTERNAL THORACIC ARTERY
The internal thoracic artery, when fully mobilized and divided, is occluded with an atraumatic bulldog clamp *after* the patient has been fully heparinized to prevent any clotting within the lumen of the vessel.

NB ***INCISING THE PERICARDIUM FOR BYPASS GRAFTING TO THE CIRUMFLEX CORONARY ARTERY***
The pericardium is divided with an electrocautery where the thoracic pedicle crosses it down to 1 cm above the left phrenic nerve. This allows the thoracic pedicle to assume a more lateral position and lie against the medial surface of the lung instead of coursing over the apex of the lung. This is especially important when the left internal thoracic artery is grafted to an obtuse marginal branch of the circumflex coronary artery.

NB ***COURSE OF THE RIGHT INTERNAL THORACIC ARTERY***
An *in situ* right internal thoracic artery can easily reach the diagonal, ramus intermedius or a proximal obtuse marginal branch of the circumflex coronary artery. The pedicle should cross the distal ascending aorta near the innominate vein. Thymic tissue and fat can be used to cover the pedicle. If the right internal thoracic artery is grafted to the left anterior descending coronary artery, its course will be across the more proximal aspect of the ascending aorta, which puts it at high risk of injury during reoperative procedures.

TECHNIQUE FOR RADIAL ARTERY HARVEST

Usually the nondominant arm is identified preoperatively for radial artery harvest. Intravenous catheters and venipunctures are avoided in this arm. Allen's test is performed using a Doppler probe to ensure adequate ulnar artery filling of the palmar arch.

In the operating room, the arm is abducted to 90 degrees and under sterile conditions prepared and draped on an armboard. An incision is made in the midportion of the forearm over the belly of the brachioradialis muscle. The opening is then extended for a variable distance proximally toward the groove between the brachioradialis and biceps tendon (Fig. 10-2). Distally the incision is extended toward the wrist crease. With expe-

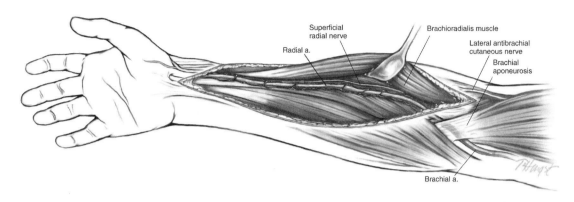

FIG. 10-2. Harvesting a radial artery.

rience, the opening in the forearm can be fairly limited in length and still allow adequate exposure to harvest the radial artery.

The dissection of the radial artery begins distally by dividing the fascia and then proceeding proximally between the belly of the brachioradialis and flexor carpiradialis muscles. A vessel loop is then passed around the radial artery to facilitate exposure. The artery is dissected along with the two venae comitantes, double clipping and sharply dividing all the branches. When the radial artery is completely mobilized, the radial recurrent artery is identified proximally and the superficial palmar artery is seen distally. These two large branches define the limits of the dissection and should be preserved (Fig. 10-2). The radial artery is divided distally and proximally and placed in a solution of heparinized blood and papaverine.

 INJURY TO THE SUPERFICIAL RADIAL NERVE
The superficial radial nerve provides cutaneous innervation to the radial aspect of the thumb and dorsum of the hand. Excessive lateral retraction of the brachioradialis muscle may lead to injury to this nerve and resultant numbness of the thumb. This may occur in 5% to 10% of the patients undergoing radial artery harvest.

The arm incision is closed in two layers with continuous absorbable suture. The deep layer includes the subcutaneous tissue distally.

 HEMATOMA FORMATION
An electrocautery is used only on the skin and subcutaneous tissue. All the radial artery branches should be clipped proximally and distally with small Ligaclips before division. In addition, the proximal stump of the divided radial artery should be oversewn with a suture ligature to prevent late bleeding and hematoma formation.

NB *PREVENTING RADIAL ARTERY SPASM*
The graft is gently flushed with heparinized blood and papaverine after harvesting. In addition, an intravenous calcium channel blocker (nicardipine) is administered in the operating room and continued postoperatively until the patient can tolerate oral medications. Diltiazem is then given orally for 6 to 12 weeks after surgery.

 COMPARTMENT SYNDROME
Compartment syndrome occurs rarely after radial artery harvest. However, if not recognized and treated promptly, extensive muscle loss and distal ischemic injury can occur. The hand must be checked for unrestricted movement and intact sensation at routine intervals in the immediate postoperative period to prevent such devastating consequences.

TECHNIQUE FOR GREATER SAPHENOUS VEIN HARVEST

An incision is made in the groin, one fingerbreadth medial to the femoral artery pulse. The subcutaneous tissue is dissected to expose the greater saphenous vein as it curves to pierce the cribriform fascia of the femoral sheath and join the femoral vein. The skin incision is then extended downward along the course of the vein. The incision can alternatively be started at the ankle, anterior to the medial malleolus, and extended upward. Many surgeons consider this approach convenient and elect to use it routinely.

The vein is harvested using the "no touch" technique. This entails handling of the vein only by its adventitia with an atraumatic vascular forceps. The vein is then gently removed from its bed by careful dissection and division of its branches.

 SKIN INFECTION OR ULCERATION
Harvesting veins from limbs with evidence of infection or ulceration should be avoided if possible.

ACCIDENTAL DIVISION OF THE VEIN

With the aid of a pair of sharp scissors, the skin incision is extended over the surgeon's index finger, which has tunneled above and parallel to the saphenous vein. This technique prevents accidental division of a more superficially placed saphenous vein and eliminates the development of unnecessary dead spaces or redundant skin flaps.

NERVE INJURY

The saphenous nerve runs a course along the greater saphenous vein. Special care should be taken not to divide it to avoid postoperative paresthesia.

SKIN INCISION ALONG THE KNEE

The incision alongside the knee joint is subjected to much strain and stretch in several directions as the joint moves. This may give the patient significant discomfort and interferes with satisfactory healing. Therefore, the skin in this location is usually left intact (Fig. 10-3).

NB *INTERRUPTED SKIN INCISIONS*

In patients who are diabetic or have peripheral vascular disease and are prone to poor wound healing, multiple skin incisions are made, leaving intervening bridges of skin intact. This allows better closure of the wound and minimizes ischemic changes along the skin edges (Fig. 10-3A).

WOUND HEALING

A wound in the lower leg tends to heal slowly; this is of particular significance in the elderly diabetic patient with peripheral vascular disease. Meticulous handling of tissues and careful wound closure are mandatory.

NB It is perhaps preferable not to harvest veins from the lower legs of elderly patients with diabetes or peripheral vascular disease.

When both greater saphenous veins have been stripped for varicosities or removed for previous bypass procedures, a search should be made for one or both lesser saphenous systems. Often, an adequate segment of vein can be procured.

In these cases, the patient should be prepared and draped in such a fashion that the back of the legs can be exposed. Cryogenically preserved homograft vein grafts are available in tissue banks in most cardiac surgery centers and can provide an alternative when no other autologous vein or arterial conduit is available. The long-term patency of these grafts is poor compared with that of native vein conduits.

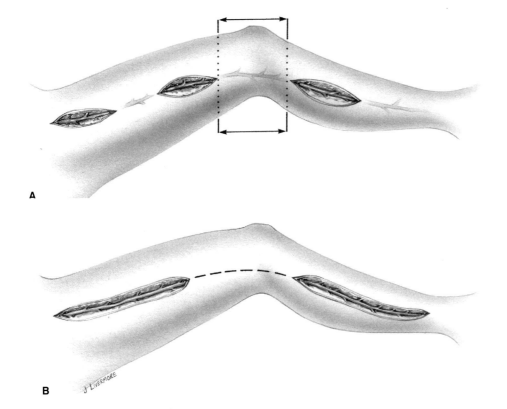

FIG. 10-3. Harvesting a greater saphenous vein. **A:** Multiple skin incisions. **B:** Long incisions leaving a skin bridge alongside the knee joint.

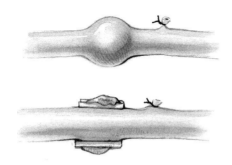

FIG. 10-4. Excluding a localized varicosity.

VARICOSITIES
Saphenous veins with varicosities should be avoided. The walls of these vessels are dilated and abnormal, and the large caliber predisposes to lower flow velocity and possibly early graft thrombosis and occlusion.

LOCALIZED VARICOSITIES
Localized varicosities can be detected along the vein wall when it is being gently distended. They may be partially excluded by application of hemostatic metal clips on the redundant tissue parallel to the vein wall (Fig. 10-4).

INTIMAL INJURY
The vein must never be pulled or stretched to facilitate dissection. The intimal layer is very delicate and may tear, giving rise to the formation of a nidus for platelet aggregation and possible subsequent early occlusion of the graft (Fig. 10-5A). This is more likely to occur when multiple skin incisions are made and the vein has to be harvested from beneath the skin bridges.

OVERDISTENTION OF THE VEIN
The vein graft should be gently distended; any excessive pressure can result in intimal tear and dis-

ruption. Devices are commercially available to prevent the intraluminal pressure from exceeding 150 mm Hg.

AVULSION INJURY
Stretching of the vein may also result in avulsion injury owing to tension on small side branches. These tears on the vein wall can be oversewn with 7-0 or 8-0 Prolene sutures to ensure adequate hemostasis; however, the vein integrity remains disrupted.

The vein can be gently retracted by means of elastic vessel bands whenever necessary (Fig. 10-5B).

The side branches are identified and ligated; alternatively, they can be occluded with metal clips and then divided (Fig. 10-6).

BRANCH STUMP
The branches should be ligated or clamped approximately 1 mm from the vein wall to minimize the presence of a stump, which may predispose to thrombus formation and early graft occlusion (Fig. 10-7A). Any stump can easily be eliminated by application of a fine hemostatic metal clip behind the tie, parallel with the vein wall (Fig. 10-7B).

GRAFT NARROWING
Conversely, the tie or metal clip should never occlude part of the vein wall itself; this gives rise to localized constriction (Fig. 10-7C). The tie or clip should be gently removed with a heavy needle driver and replaced appropriately.

ADVENTITIAL CONSTRICTION
The adventitial tissue may at times be caught in the tie around one of the branches, creating a localized constriction. The adventitial band should be carefully divided with Potts scissors (Fig. 10-8).

When an adequate segment of vein is dissected free, it is divided at each end and removed. The vein stumps in

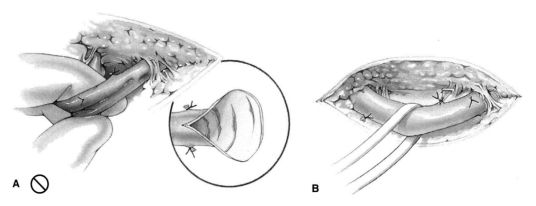

FIG. 10-5. A: Pulling or stretching vein injures the intima. **B:** Gentle retraction with an elastic band.

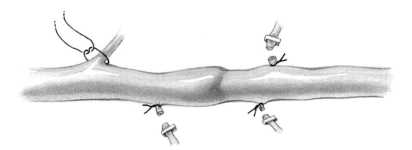

FIG. 10-6. Ligating or clipping vein branches.

the groin and the ankle are then securely ligated. An olive-tipped cannula is introduced into the distal end of the vein, which is then distended gently with *autologous, heparinized blood.* Any avulsed branches are identified and securely ligated with 4-0 silk or oversewn with 7-0 or 8-0 Prolene sutures, taking all the aforementioned precautions into consideration (Fig. 10-9).

 SUTURING THE VEIN WALL
At times, the wall of the vein itself at the site of the avulsion of its branches requires suture closure; this can be accomplished by taking longitudinal bites of the vein wall with 7-0 or 8-0 Prolene when it is being distended. Transverse suturing gives rise to localized constriction (Fig. 10-10).

The end of the vein is then cut, avoiding any intimal valvular remnant, and trimmed so that is has a smooth, hood-shaped orifice for anastomosis to the coronary artery (Fig. 10-11).

 VEIN END
If the caliber of the vein is small, the opening may be further enlarged by incising the vein orifice at the heel.

 VALVULOTOME INJURY
Some surgeons have advocated the use of a valvulotome to cut away the valve leaflets in the saphenous veins. Although this appears to be useful at times, it may create buttonhole defects in the vein wall. Therefore, if the device is used, great caution must be exercised. We do not routinely remove the valve leaflets unless they are located at the anastomotic sites.

NB *LOWER VERSUS UPPER LEG VEINS*
Traditionally, the vein procured from the ankle region conforms more to the caliber of the coronary arteries, has few if any valves, and can withstand higher intraluminal pressure. It is therefore more

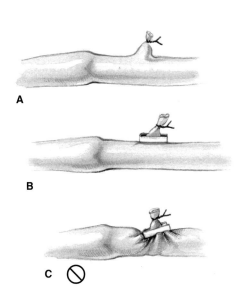

FIG. 10-7. A: Leaving excess stump on a vein branch. **B:** A metal clip eliminates stump. **C:** A clip constricting vein.

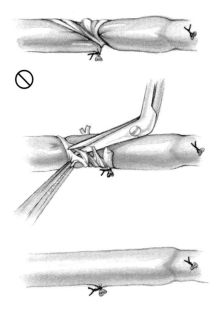

FIG. 10-8. Dividing the adventitial band to relieve constriction.

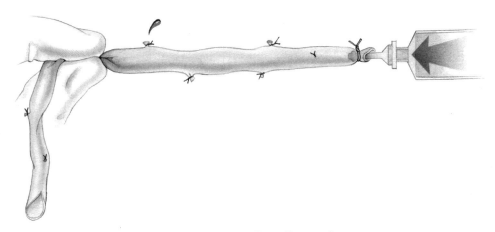

FIG. 10-9. Gently distending a vein.

suitable for bypass grafting of the smaller coronary arteries. However, the normal arterialization process and intimal hyperplasia may result in higher early graft closure of small saphenous vein conduit.

Despite all its advantages, the proximal end of a narrow-caliber vein graft may be too small for a standard aortic anastomosis. The proximal anastomosis will have to be carried out to a smaller aortic opening rather than a regular punched-out hole.

Skin Closure

The leg wound is closed in layers with absorbable sutures. In the groin region or where the wound is deep, an extra layer of closure may be necessary. The skin is closed with fine absorbable suture material in a subcuticular fashion (3-0 Dexon, Vicryl, or PDS).

🚫 **WOUND DRAINAGE**

If the wound is deep or continues to ooze blood, closed-system drainage for 24 hours should be used. This prevents hematoma formation and possible infection.

🚫 **WOUND INFECTION**

Patients with diabetes and patients with peripheral vascular disease are at increased risk of this complication. Therefore, the wound must be closed atraumatically and without leaving any dead space. Absolute hemostasis must be achieved before closure is begun. The subcuticular skin closure may be reinforced with deeply placed, interrupted horizontal mattress monofilament sutures that are left in place until satisfactory healing has been completed, usually for at least 2 to 3 weeks.

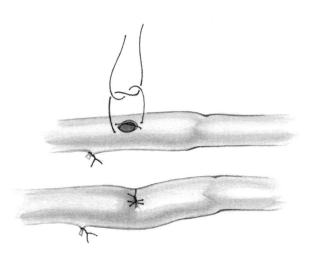

FIG. 10-10. Transverse closure of an avulsed branch leads to constriction of a vein.

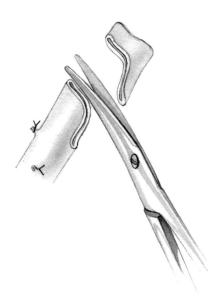

FIG. 10-11. Trimming the end of a vein to create a hood.

ENDOSCOPIC SAPHENOUS VEIN HARVESTING

Traditional open vein harvesting through one long incision or multiple interrupted incisions can result in significant wound morbidity including infection and chronic leg edema. The endoscopic approach avoids the healing problems associated with a long leg incision and may in particular benefit patients with diabetes, obesity, or peripheral vascular disease.

A 2-cm incision is made at the knee over the greater saphenous vein. An endoscope is then introduced using carbon dioxide insufflation to dissect a plane superficial to the vein. A specialized cautery device, clip applier, and scissors are introduced to obtain hemostasis and divide the vein branches. Once the proximal extent of the dissection is reached, a counterincision is made to facilitate division of the vein and oversewing of the stump. The vein is then gently withdrawn through the knee incision. The vein is prepared as described previously.

If two vein graft segments are required, the thigh vein is harvested as described. For additional conduit, the lower leg vein can be harvested by directing the endoscope inferiorly through the same knee incision.

The two incisions are then closed in two layers, and an elastic bandage is snugly wrapped around the leg and kept in place for 24 hours.

INTRALUMINAL CLOT
Endoscopic dissection with carbon dioxide insufflation causes vein compression and can lead to stasis of blood flow. Heparin should be administered intravenously before endoscopic vein harvest to prevent intraluminal thrombus formation.

HEMATOMA FORMATION
Hemostasis must be meticulously achieved using an electrocautery to avoid the development of a hematoma. If a large area of dead space has been created by the dissection, a soft drain connected to a closed drainage system should be placed along the endoscopic tract and left in place for 24 hours.

TRACTION INJURY TO THE VEIN
Excessive traction on the vein to mobilize it and withdraw it from the endoscopic tract can lead to intimal injury and avulsed branches. This must be avoided by extensive dissection with the cautery device and endoscopic scissors.

The learning curve for using endoscopic equipment is significant. With experience, it adds little time to the overall operation. Endoscopic vein harvesting is our procedure of choice when two or more vein conduits are required.

CORONARY ARTERY BYPASS GRAFTING WITH CARDIOPULMONARY BYPASS

Although many approaches have been used in the past decade for coronary artery bypass surgery, including limited thoracotomy incisions and endoscopic techniques, a median sternotomy is considered the incision of choice in most cases today. An increasing number of coronary bypass cases is now being performed without the use of cardiopulmonary bypass (see later). However, cardiopulmonary bypass is often preferred or required.

Venous drainage is accomplished through a single atriocaval cannula in most patients undergoing coronary artery bypass surgery. Bicaval cannulation is used when concomitant procedures necessitating an opening into the right side of the heart is indicated. Oxygenated blood is returned to the patient by direct cannulation of the ascending aorta. In rare instances when aortic cannulation is not feasible because of an ascending aortic aneurysm or extensive aortic wall calcification, the femoral arterial route is chosen instead (see Chapter 2).

Venting of the left side of the heart through the right superior pulmonary vein or through the pulmonary artery has been used, but it is unnecessary in most instances (see Chapter 4 for techniques of venting of the heart). In rare instances, when reoperative surgery for a single bypass to the circumflex coronary artery is needed, a left thoracotomy is an alternate approach. In such instances, cardiopulmonary bypass is achieved by both femoral artery and femoral vein cannulation (see technique described in Chapter 2).

Myocardial Preservation

Cold blood cardioplegia is infused into the aortic root to achieve cardioplegic arrest of the heart initially and repeated every 10 to 15 minutes during the cross-clamp time. Additional cardioplegic solution is infused directly into the vein graft after the distal anastomosis is completed. Core cooling to 34°C and topical cold or iced saline supplement myocardial protection. Critical proximal disease of major coronary arteries may interfere with the uniform distribution of cardioplegia and prevent complete cardioplegic arrest of the myocardium. Retrograde cardioplegic perfusion through a coronary sinus catheter may be useful in a select group of patients with several critically stenosed or diffusely diseased vessels (see Chapter 3).

In patients with acute coronary occlusion and impending infarction, the culprit vessel is grafted first to allow cardioplegic solution to be delivered through the vein graft to the involved myocardial territory.

NB Retrograde administration of cardioplegia may be particularly useful when arterial conduits are used because cardioplegia cannot be delivered through the graft.

NB Patients undergoing redo coronary artery bypass procedures with patent but diseased vein grafts are at risk of embolization of graft debris into the distal coronary artery bed. When patent *in situ* arterial grafts are present, antegrade cardioplegia will not reach the myocardium that these grafts supply. In these cases, retrograde cardioplegia is indicated.

NB Cardioplegic solutions containing high potassium must never be infused directly into the vein grafts because this may cause injury to the vein wall intima.

General Principles of Arteriotomy

On cardiopulmonary bypass with a quiet, decompressed heart, the coronary arteries are digitally palpated for evidence of disease and calcification. An appropriate site for arteriotomy is selected. This site should be, as much as possible, free of any gross disease. The epicardium overlying the coronary artery is incised and spread sideways with a special knife, a stroker blade (e.g., Beaver Mini-Blade A6400, Fig. 10-12A). This allows better inspection of the coronary artery wall. After the exact site of arteriotomy has been established, a poker blade (e.g., Beaver Micro-Sharp Blade A7513) is used to incise the anterior wall of the coronary artery (Fig. 10-12B).

NB The surgeon must memorize the precise anatomy of the coronary arteries as depicted in the angiogram so that the bypass graft is placed *distal* to the site of obstruction of the coronary artery.

🚫 ***PLACEMENT OF THE ARTERIOTOMY***
Care must be taken to perform the arteriotomy in the midline of the coronary artery. An oblique incision results in distortion of the artery at the heel or toe of the anastomosis. If an attempt is made to correct the direction of the arteriotomy, a flap of arterial wall is created. This leads to a less than perfect anastomosis (Fig. 10-13).

🚫 ***INJURY TO THE POSTERIOR ARTERIAL WALL***
Special precautions must be taken not to damage the posterior wall of the coronary artery. This can happen if the angle of the blade is perpendicular to the vessel. The angle should always be approximately 45 degrees with respect to the coronary artery (Fig. 10-14). If the posterior wall has been incised through the adventitia by the blade, it should be approximated with a fine suture of 8-0 Prolene tied on the outside of the vessel (Fig. 10-15).

🚫 ***CALCIFIED, NONPLIABLE ARTERIAL WALL***
Sometimes the arterial wall is inflexible and heavily calcified, making it impossible to tailor a satisfactory arteriotomy to perform a functioning anastomosis. A button of anterior wall is removed at the arteriotomy site. The technique essentially

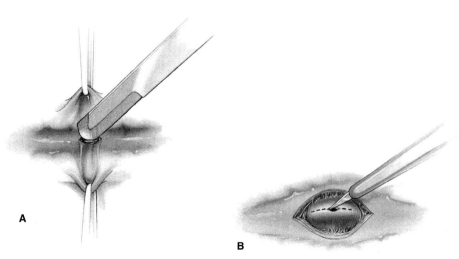

FIG. 10-12. A: A stroker blade is used to expose coronary artery. **B:** A poker blade is used to incise the anterior wall of a coronary artery.

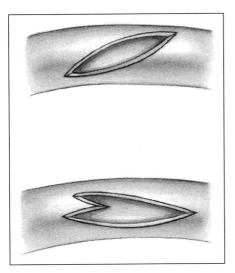

FIG. 10-13. Oblique arteriotomy and attempted correction create a flap of arterial wall.

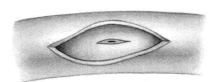
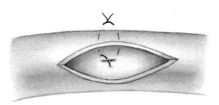

FIG. 10-15. Incision through the posterior wall of a coronary is repaired with a suture tied outside the vessel.

entails the removal of a triangular segment of anterior arterial wall from the site of the anastomosis. The calcified arterial wall would otherwise restrict the lumen of the graft anastomosis (Fig. 10-16).

The arteriotomy is then enlarged both proximally and distally (Fig. 10-17). A special modification of Potts scissors is available to enlarge a coronary artery in particularly difficult locations. The diameter of the coronary artery lumen as well as the presence of distal

obstructive plaques may be evaluated by gently inserting calibrated probes through the arteriotomy site (Fig. 10-18).

⊘ *DISTAL OBSTRUCTIVE PLAQUE*
Although every attempt is made to identify a relatively normal site for the anastomosis, at times localized plaques at the toe of the anastomosis may limit the flow and cause early occlusion of the graft. It is therefore important to enlarge the arteriotomy by cutting across the obstructive plaque (Fig. 10-19). Similarly, the distal opening of the conduit is enlarged and an anastomosis is then carried out. If the obstructing segment is too long and this procedure is not feasible, a second bypass graft must be placed distal to the site of obstruction.

⊘ *INTIMAL INJURY*
Probing must be performed gently, taking every precaution not to force too large a probe into the arterial lumen to prevent intimal tear.

⊘ *INTRAMYOCARDIAL COURSE OF THE CORONARY ARTERY*
The artery may follow an intramyocardial course. It must be followed into the muscle, and the myocardial bridge over the artery must be divided with great caution. The intramyocardial segment of the artery is nearly always disease free. The division of the myocardial bridge must be limited to the extent needed to perform a satisfactory anastomosis. Low-

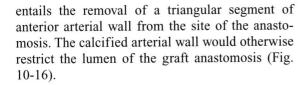
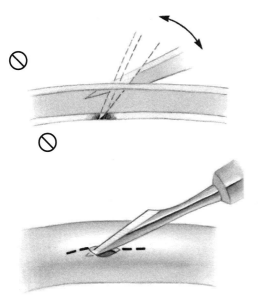

FIG. 10-14. Perpendicular angle of a blade damages the posterior wall of a coronary artery.

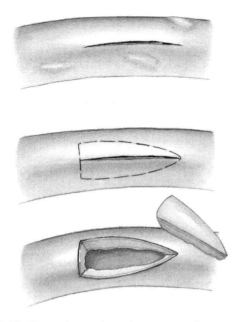

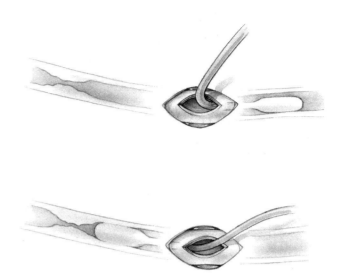

FIG. 10-18. Calibrating the lumen of a coronary artery with a probe.

FIG. 10-16. Removing a triangular segment from a calcified coronary artery.

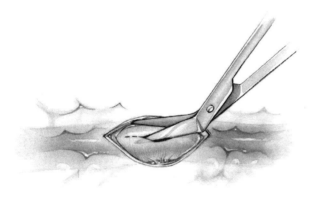

current electrocoagulation is used to cauterize the edges of the muscular bridge.

🚫 ***DIFFICULTY IDENTIFYING CORONARY ARTERIES***
In some patients, epicardial fat along the course of the coronary artery prevents the precise identification of the vessel. Under such circumstances, the side branches of the artery are identified first and then followed toward the parent trunk. The artery is then dissected clear of the fatty tissue. When the left anterior descending coronary artery cannot be identified, it may be useful to locate the posterior descending artery and follow it to the apex of the heart. The distal anterior descending coronary artery should be near this site.

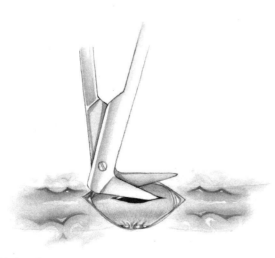

FIG. 10-17. Enlarging an arteriotomy with Potts scissors.

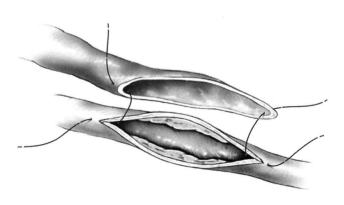

FIG. 10-19. Enlarging an arteriotomy across obstructive plaque.

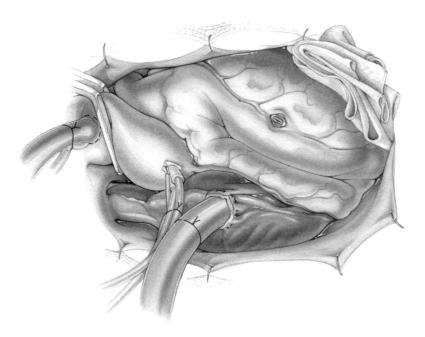

FIG. 10-20. Positioning the heart to expose anterior coronary artery branches.

POSITIONING THE HEART TO EXPOSE CORONARY ARTERIES

Exposure of the Anterior Surface of the Heart

A laparotomy pad soaked in ice-cold saline solution is placed into the pericardium behind the empty and flaccid heart. This maneuver usually exposes the anterior surface of the heart quite well. The left anterior descending, diagonal, and, with some minor adjustments, ramus intermedius coronary arteries can be viewed with ease (Fig. 10-20).

EXPOSURE OF THE RIGHT CORONARY ARTERY AND BRANCHES

The right coronary artery is usually a large vessel and is covered by epicardial fat in the right atrioventricular groove. Its distal branches, the posterolateral and right posterior descending arteries, tend to be more superficial as they course toward the apex of the heart.

The operating table is elevated, and the patient is placed in a slight Trendelenburg position. The acute margin of the right ventricle is gently elevated and held in position by the assistant surgeon's hand. The distal right coronary artery and the proximal segment of its branches are brought into view (Fig. 10-21). The epicardium over the atrioventricular groove is incised. The distal right coronary is identified and dissected for a short distance. To provide exposure for the posterior descending or posterolateral arteries, the apex of the heart is elevated toward the patient's right shoulder (Fig. 10-22).

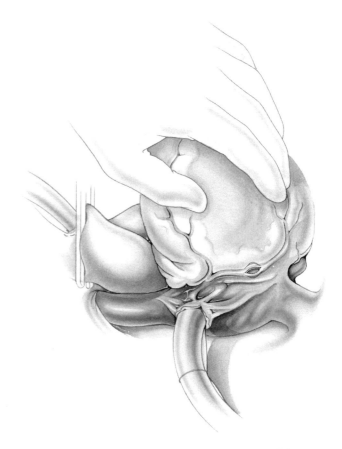

FIG. 10-21. Positioning the heart to expose the right coronary artery and branches.

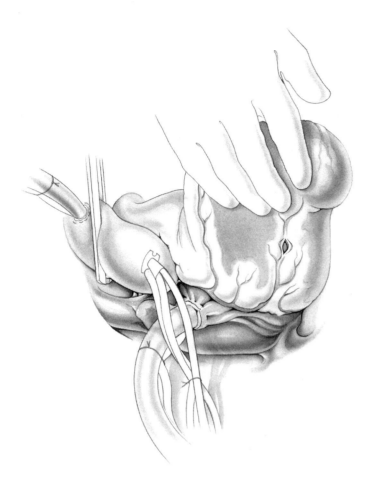

FIG. 10-22. Exposing posterior descending and posterolateral arteries.

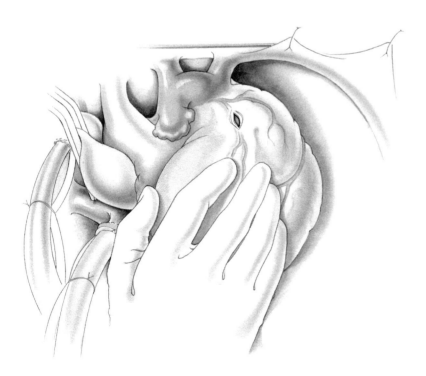

FIG. 10-23. Positioning the heart to expose the circumflex coronary artery and branches.

EXPOSURE OF THE CIRCUMFLEX CORONARY ARTERY AND BRANCHES

The operating table is lowered slightly and its left side raised. The empty, flaccid heart is gently elevated and held by the assistant surgeon's right hand. This maneuver, with some minor adjustments, brings all the obtuse marginal and posterior lateral branches of both the circumflex and right coronary arteries into view (Fig. 10-23).

Anastomotic Techniques

The technique for anastomosis to all the coronary arteries is essentially the same. The arteriotomy is made at the selected site. It is enlarged to a length of 5 to 7 mm with Potts scissors. The distal end of the conduit must be tailored to have an oblique, hood-shaped lumen with a circumference at least 25% larger than that of the arteriotomy (Fig. 10-11). The distal anastomosis is started with 30-in. long, 7-0 or 8-0 Prolene sutures double-armed with tapered needles. The first needle is passed from the outside of the graft 2 mm to the surgeon's side of the heel. It is then passed from the inside to the outside of the lumen of the coronary artery, 2 to 3 mm to the right of its heel (Fig. 10-24). The same needle is now passed again from the outside to the inside of the graft, adjacent to the previous suture in a clockwise direction. The needle is then passed from the inside to the outside of the coronary artery, adjacent to the previous stitch and similarly in a clockwise direction (Fig. 10-25). This sequence is repeated until four rounds of sutures have been placed in the internal mammary artery graft or the vein graft. By gently pulling on both ends of the suture in a seesaw fashion, the graft is lowered into position (Fig. 10-26).

Traditionally, the vein or the mammary artery is held by the assistant surgeon with two atraumatic forceps (Fig.

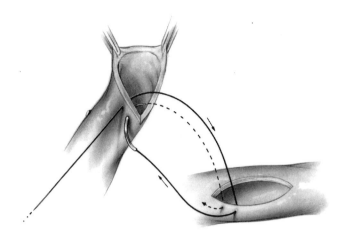

FIG. 10-25. Stepwise technique for a distal anastomosis.

10-24). The forceps ideally should hold the adventitial tissue of the conduit. This may be difficult, and the whole wall thickness including the intima is often grasped by the forceps. This damages the wall of the conduit and may lead to early graft closure.

The conduit can be held between the surgeon's left thumb and index finger; the anastomosis is carried out with the right hand (Fig. 10-27). This technique eliminates any possible forceps injury to the conduit and does not require the expertise of an assistant surgeon. Moreover, although initially it may appear to be somewhat clumsy and difficult, with a little experience, this technique becomes easy and actually expedites the anastomosis. Alternatively, the conduit is placed on the heart adjacent and parallel to the anastomotic site on the coronary artery (Fig. 10-28). The sequence of suturing remains the same for all the techniques described.

 ANASTOMOTIC LEAK AT THE HEEL
The sutures at the heel must be extremely close to each other to minimize the possibility of leaks. Subsequent placement of reinforcing sutures in this

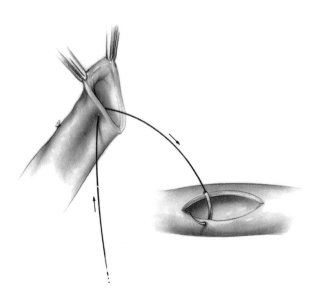

FIG. 10-24. Stepwise technique for a distal anastomosis.

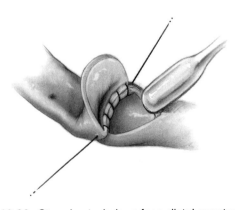

FIG. 10-26. Stepwise technique for a distal anastomosis.

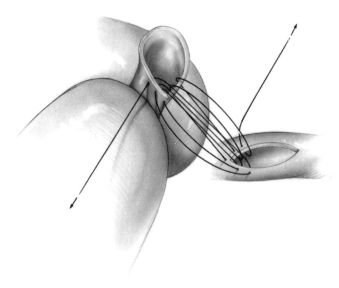

FIG. 10-27. Holding a vein graft between the left thumb and index finger.

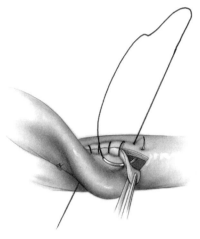

FIG. 10-29. Completing a distal anastomosis.

area is difficult and may compromise the lumen of the anastomosis.

🚫 ***PATENCY OF THE LUMEN AT THE HEEL OF THE ANASTOMOSIS***
An appropriately sized ballpoint probe is now introduced into the lumen of the coronary artery and the internal mammary artery for a short distance to ensure a satisfactory anastomosis at the heel (Fig. 10-26).

NB This probe can be left in the lumen of the coronary artery to stop the flow of blood and allow accurate placement of stitches.

The left arm of the suture is tagged with a rubber-shod clamp to provide gentle traction. The needle at the other end of the suture is now continued as an over-and-over stitch, outside in on the conduit and inside out on the coronary artery (Fig. 10-29). This is continued forward, passing well around the toe of the anastomosis (Fig. 10-30).

The needle should take small and superficial bites very close to each other on the coronary artery at the toe.

NB The needle may include a very thin segment of the surrounding epicardium to minimize anastomotic leaks.

At this time, an appropriately sized probe is passed through the toe of the anastomosis to ensure its patency. The suturing is continued until the other suture end is reached.

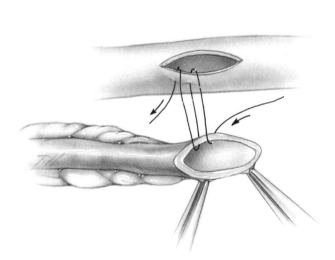

FIG. 10-28. Placing conduit on the heart next to the anastomotic site on a coronary artery.

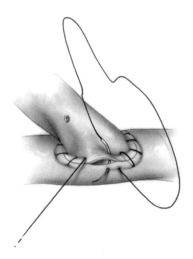

FIG. 10-30. Completing distal anastomosis.

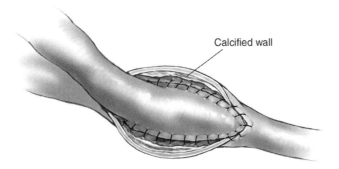

FIG. 10-31. Sewing a vein graft within an arterial lumen excluding a calcified segment.

 CALCIFIED ARTERIAL WALL

When the wall of the coronary artery is heavily calcified, a diamond-tipped needle swaged on 7-0 Prolene suture is used to perform the anastomosis. These needles are much stronger and can pierce the calcified plaques with minimal difficulty. Alternatively, when the edge of the coronary arterial wall is calcified, the vein graft can be sewn in place within the arterial lumen, excluding the calcified segment. Because the diameter of the vein is larger than that of the artery, the lumen of the anastomosis will be adequate (Fig. 10-31).

 INADVERTENT SUTURING OF THE POSTERIOR WALL

The toe of the anastomosis is its most critical part because it determines the outflow capacity of the graft. When the lumen of the artery is small or the visibility and exposure are suboptimal, the needle may pick up the posterior wall of the artery (Fig. 10-32). An appropriately sized ballpoint probe or a disposable plastic probe passed for a short distance into the distal artery may allow the precise place-ment of sutures and prevent the occurrence of this complication.

 CONSTRICTION AT THE TOE OF THE ANASTOMOSIS

Although passing the needle from inside the coronary artery at the toe of the anastomosis certainly minimizes the possibility of incorporating the posterior wall of the artery in the stitch, nevertheless, it is difficult to predict exactly where the needle will exit the artery, and a longer and larger segment of arterial wall may become included in the stitch. When tightened, the stitch produces some dimpling and stenosis of the anastomosis at the toe. Every precaution must be taken to avoid this complication (Fig. 10-33).

NB *APPEARANCE OF THE ANASTOMOSIS AT THE TOE*

Sutures should be placed farther apart on the graft compared with the coronary artery at the toe of the anastomosis so that when blood flow is established,

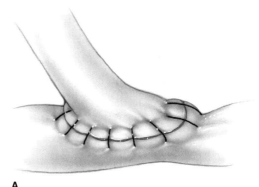

A

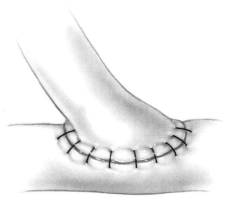

B

FIG. 10-33. A: Dimpling and narrowing at the toe of the anastomosis. B: Small, close-together suturing at the toe prevents narrowing of the anastomosis.

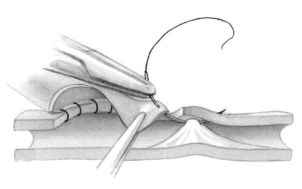

FIG. 10-32. A needle inadvertently picking up the back wall at the toe of an anastomosis.

the graft will bulge and provide a "hood" over the anastomosis.

Blood cardioplegic solution is gently infused through the graft before tightening the suture line to allow air to escape and prevent any air embolization to the coronary arteries. The sutures are tightened with care and securely tied (Fig. 10-34). Similarly, in the case of the internal thoracic artery, the bulldog clamp is removed. It is reapplied after the sutures have been tied if other coronary anastomoses are still to be done.

NB *INCORPORATION OF THE EPICARDIUM INTO THE ANASTOMOSIS*
The epicardial tissue on each side of the coronary arteriotomy is very often incorporated into the suturing process to ensure a more secure anastomosis.

The pedicle of the internal thoracic artery is tacked to the epicardium on each side of the anastomotic site with simple 6-0 Prolene sutures. This prevents the pedicle from twisting on itself and therefore obstructing flow through the vessel.

 FLATTENING OF THE THORACIC PEDICLE
If the tacking sutures are placed too far from the coronary artery, the pedicle may be stretched when the heart fills. This lateral traction may compress the internal thoracic artery and compromise the graft flow.

ANASTOMOTIC LEAK
Infusion of blood cardioplegic solution through the vein graft reveals any anastomotic leaks. These are

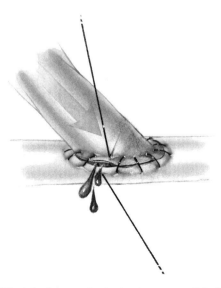

FIG. 10-34. Infusing cardioplegia down a graft before tying the suture.

best controlled at this time with a separate suture, taking care not to impinge on the lumen of the anastomosis. The surrounding epicardial tissue can be incorporated in the suture over the leak site.

ALTERNATE DISTAL ANASTOMOTIC TECHNIQUES

Interrupted Suture Technique

The anastomosis can also be accomplished with interrupted sutures; this is considered a superior technique, at least on theoretical grounds. Many surgeons combine both continuous and interrupted techniques, reserving the latter for the toe of the anastomosis. The general principles are the same as described previously for the continuous suture technique, but the incidence of anastomotic leaks is considerably higher, requiring additional reinforcing sutures.

Sequential Anastomosis

When the availability of conduits is limited, the technique for sequential anastomosis may be helpful. Although the technique can be applied to any combination of vessels, it is most applicable to the left anterior descending and diagonal coronary arteries or the posterior descending and distal right coronary arteries. Occasionally, multiple sequential distal anastomoses with only one proximal anastomosis are used, but this is not generally considered ideal.

 DISTAL GRAFT OCCLUSION
The patency of the most distal coronary artery anastomosis depends on the flow characteristics of the more proximal coronary artery. If the flow in the most proximal coronary artery is significantly more than the most distal coronary artery, the graft segment to the more distal coronary artery may gradually occlude.

 KINKING OF THE GRAFT
The length of the intervening graft between the anastomoses must be correct and must lie comfortably on the heart without kinking.

If all these technical details are accomplished and adhered to, excellent long-term results can be achieved with the technique for sequential anastomosis.

TOE-FIRST ANASTOMOSIS

This technique may be useful when grafting branches of the right coronary artery. The first suture needle is passed from the outside into the lumen of the artery at the

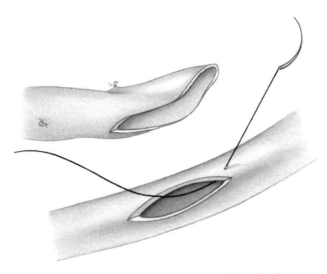

FIG. 10-35. Stepwise technique for a toe-first distal anastomosis.

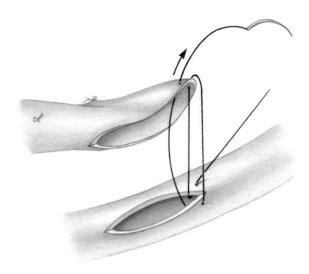

FIG. 10-37. Stepwise technique for a toe-first distal anastomosis.

toe of the anastomosis (Fig. 10-35). It is then passed from the inside to the outside of the conduit. The same needle is now passed again from the outside into the arterial lumen adjacent to, but to the surgeon's right of, the previous suture (Fig. 10-36) and through the conduit from the inside to the outside (Fig. 10-37). This arm of the suture is clamped. The graft is now lowered into position. At this point, an appropriately sized probe is introduced into the lumen of the coronary artery to ensure a patent anastomosis at the toe.

The needle at the other end of the suture is passed through the graft wall and then through the arterial wall from the inside to the outside (Fig. 10-38). The suturing is thus continued as an over-and-over stitch to a point well around the heel of the anastomosis (Figs. 10-39 through 10-42). The needle is then clamped. The other needle is

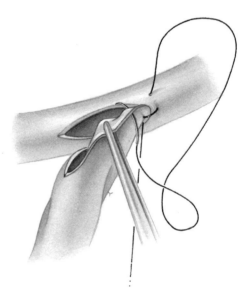

FIG. 10-38. Stepwise technique for a toe-first distal anastomosis.

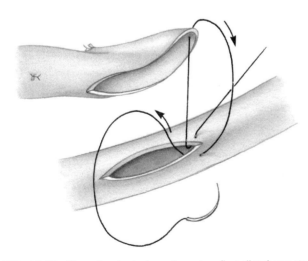

FIG. 10-36. Stepwise technique for a toe-first distal anastomosis.

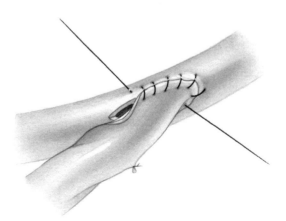

FIG. 10-39. Stepwise technique for a toe-first distal anastomosis.

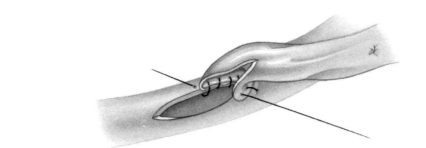

FIG. 10-40

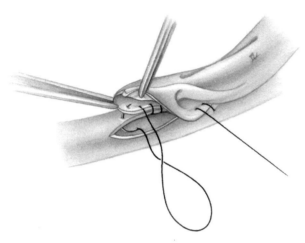

FIG. 10-41

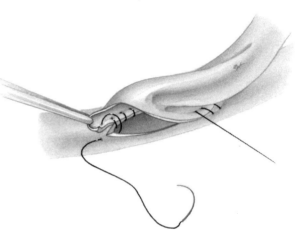

FIG. 10-42

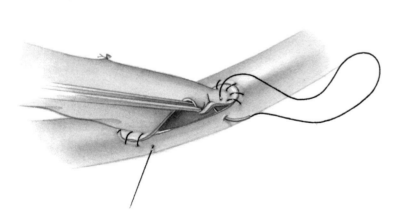

FIG. 10-43

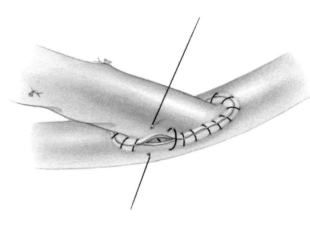

FIG. 10-44

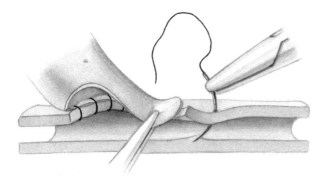

FIG. 10-45. A needle picking up the back wall of a coronary artery at the toe.

passed through the arterial wall from the outside to the inside and then from the inside to the outside of the graft (Fig. 10-43). The anastomosis is then completed and the suture ends tied after deairing by infusion of cardioplegic solution into the graft (Fig. 10-44).

 INADVERTENT SUTURING OF THE POSTERIOR WALL
The needle may pick up the posterior wall of the coronary artery (Fig. 10-45). This complication can be prevented if the lumen at the toe is fully visualized before passing the needle through the graft (Fig. 10-46). This part of the anastomosis can also be accomplished with interrupted sutures.

ENDARTERECTOMY

The role of endarterectomy in coronary artery disease is controversial. Many surgeons have achieved excellent results with the technique and use it when dealing with all the main branches of coronary arteries. Others are less enthusiastic and reserve the technique for the distal right coronary artery, whereas still others refrain from using endarterectomy at all. Nevertheless, in many cases, endarterectomy is the only way to provide a suitable lumen that accepts a bypass graft. It may well be that endarterectomized coronary arteries have decreased late patency and that the technique leads to increased perioperative myocardial infarction. It is nonetheless a useful technique and, when used appropriately, does provide excellent results.

Technique

The epicardium over the diseased segment of the coronary artery is incised. A 1-cm arteriotomy is made on the anterior surface of the vessel in the usual fashion. With a fine endarterectomy elevator, a plane is developed between the calcified media and the elastic adventitial segment of the coronary artery wall. The calcific core is dissected free

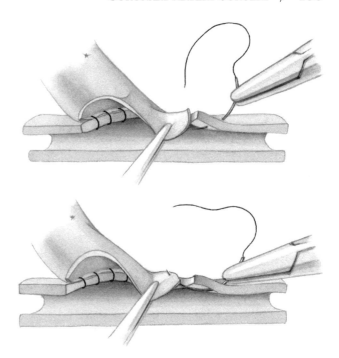

FIG. 10-46. Correct needle placement at the toe.

from the arterial wall circumferentially as well as distally and proximally (Fig. 10-47). With peanut dissectors providing traction and countertraction, the calcified plaque is gently withdrawn with a clamp or a pair of forceps (Fig. 10-48). The calcific core is withdrawn proximally and then divided with scissors. The distal segment is gently pulled and withdrawn until it becomes detached.

 TEAR OF THE CORONARY ARTERIAL WALL
Often the calcific core is adherent to the arterial wall to such an extent that its removal may create a tear in the arterial wall. Dissection must therefore be carried out with great caution. If a tear occurs, it should be directly sutured, *provided that the lumen is adequate.* Alternatively, the injured site is incor-

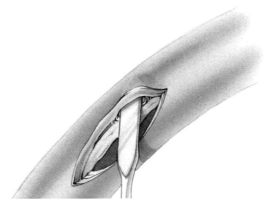

FIG. 10-47. Stepwise technique for a coronary endarterectomy.

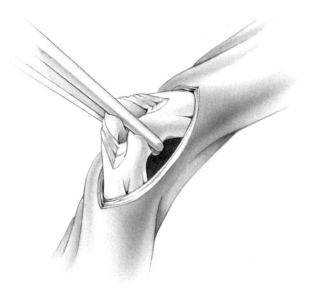

FIG. 10-48. Stepwise technique for a coronary endarterectomy.

porated into the arteriotomy and the vein graft anastomosis.

The lumen of the endarterectomized coronary artery is irrigated profusely to remove any debris, and the vein graft is anastomosed to it in the usual fashion.

 CONSTRICTION OF THE ANASTOMOTIC SITE
Often the length of the anastomosis may be quite extensive. Care should be taken to prevent the purse-string constrictive effect of the continuous suture technique.

 SEPTAL BRANCH OCCLUSION
Detachment of calcific plaque may occlude some of the arterial branches. This is particularly important whenever the left anterior descending coronary artery is endarterectomized because total occlusion of the septal branches may result in perioperative myocardial infarction.

NB The internal mammary artery should preferably *not* be used as a conduit when endarterectomy is performed because the internal mammary artery is prone to distortion at the heel and compromised inflow when a long arteriotomy is required.

PROXIMAL ANASTOMOSES

Increasingly, all proximal anastomoses are being performed with the aortic cross-clamp in place. This technique appears to be associated with a reduced incidence of intraoperative stroke owing to detachment of calcific plaques caused by clamp injury to the aorta. It is impor-

tant for a surgeon to commit to memory the size of the heart before the initiation of cardiopulmonary bypass and to envision how the vein grafts are to lie. With the heart empty and flaccid, estimation of the correct length of the vein graft may be difficult. A good rule is to estimate the length of the vein graft by the contour of the parietal pericardium. Alternatively, the heart can be filled and the correct length of the conduit be ascertained.

Another technique is to remove the aortic cross-clamp and allow the heart to beat normally. The vein grafts are cut to the optimal length, and the proximal anastomoses are performed with a side-biting clamp applied to the aorta.

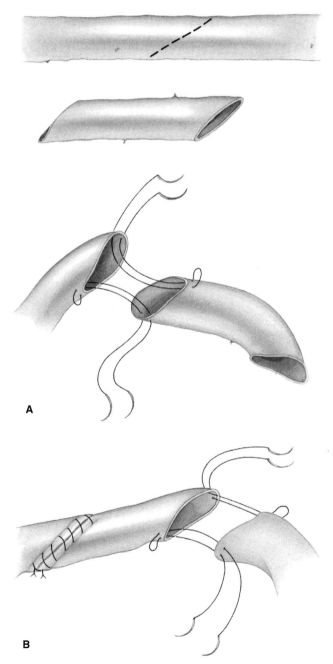

FIG. 10-49. Lengthening a vein graft with an extra vein segment.

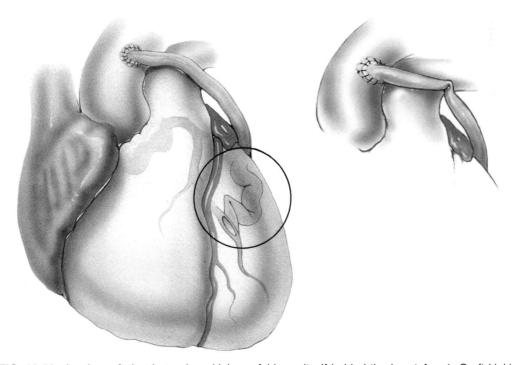

FIG. 10-50. A vein graft that is too long kinks or folds on itself behind the heart. **Inset:** Graft kinking when the chest is closed.

 LENGTH OF THE VEIN GRAFT

Saphenous vein grafts tend to shrink a little over time. If the length is a little short, shrinkage may cause tension on the anastomosis and predispose the graft to premature failure. The vein graft must be divided at a point that ensures a comfortable length of the graft when the heart is fully filled. This necessitates an extra length of 1 to 2 cm.

If the graft is noted to be too short, it should be repositioned on the aorta. Alternatively, the vein should be divided obliquely and lengthened with an extra segment of vein (Fig. 10-49).

Leaving the vein graft too long may result in kinking or folding of the conduit on itself when the heart is placed back in the pericardial well (Fig. 10-50). Sometimes the graft appears to be the appropriate length but kinks when the chest is closed (Fig. 10-50, inset). This occurs most frequently with circumflex grafts. In this case, the graft should be shortened by taking down the proximal anastomosis and excising the extra length before resuturing the graft to the aorta. Alternatively, if the aorta is extensively diseased, the appropriate length of vein may be excised and the two resulting vein ends reanastomosed, taking care not to twist the graft. Often a graft that is slightly too long can be positioned well behind the left atrial appendage and kept in place with a piece of Surgicel (Fig. 10-51).

 TWIST OF THE GRAFT

Every precaution should be taken to ensure the proper lie of the graft without any twisting along its length, which may occur particularly with vein grafts at the back of the heart (Fig. 10-52). In rare cases when this occurs, the proximal anastomosis must be redone. If for any reason this is not feasible, the vein graft may be divided and reanastomosed after being untwisted. Some surgeons prefer to mark the vein graft with a methylene blue stripe to prevent this complication.

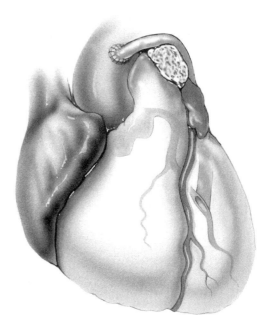

FIG. 10-51. Positioning a slightly long vein graft behind the left atrial appendage with a piece of Surgicel.

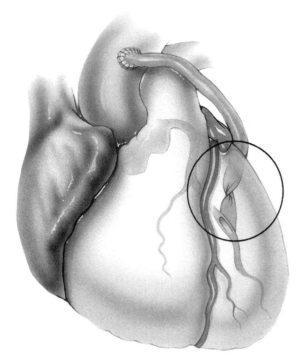

FIG. 10-52. Twisting of a vein graft.

The vein end is tailored to have a large, wide, hood-shaped opening (Fig. 10-11). This can be accomplished by dividing the vein approximately 30 degrees obliquely with respect to its length and then extending the incision generously downward at the heel to create a vein graft opening that is at least 20% larger than the aortic opening.

 MISMATCH BETWEEN THE VEIN GRAFT AND AORTIC OPENING
The circumference of the vein graft must be at least 20% larger than the aortic opening; otherwise, the vein stretches out flat and compromises the lumen (Fig. 10-53).

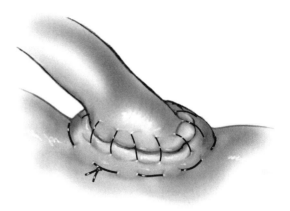

FIG. 10-54. Narrowing a too large an aortic opening with a purse-string suture.

NB If the vein caliber is small, the aortic opening should be limited to a narrow slit corresponding to the incision at the heel of the graft.

NB If the aortic opening is inadvertently made too large, the opening can be narrowed to the appropriate diameter with a purse-string 4-0 Prolene suture (Fig. 10-54).

With a no. 11 blade, a 3- to 4-mm slit-like incision is made at a precise site for each proximal anastomosis. The opening is dilated slightly with the tip of a fine forceps. A disposable punch is introduced into the slit-like opening, and a circular part of the aortic wall, 4.0 to 4.8 mm in diameter, is removed (Fig. 10-55).

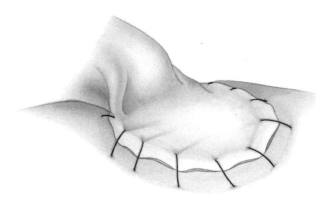

FIG. 10-53. The hood of a vein graft is flattened owing to too large of an aortic opening.

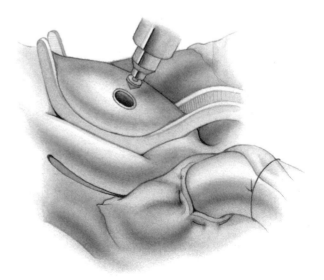

FIG. 10-55. Creating aortic openings with a disposable punch.

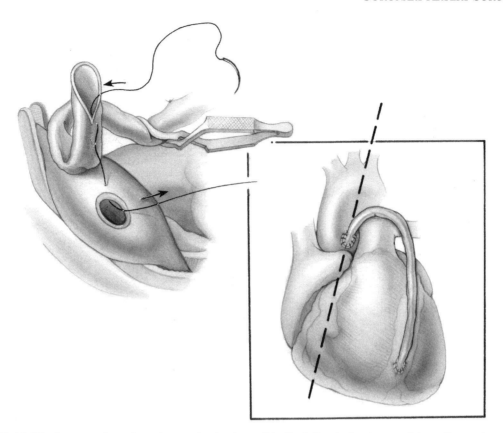

FIG. 10-56. Correct orientation of a proximal vein graft to the left anterior descending or diagonal coronary artery.

 INTIMAL WALL DETACHMENT
The introduction of the punch into the aortic lumen must be performed meticulously to avoid intimal detachment, which could lead to subsequent dissection of the aorta. When the aortic wall is thick and calcified, the separated segment of the aortic wall should be included in the suturing process.

Technique for Proximal Anastomosis

The lie of the left anterior descending or diagonal vein grafts should take a deep concave course to join the aorta in an oblique fashion at the 2-o'clock position at the anastomotic site (Fig. 10-56). Positioning this graft with the heel of the anastomosis between the 3- and 5-o'clock positions may result in kinking of the graft by the pulmonary artery (Fig. 10-57). The ramus and obtuse marginal grafts join the aorta horizontally at the

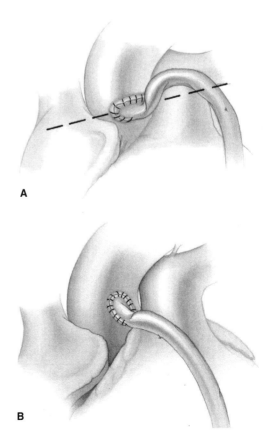

FIG. 10-57. Incorrect orientation of a proximal vein graft leading to kinking by the pulmonary artery. **A:** A graft to the left anterior descending artery. **B:** A graft to the right coronary artery.

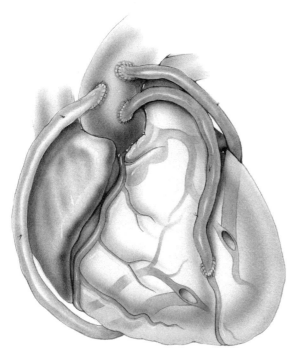

FIG. 10-58. Correct placement and orientation of a proximal vein grafts.

3-o'clock position. The distal right vein graft takes a course along the atrioventricular groove and joins the ascending aorta at the 6- to 7-o'clock position, and the posterior descending artery grafts take a course lateral to the atrium and join the aorta at approximately the 8-o'clock position. The right-sided grafts are anastomosed

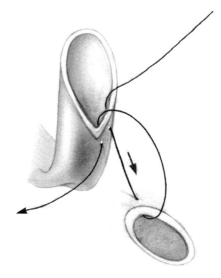

FIG. 10-60. Stepwise technique for a proximal anastomosis.

to the anterior right lateral aspect of the aorta relatively high on the aorta (Fig. 10-58). This prevents the graft from being kinked by the superior vena cava or the right ventricular outflow tract (Fig. 10-57B). Under special circumstances, the left-sided grafts can be passed behind the aorta through the transverse sinus and be anastomosed to the right side of the aorta (Fig. 10-59). The latter technique is particularly useful when there is calcification of the left side of the ascending aorta or when the vein is short. Nevertheless, this technique predisposes the vein graft to possible twisting behind the aorta and makes control of any bleeding from a side branch difficult.

NB *The surgeon must always anticipate the possibility that the patient may require aortic valve replacement at some time in the future. Thus, the*

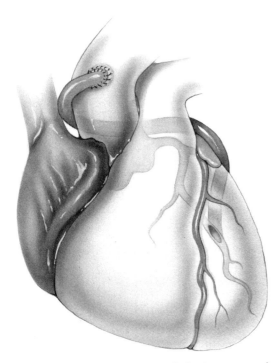

FIG. 10-59. Routing a graft through the transverse sinus.

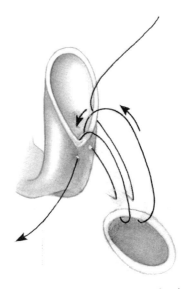

FIG. 10-61. Stepwise technique for a proximal anastomosis.

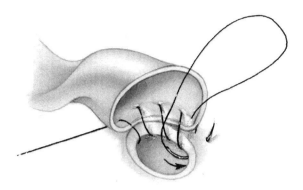

FIG. 10-62. Stepwise technique for a proximal anastomosis.

proximal anastomoses should be placed high on the aorta to allow a subsequent aortotomy to be made without interfering with the proximal graft sites.

The proximal anastomosis is started with a 30-in. long 5-0 or 6-0 Prolene double-armed suture. The precise lie and course of direction of the vein graft are envisioned. The first stitch is passed from the inside of the graft to the outside and then passed from the outside to the inside of the aorta in an counterclockwise direction (Fig. 10-60). After three to five rounds of suturing, the graft is lowered into position, and the needle is clamped (Fig. 10-61). The needle at the other end of the suture is now passed in a backhand fashion, from the inside to the outside of the aorta (Fig. 10-62), followed by outside to inside of the vein graft in a clockwise direction (Fig. 10-63). This over-and-over suturing is continued to meet the other arm of the suture (Fig. 10-64). When all the proximal anastomoses are completed, the vein grafts are each occluded with atraumatic bulldog clamps. The perfusion pressure is temporarily reduced, and the aortic clamp is removed. Blood is allowed to distend the vein grafts and to leak through the anastomoses (Fig. 10-65). This maneuver displaces air, allows the vein graft to

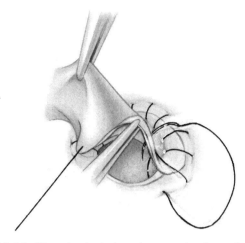

FIG. 10-64. Stepwise technique for a proximal anastomosis.

assume its hood shape, and prevents purse-string constriction of the anastomosis. The suture ends are now tied securely. Normal perfusion pressure is resumed when all sutures have been tied.

NB *CALCIFIED AORTA*
Placement of proximal anastomoses should be on the normal aortic wall. Calcific sites should be avoided. However, aortic walls are sometimes very diseased and at times calcified. Often, "toothpaste" material is squeezed out of the aortotomy site; at other times, there are calcific plaques within the aortotomy. The edges of the aortotomy should be free of any debris. It is cleaned with dry gauze, and the aortic clamp is loosened slightly to allow blood to gush out of the aortotomy and wash away any debris or particles.

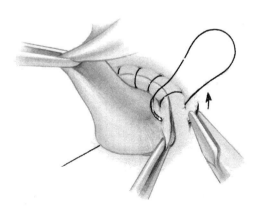

FIG. 10-63. Stepwise technique for a proximal anastomosis.

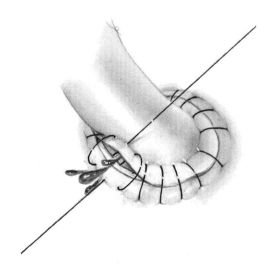

FIG. 10-65. Stepwise technique for a proximal anastomosis.

Technical points to ensure good proximal anastomoses include tailoring a generous opening in the proximal vein because the aortic wall is not pliable. In addition, deep bites of all the layers of the aortic wall must be taken.

NB *SURFACE ECHOCARDIOGRAPHY*
Atherosclerotic changes of the aorta are very common in elderly patients. Surface echocardiography has been used to detect localized atheromatous areas when digital palpation fails. At times, the aorta may be so diseased that proximal vein grafts may have to be placed on the innominate artery. A totally calcified lead pipe aorta may have to be replaced (see Chapter 2).

NB *FREE INTERNAL THORACIC AND RADIAL ARTERIAL GRAFTS*
If a free internal thoracic or radial arterial graft is used, a small aortic opening must be made. Unless the aortic wall is fairly thin, it may be preferable to anastomose the proximal arterial conduit to a vein graft hood or to a patch of vein or pericardium that has already been sewn to an aortic opening.

🚫 *AORTIC WALL ADVENTITIAL TISSUE*
In preparing the site for proximal anastomosis, adventitial tissue on the aortic wall should be incorporated in the suturing process. This is particularly important in elderly patients with delicate aortic walls. The adventitial tissue acts as "natural" pledgets, providing a secure anastomosis and adding strength to the aortic wall.

OFF-PUMP CORONARY ARTERY BYPASS GRAFTING

For the past 30 years, coronary artery bypass grafting has relied on the aid of cardiopulmonary bypass to obtain a bloodless and stationary operating field. However, despite the many advances made, blood contact with the artificial surfaces of the cardiopulmonary bypass circuit continues to produce a well-documented diffuse inflammatory response that affects multiple organ systems and is responsible for much of the noncardiac morbidity (consequently cost) after open heart surgery. Although beating heart surgery is not a new concept, critics of this technique have questioned the quality of the distal anastomoses, which may result in lower graft patency rates. Concerns have also been raised regarding the possibility of incomplete revascularization owing to the greater hemodynamic instability for exposure of posterior and lateral vessels. However, with the development of innovative stabilizing instruments that have made possible complete multivessel coronary bypass through a sternotomy, there has been a resurgence of interest in performing coronary bypass grafts without cardiopulmonary bypass or off-pump coronary artery bypass.

Anesthetic Considerations

The main goal of anesthesia management is to maintain hemodynamic stability during the various manipulations of the heart during off-pump coronary surgery. Ideally, an oximetric pulmonary artery catheter is used to continuously measure mixed venous oxygen saturation and cardiac output. Transesophageal echocardiography may have limited value when the heart is displaced to a vertical position. The key to avoiding emergent conversion to cardiopulmonary bypass is to be proactive, rather than reactive, in optimizing surgical conditions to prevent hypotension and low cardiac output. Intravascular volume should be replenished because the most common cause of low blood pressure is decreased venous return with positioning of the heart. Hemoglobin level, electrolytes, and arterial blood gases should be maintained within a normal range. Although inotropic support may be necessary, it is kept to a minimum to prevent tachycardia, which can interfere with optimal suture placement and increase myocardial oxygen consumption. Most important, continuous communication is needed between the operating surgeon and the anesthesiologist.

NB *POSITIONING THE HEART*
The most critical aspect of off-pump coronary bypass surgery is the positioning of the heart to expose the target vessel adequately without hemodynamic compromise. This can be accomplished via strategic placement of four deep pericardial sutures (Fig. 10-66) and appropriately placing the patient in various positions. The first pericardial suture is placed above the left inferior pulmonary vein well below the phrenic nerve, the second near the inferior vena cava, and the last two equidistant in a line drawn between the first two sutures. Rommel tourniquets are used to avoid abrasions on the epicardium by the pericardial sutures. By sequentially increasing the tension on each suture from the pulmonary vein to the inferior vena cava, coupled with steep Trendelenburg positioning of the operating table rotated toward the surgeon, the heart can be lifted out of the pericardial sac to expose even the most posterior vessel for grafting. Generally, lifting the heart to a vertical position is relatively well

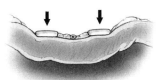

FIG. 10-68. Target stabilization using compressive forces.

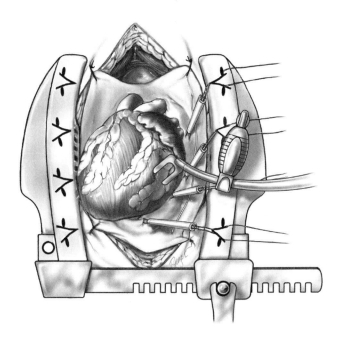

FIG. 10-66. Strategic placement of deep pericardial sutures.

tolerated. Alternatively, commercially available apical suction devices (Fig. 10-67) can be used to lift the heart instead of deep pericardial sutures. The flexible joint at the hinge point of the apex device allows the heart to freely twist about its long axis.

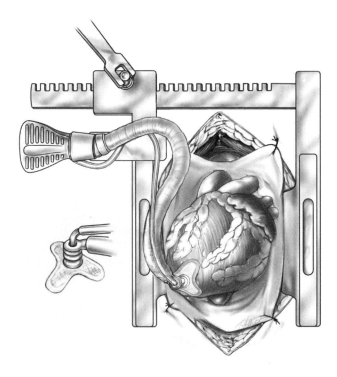

FIG. 10-67. An apical suction device for exposing lateral and posterior vessels.

NB *MECHANICAL STABILIZATION*

There are three basic types of devices designed to locally immobilize the target coronary artery during off-pump surgery. The CTS Ultima system (Cardio-Thoracic Systems, Cupertino, CA) (Fig. 10-68) stabilizes the vessel by applying downward pressure on each side of the vessel. The degree of stabilization correlates with the amount of pressure applied. It is easy to use and has a relatively low profile. However, excessive force on the heart can cause hemodynamic instability. Therefore, it is important to apply the minimal pressure to achieve immobilization without compression of the heart. The Octopus system (Medtronic, Inc., Minneapolis, MN) (Fig. 10-69) obtains stabilization by applying high-pressure suction to the surrounding tissue via multiple suction cups. Compressive forces are therefore not required for vessel immobilization. However, it is bulkier, has a higher profile, and may cause suction injury to the surrounding epicardium. A more recently developed device, the Estech Synergy (Estech, Danville, CA), is a hybrid device that combines both compression and suction technology to stabilize the target vessel.

STABILIZER MYOCARDIAL INJURY

It is important that the stabilizer is used for local immobilization of the myocardium only. It should not be used as a retraction device, which may cause hemodynamic compromise.

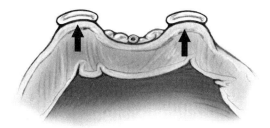

FIG. 10-69. Target stabilization using high-pressure suction.

ANTERIOR VESSELS

Left Anterior Descending and Diagonal Branch

Generally, the anterior vessels are grafted first. Revascularization of the left anterior descending artery with the internal thoracic artery allows immediate perfusion of a sizable portion of the myocardium.

NB Sometimes the diagonal artery may need to be grafted before the left anterior descending artery because the internal mammary pedicle can make placement of the stabilizer for immobilization of the diagonal branch difficult.

These anterior branches are exposed by gentle traction on the deep pericardial sutures to rotate the apex of the heart into the surgical field. The stabilizer is placed on the target site with the tips toward the base of the heart (Fig. 10-70).

NB The left anterior descending artery is usually grafted at the distal one-third to one-half where the vessel normally emerges from its intramyocardial location. Occasionally, grafting of the artery is required more proximally. Test occlusion with a soft Silastic tape (see below) is performed before arteriotomy as significant myocardial ischemia may occur, thereby causing left ventricular distention and hypotension. In this case, intraluminal shunting is recommended.

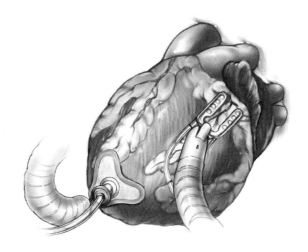

FIG. 10-71. Exposure and stabilization of the ramus intermedius and high obtuse marginal branches.

Ramus Intermedius and High Obtuse Marginal Branches

These are often intramyocardial and require grafting near the base of the heart that cannot be mobilized into the field. However, displacement of the heart into a vertical position allows easier access for arteriotomy and suturing. The stabilizer is placed with the tips toward the base of the heart (Fig. 10-71). Placing the patient in Trendelenburg position and rotating the table toward the surgeon may facilitate exposure.

⊘ ***INJURY TO THE LEFT ATRIAL APPENDAGE***
Although the stabilizer can be positioned with the heel toward the base of the heart, bleeding from the left atrial appendage can occur if it is allowed to rub against the stabilizer arm (Fig. 10-72).

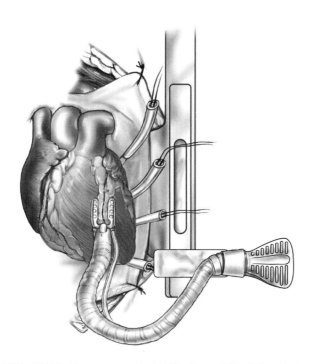

FIG. 10-70. Exposure and stabilization of the left anterior descending artery.

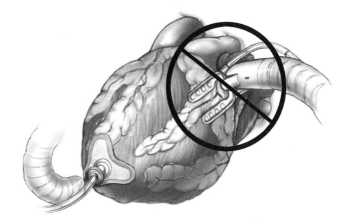

FIG. 10-72. Injury to the left atrial appendage from inappropriate placement of a stabilizer.

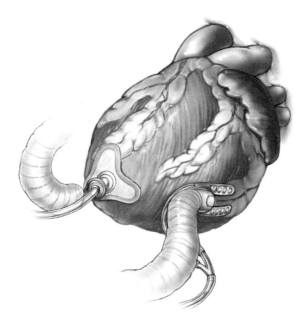

FIG. 10-73. Exposure and stabilization of obtuse marginal branches.

POSTERIOR VESSELS: OBTUSE MARGINAL BRANCHES

Other lower obtuse marginal branches can be best accessed with the heart in the vertical position and slightly rotated to the right. The stabilizer is attached on either the crossbar or the right side of the retractor and placed with the tips toward the base of the heart (Fig. 10-73).

 OBSTRUCTION OF VENOUS RETURN
The heart should not be rotated excessively in an attempt to provide better target exposure because this may cause obstruction of venous return.

POSTERIOR VESSELS

Posterior Descending Artery

Exposure of this vessel is usually very well tolerated without hemodynamic instability. The heart is displaced vertically without any rotation. The stabilizer is attached to the left side of the retractor and placed toward the base of the heart (Fig. 10-74).

Distal Right Coronary Artery

Adequate exposure can usually be accomplished without lifting the heart out of the chest. The stabilizer is attached to the right side of the retractor with the tip directed downward along the course of the artery (Fig. 10-75).

 RIGHT VENTRICULAR DISTENTION AND BRADYCARDIA
It is not uncommon for bradycardia and right ventricular distention to occur with proximal occlusion of the right coronary artery. Therefore, alligator clips should be applied to the epicardium and attached to a pacemaker before coronary occlusion. Alternatively, an intraluminal shunt can be used.

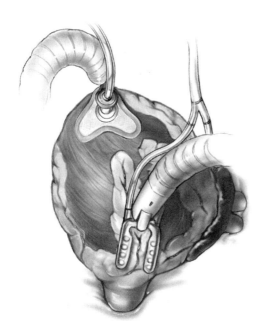

FIG. 10-74. Exposure and stabilization of the posterior vessels.

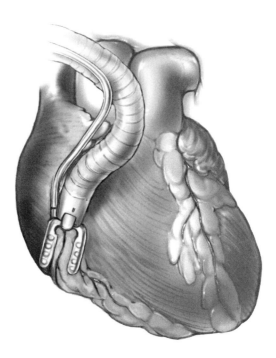

FIG. 10-75. Exposure and stabilization of the distal right coronary artery.

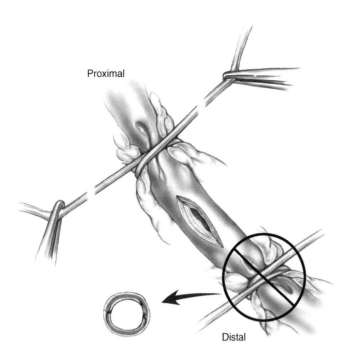

FIG. 10-76. Avoid the use of distal occlusion.

Conduct of the Operation

As in on-pump coronary artery surgery, the heart is exposed via a median sternotomy and all conduits are harvested in the usual fashion. The operative technique for grafting vessels during an off-pump case is similar to that used with on-pump surgery. After an arteriotomy is made, bleeding is controlled either with the use of an intraluminal shunt or with a soft Silastic tape placed proximally around the vessel and placed on gentle traction.

⊘ ***INJURY TO THE ARTERY DISTAL TO THE ANASTOMOSIS***
Avoid the use of distal vessel occlusion because it may cause intimal injury and subsequent stenosis (Fig. 10-76).

A bloodless field is obtained with a CO_2 mist blower.

⊘ ***LIFTING AN INTIMAL PLAQUE***
Vigorous spraying with the CO_2 blower can either lift an intimal plaque or separate the intimal layer to cause a localized dissection (Fig. 10-77). Use of the CO_2 blower should be limited to the time that the needle passes through the target vessel and only when sufficient blood is present to obscure the field. Focus should be on the site of each needle passage with attention to the back wall and edges. A completely bloodless field is not necessary.

NB After each distal anastomosis, the graft is deaired by gently flushing with warm blood (or removing the internal thoracic artery occluder) before tightening and securely tying the suture.

With a relatively disease-free aorta, proximal vein graft anastomoses are performed using a partial occlusion clamp. The systemic arterial blood pressure is lowered to a systolic level of approximately 100 mm Hg before the clamp is applied. The clamp should be tightened just enough for hemostasis but securely enough to not slip off.

⊘ ***AORTIC DISSECTION***
Applying the clamp too tightly or during hypertension can cause aortic dissection, especially in the elderly with a fragile aorta.

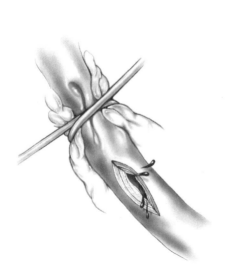
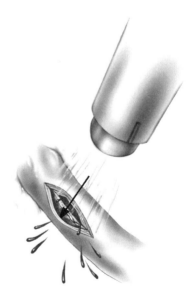

FIG. 10-77. Separation of intimal plaque from vigorous spraying with a CO_2 blower.

The use of commercially available proximal anastomotic stapling devices may be considered in patients with diseased ascending aortas.

TRANSMYOCARDIAL REVASCULARIZATION

Transmyocardial laser revascularization is used to treat ischemic areas of viable myocardium that cannot be directly revascularized. A holmium:YAG laser is used to create 1-mm wide channels into the left ventricular cavity. Although these laser channels close, angiogenesis results in improved perfusion to treated areas of myocardium.

NB Patients with ejection fractions less than 30% or acute ischemia are generally not candidates for transmyocardial revascularization.

NB Although transmyocardial revascularization is usually applied only to areas of myocardium that cannot be directly revascularized, patients with diffusely diseased coronary arteries may benefit from combined treatment.

Technique

Transmyocardial revascularization is performed typically after bypass grafting is completed during cardiopulmonary bypass. The viable ischemic area is exposed and the ventricle is filled. The laser is fired to create between 15 to 20 channels 1 cm apart extending from revascularized myocardium to ischemic regions. Bubbles are seen by transesophageal echocardiography when the laser beam reaches the ventricular cavity, confirming a completed channel. After cardiopulmonary bypass is discontinued and protamine administered, most channels readily seal at the epicardial surface with gentle digital pressure. Occasionally, a figure-of-eight 6-0 Prolene suture may be required for hemostasis.

CONSIDERATION IN REOPERATIVE CORONARY ARTERY BYPASS SURGERY

The operative strategy for performing redo coronary surgery is similar to the primary procedure. Some important points need to be considered.

General precautions for repeat sternotomy need to be followed (see Chapter 1). In particular, if a patent *in situ* right internal thoracic graft is present and crossing the midline or if a redundant left internal thoracic artery lies directly beneath the sternum, great care must be exercised to prevent injury to these grafts.

NB If a thoracic pedicle is injured or divided, it may be cannulated with an olive-tipped catheter and perfused with a line connected to a femoral arterial catheter. Alternatively, cardiopulmonary bypass is rapidly achieved using the femoral vessels, and the internal thoracic graft is perfused from the pump circuit.

Patent but diseased saphenous vein grafts should not be manipulated to prevent embolization of debris into the distal coronary artery bed. Some controversy exists as to whether antegrade cardioplegia should be administered down diseased vein grafts. Some surgeons divide all old, patent vein grafts once on cardiopulmonary bypass and flush debris out of them with retrograde cardioplegia. The two ends are oversewn after the distal anastomosis of the new graft is completed.

 INADEQUATE FLOW THROUGH INTERNAL THORACIC ARTERY
An internal thoracic artery may not provide sufficient flow to a previously grafted coronary artery with a diseased but patent vein graft. This is especially true if the surgeon elects to divide and oversew the old graft to prevent embolization of debris. In this case, another vein graft is preferred.

If a patent *in situ* internal thoracic graft is present, the pedicle must be identified and mobilized if the redo procedure is to be done on cardiopulmonary bypass with cardioplegic arrest of the heart. The pedicle must be occluded with an atraumatic bulldog clamp during the cross-clamp interval. The safest technique for identifying the left internal thoracic pedicle is to begin the dissection from the diaphragm and proceed superiorly. The anastomotic site is thus encountered first, and the pedicle then can be gently encircled for later clamping.

Injury to the Lung

The internal thoracic pedicle often lies between the lung and the heart. If dissection is carried out superiorly to locate the pedicle, the lung tissue is frequently injured in multiple locations. This results in air leaks that may persist for several days postoperatively.

NB If the internal thoracic pedicle cannot be safely found, the operation may be performed as an off-pump procedure or on cardiopulmonary bypass with deep hypothermic arrest.

The ascending aorta is often quite thickened and diseased in patients undergoing redo coronary artery procedures. Therefore, it is generally safer to perform all distal and proximal anastomoses under a single aortic cross-clamp period. The hood of the old vein graft is usually free of disease and provides a good location for a proximal anastomosis.

CHAPTER 11

Surgical Correction of Mechanical Complications of Myocardial Infarction

The mechanical complications of acute myocardial infarction have serious clinical implications and are generally associated with a poor prognosis. The onset of ischemia is usually heralded by pain that may be followed by shock and ventricular failure owing to significant myocardial injury. The severity of symptoms and clinical manifestations are intimately related to the magnitude of myocardial necrosis and loss of contractile strength.

Necrosis of the ventricular free wall may cause acute myocardial rupture and death or late development of a left ventricular aneurysm. Necrosis of the ventricular septum may result in an acute septal defect and thus sudden hemodynamic instability requiring urgent surgical intervention. Necrosis of papillary muscles will result in papillary muscle dysfunction or rupture causing mitral valve insufficiency requiring urgent surgical intervention.

Most patients will require emergent surgery because of intractable and progressive cardiogenic shock. Some may stabilize with medical management and intraaortic balloon counterpulsation to undergo cardiac catheterization and coronary angiography before urgent surgical intervention. A few will compensate and present late with a left ventricular aneurysm, ventricular septal defect, or mitral valve insufficiency. In most cases, concomitant coronary artery bypass grafting should always be contemplated, whenever possible, to achieve complete myocardial revascularization.

EXPOSURE AND CANNULATION OF THE HEART

The heart is exposed through a median sternotomy. Venous drainage is accomplished through bicaval cannulation, although a single, large atrial cannula is adequate whenever the right heart remains a closed system during the procedure. Arterial blood is returned by direct aortic cannulation.

NB *CONTAINED BLEEDING WITHIN THE PERICARDIUM*
When there is evidence for contained bleeding within the pericardium owing to a pseudoaneurysm or rupture of the heart, it is prudent to cannulate the aorta through a small enough opening in the pericardium overlying the aorta to allow volume replacement during venous cannulation and initiation of cardiopulmonary bypass. Alternatively, femoral cannulation should be contemplated.

NB *CARDIOGENIC SHOCK*
Most patients requiring surgical intervention for management of *acute* mechanical complications of myocardial infarction are in cardiogenic shock. Many may be on intraaortic balloon pump support, and a few may already be on a portable cardiopulmonary support system.

Cardiopulmonary bypass is initiated, and the heart is decompressed. Both antegrade and retrograde routes of administration of blood cardioplegic solution are established. Core cooling to 30° to 32°C is carried out, and the aorta is clamped. Cold blood cardioplegic solution is then administered through the aortic root followed by retrograde cardioplegia into the coronary sinus (see Chapter 3).

ACUTE MYOCARDIAL RUPTURE

Cardiorrhexis is a dramatic and lethal event. It is virtually always associated with a transmural infarction. Through a rent in the ventricular endocardium, blood gradually leaks into the area of infarction and distends the necrotic tissue. This hematoma continues to expand and finally ruptures the myocardium. The incidence of myocardial rupture after myocardial infarction is 10 times greater than either a ventricular septal defect or papillary

166

muscle tear. The left ventricle is involved in 90% of all ruptures.

The sudden onset of cardiogenic shock 3 to 4 days after acute myocardial infarction may herald the development of cardiac tamponade owing to myocardial rupture. Equalization of pressures in the right atrium, right ventricle in diastole, and pulmonary artery wedge, as measured with a Swan-Ganz catheter; and aspiration of blood from the pericardial cavity are significant clues to the accurate diagnosis. Immediate surgery should be undertaken. Infarctectomy followed by patch closure of the defect with a Hemashield patch or bovine pericardium should be securely performed.

RESECTION OF A LEFT VENTRICULAR ANEURYSM

Cardiopulmonary bypass is initiated in the standard fashion. Usually a single atriocaval cannula is adequate for venous return. Cardioplegic arrest of the heart is accomplished by infusion of cold blood cardioplegic solution through the aortic root after clamping the aorta. This is complemented by infusion of cold blood cardioplegia into the coronary sinus by the retrograde technique (Chapter 3, Myocardial Protection). Venting of the left ventricle through the right superior pulmonary vein helps to keep the field dry. When the heart is still and vented empty, the extent of the aneurysm is evaluated. The scar segment of the left ventricular wall, devoid of myocardium, tends to be sucked in by the vent. The aneurysm is carefully dissected free from the pericardium. Traction sutures are placed in the aneurysm, and an incision is made through the scar tissue (Fig. 11-1). The opening is then enlarged, and some *excess* scar tissue is excised to provide easy access for removal of blood clots from within the left ventricle and aneurysm wall (Fig. 11-2).

⊘ *ADHERENT CALCIFIED ANEURYSM WALL*
Occasionally, there may be marked fibrous reaction or even calcification of the aneurysm wall, making its mobilization tedious and time-consuming. The involved segment of the aneurysm can be amputated free from the heart and left adherent to the pericardium and pleura (Fig. 11-3).

⊘ *DISLODGMENT OF BLOOD CLOTS FROM THE ANEURYSM*
Manipulation and dissection to free the left ventricular aneurysm from the pericardium are performed after the aorta has been cross-clamped to avoid dislodgment and systemic embolization of blood clots.

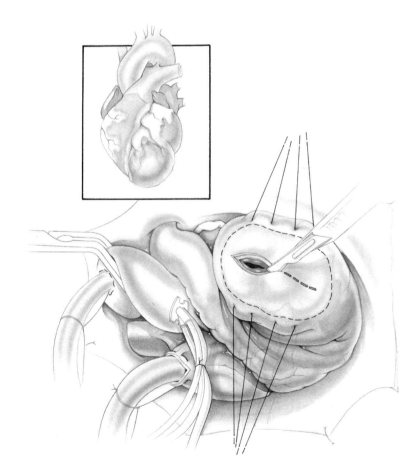

FIG. 11-1. Ventriculotomy through scar tissue.

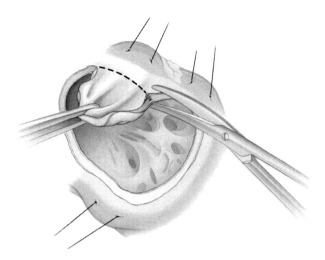

FIG. 11-2. Excision of a scarred ventricular wall.

⊘ *LOOSE BLOOD CLOTS*

There are often loose blood clots in the ventricular cavity. A sponge should be placed in the outflow tract of the left ventricle near the aortic valve before attempting to remove blood clots and debris from the aneurysmal cavity. The sponge will prevent the escape of blood clots into the aortic root and possible embolization into the coronary arteries. The interior of the left ventricle is then thoroughly irrigated with cold saline solution to wash away any debris.

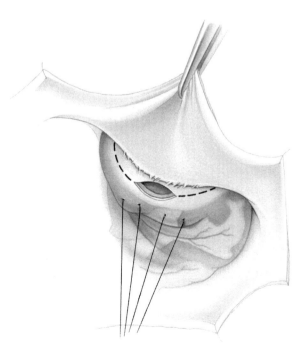

FIG. 11-3. Technique for leaving a scarred ventricular wall adherent to the pericardium.

With sharp scissor dissection, a 3-mm-thick layer of the endocardial fibrous lining of the left ventricular cavity is stripped en masse for approximately 1 to 2 cm from the edge of the aneurysm. This *theoretically* removes any abnormal foci of electrical activity.

NB *RADICAL ENDOCARDIAL DISSECTION*

If a patient has a history of ventricular arrhythmia, it is advisable to carry out a radical endocardial resection while performing the left ventricular aneurysmectomy. The procedure entails the dissection of a 2- to 3-mm thickness of the endocardium of the left ventricle. The resection should be extensive, reaching to the base of the papillary muscle and the aortic root, to ensure complete removal of any scattered arrhythmogenic foci. Cryoablation of the transitional zone between the scar tissue and myocardium in patients with ventricular aneurysm may be helpful. Care must be taken not to damage the papillary muscle to avoid causing mitral insufficiency. Most of these patients are candidates for implantation of an internal cardioverter-defibrillator device.

NB The liberal use of internal cardiac defibrillators and antiarrhythmic drugs has markedly decreased the indication for endocardial resection.

NB *CONCOMITANT MITRAL VALVE REPLACEMENT*

Occasionally, patients with left ventricular aneurysms have hemodynamically significant mitral regurgitation owing to papillary muscle dysfunction and mitral valve disease. If the valve is grossly diseased and unsuitable for repair, it is replaced through the ventriculotomy. Pledgeted sutures of 2-0 Ticron are used to anchor the prosthesis in position (Fig. 11-4).

⊘ *CHOICE OF PROSTHESIS*

Only a bileaflet mechanical or bioprosthesis should be used in the mitral position, especially if implanted through the left ventriculotomy. Particular attention should be given to the orientation of the prosthesis, which is not as familiar from the left ventricular aspect.

An attempt is made to leave the subvalvular apparatus intact. Excess leaflet tissue can be excised or incorporated in the sutures. The direction of the sutures is from the left atrium toward the left ventricular cavity. The sutures are then passed from the superior aspect of the prosthetic sewing ring to its inferior aspect so that when the sutures are tied, the knots are on the left ventricular side (Fig. 11-4). Care must be taken to ensure that the knots of the sutures do not interfere with the occlusive mechanism of the prosthesis.

The ventricle should be closed in such a fashion as to restore its normal geometry. This can be achieved by

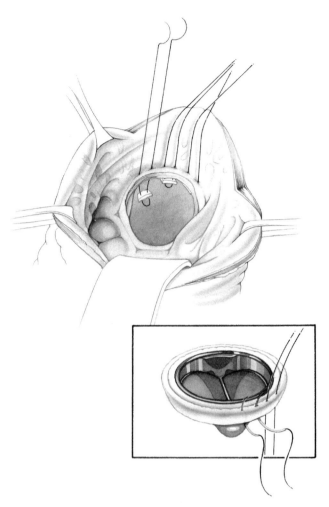

FIG. 11-4. Technique for mitral valve replacement through a left ventriculotomy.

Hemashield patch closure of the wall defect with approximation of the left ventricular wall over it. A continuous 2-0 monofilament suture is placed deep into the scar along the margin of the aneurysm wall (the edge of the normal left ventricular wall) and tied to create a purse-string effect (Fig. 11-5A). This reduces the size of the defect in the left ventricular wall to a great extent and gives the left ventricular cavity a relatively normal shape and geometry (Fig. 11-5B).

A Hemashield patch is cut into the appropriate shape of the defect and sewn into place with a continuous suture of 3-0 Prolene, taking deep bites of the surrounding scar tissue. The suture line may have to be tightened with a nerve hook and reinforced with a few interrupted sutures buttressed with felt pledgets. BioGlue (CryoLife, Inc., Kennesaw, GA) can be applied to the suture line for added security. Only when the patient has been weaned off cardiopulmonary bypass and there is no bleeding from the patch site should the excess aneurysmal wall be approximated over the patch to prevent accumulation of blood and clot between the patch and aneurysm wall (Fig. 11-5C).

NB *TISSUE COVERING THE LEFT VENTRICULAR PATCH*
Covering the left ventricular patch with aneurysmal wall minimizes the possibility of graft infection should mediastinitis occur.

Coronary artery bypass grafting to diseased vessels is performed when possible to achieve maximal revascularization of the heart. Special care is taken to deair the heart

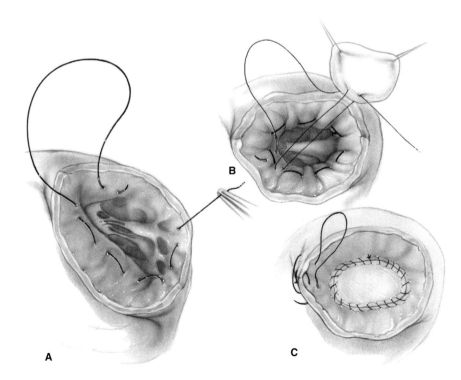

FIG. 11-5. A: Suture placed in the scar along the edge of the normal left ventricular wall. **B:** Purse-string effect of a suture reducing the size of the defect. A small Hemashield patch is sutured in place to cover the defect. **C:** The defect in the left ventricular wall is closed, and the scarred aneurysmal wall is approximated over the patch when absolute hemostasis is achieved.

before removing the patient from cardiopulmonary bypass (see Chapter 4).

PSEUDOANEURYSM

Postinfarction false aneurysm is a rare phenomenon. It occurs when blood leaking from a myocardial rupture slowly accumulates in the pericardial cavity. Reactionary adhesions limit the size of the pseudoaneurysm. Two-dimensional echocardiography and ventricular angiography delineate the lesion quite vividly. Unlike left ventricular aneurysms, eventual rupture of the pseudoaneurysm is virtually certain. Therefore, surgical management must always be carried out on a semiurgent basis.

The surgical technique is similar to that described for true aneurysms. However, false aneurysms are often very thin walled and may rupture easily during dissection and manipulation of the heart. Therefore, it is prudent to initiate cardiopulmonary bypass by cannulating the femoral artery and vein (see Chapter 2). A median sternotomy is then performed; the aorta is cross-clamped and cardioplegic arrest of the heart achieved before addressing the pseudoaneurysm. If the pseudoaneurysm ruptures, blood is removed from the field and returned to the pump by suckers. The aorta is quickly clamped, bleeding is brought under control, and cardioplegic arrest of the heart is then accomplished.

Pseudoaneurysms usually have small openings. The defect is closed with a patch of Hemashield using interrupted 3-0 Ticron sutures buttressed with felt pledgets. The suture line is reinforced with a continuous suture of 3-0 Prolene. Absolute hemostasis is obtained, and the heart is deaired (see Chapter 4).

VENTRICULAR SEPTAL RUPTURE

The ventricular septum receives blood from perforating branches of the left anterior descending artery as well as perforating branches of the posterior descending artery. Despite this dual blood supply, there is frequently no septal collateral flow. Consequently, the interventricular septum remains quite vulnerable to ischemia and occasionally ruptures after myocardial infarction. This is seen notably in patients whose infarction is owing to single-vessel disease. As with ventricular aneurysm, the anteroapical area is the most common site; it is involved in 65% of patients with ventricular septal rupture. The posterior segment of the septum is involved in 17% of the cases, and the middle segment in 13% of the cases; only 4% of the ruptures involve the inferior segment of the septum.

The optimal time for operative repair of a septal rupture is at least 3 to 4 weeks after acute myocardial infarction; during this time, some fibrosis occurs in the necrotic areas so that tissues can accept sutures safely and surgical repair can be attempted with relative ease. Neverthe-

less, there is frequently rapid progressive hemodynamic deterioration with myocardial failure making emergency surgical intervention mandatory. An intraaortic balloon pump, inotropic agents, and diuretics are helpful for temporary stabilization of these very critically ill patients. The goal of preoperative management of these patients is to reduce the left-to-right shunt by reducing systemic vascular resistance at the same time ensuring adequate systemic blood pressure and cardiac output. The operative mortality in this subgroup of patients is exceedingly high, but without surgery, they would not survive at all.

Technique for the Surgical Treatment of a Ventricular Septal Defect

The septal defect is approached through the left ventricular infarct (Fig. 11-6). The ventricular septal infarct and the extent of surrounding friable necrotic involvement are identified. With a continuous 3-0 Prolene suture, a generous patch of bovine pericardium is sewn to the left ventricular side of the septum, taking deep bites of normal, healthy muscular tissue as far away from the necrotic rim of the defect as possible. At times, this may necessitate sutures being placed close to the mitral valve annulus. The septal necrosis often extends to the ventriculotomy. The pericardial patch is then allowed to pro-

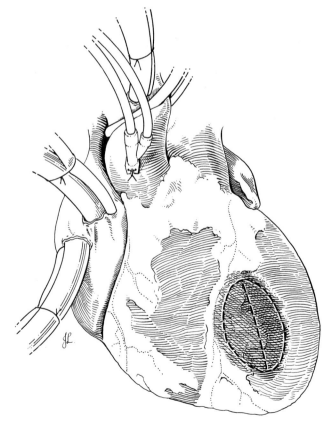

FIG. 11-6. Technique for surgical treatment of a ventricular septal defect.

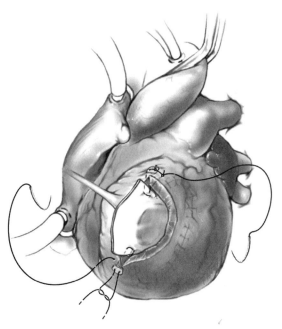

FIG. 11-7. A generous patch of bovine pericardium is sewn to the septal wall of the normal ventricle away from the defect.

trude outside the heart and be incorporated in the ventriculotomy closure (Fig. 11-7). This technique essentially excludes the infarcted area. The suture line on the septum is inspected and checked for any residual defects. This is reinforced with multiple interrupted sutures buttressed with felt pledgets. The patch is anchored to the anterior edge of the left ventricular wall with a felted suture. This technique is based on the concept that the higher left ventricular pressure will force the pericardial patch against the entire septum, thus obliterating the sep-

tal defect. Because sutures are placed on the normal, healthy tissue, well away from the defect edges, the repair should be secure.

The ventriculotomy is then closed with interrupted sutures of 3-0 Prolene with a layer of Teflon felt strip on each side of the incision. This is reinforced with a continuous suture of 3-0 Prolene.

When the septal defect is a narrow, slit-like opening in close proximity to the anterior wall of the right ventricle, the sutures are first passed through a strip of Teflon felt, then through the viable septal tissue along the posterior edge of the defect, and again through another strip of Teflon felt on the right ventricular side of the septum (Fig. 11-8A). The sutures are brought out through the anterior wall of the right ventricle before they are passed through another strip of Teflon felt. Finally, the sutures are tied down, and the ventriculotomy is closed as described previously (Fig. 11-8B). Alternatively, the single pericardial patch technique could be used.

If the apex of the heart has infarcted and is necrotic, it is amputated. The viable tissue is then reapproximated in a sandwich fashion by means of four strips of Teflon felt, one on each side of the septum and one each on the right and left exterior ventricular walls, with a series of interrupted horizontal mattress sutures (Fig. 11-9).

The approach to a rupture of the posteroinferior aspect of the septum through the infarcted inferior left ventricular wall is most hazardous. Often the posteromedial papillary muscle is also involved, and concomitant mitral valve replacement may be indicated. Closure of the ventricular septal defect is performed in the same fashion as described above. Most often, the inferior wall of the ventricle is closed using an appropriately sized Hemashield patch so as not to interfere with the normal geometry of the left ventricle. Coronary bypass grafting is performed judiciously on all bypassable vessels to ensure full revascularization of the remaining myocardium.

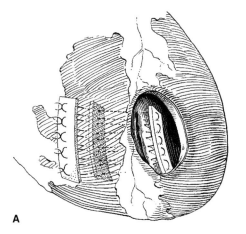

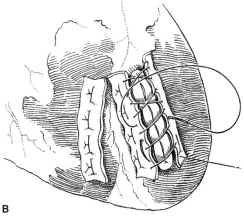

A   **B**

FIG. 11-8. A: The slit-like ventricular septal defect is closed with interrupted sutures incorporating strips of Teflon felt on both sides of the septum and anterior wall of the right ventricle. **B:** The knots are then tied, and the ventriculotomy is closed.

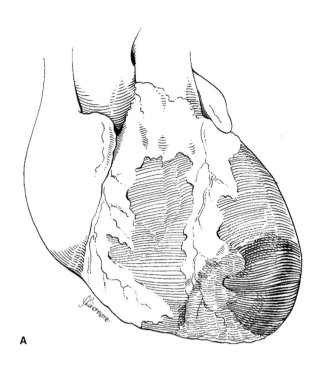

A

FIG. 11-9. A: Ventricular septal defect as the result of apical infarction. B: The necrotic apex of the left ventricle is amputated. C: The septal defect and ventricular walls are reconstructed with interrupted sutures incorporating strips of Teflon felt.

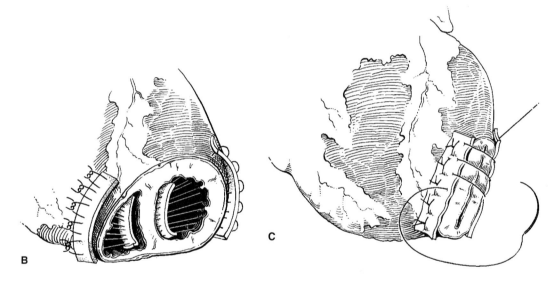

B

C

PAPILLARY MUSCLE RUPTURE

The anterolateral papillary muscle has a rich blood supply from both the left anterior descending and left circumflex coronary arteries. In 90% of hearts, the right coronary artery is dominant and supplies the posteromedial papillary muscle. In the remaining 10%, its blood supply is provided by branches of the left coronary artery system. Therefore, infarction of the posterior wall of the left ventricle frequently results in necrosis of the posteromedial papillary muscle. A papillary muscle rupture usually occurs during the first week after infarction or later with reinfarction. Because both leaflets of the mitral

valve are attached to each papillary muscle by chordae tendineae, complete disruption of either one, usually the posteromedial papillary muscle, results in massive mitral regurgitation, acute pulmonary edema, and death unless surgical intervention is prompt. A tear of the apical head of a papillary muscle that supports a small segment of only one of the mitral leaflets may result in a milder degree of mitral regurgitation (Fig. 11-10). Dysfunction of the papillary muscle is probably more common. If myocardial infarction is not massive and left ventricular function is not severely impaired, these subgroups of patients can compensate long enough to be studied and can undergo surgical treatment semiurgently.

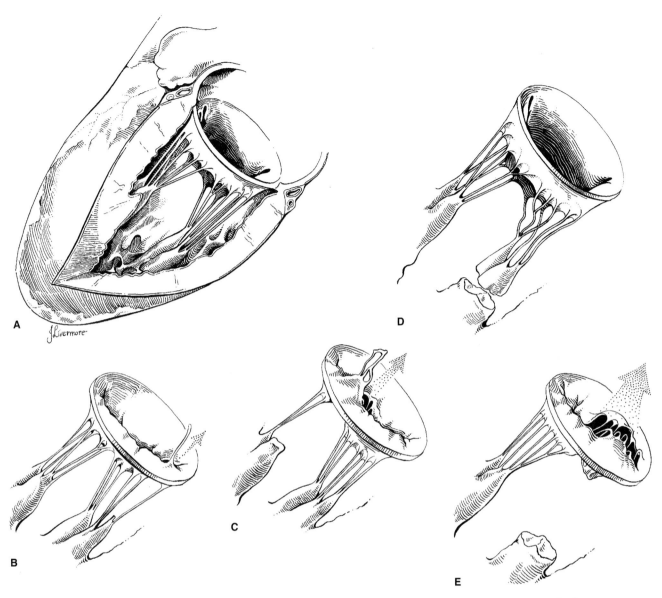

FIG. 11-10. A: Spatial relationships of the anatomic components of the mitral valve apparatus. **B:** Rupture of chordae tendineae. **C:** Partial rupture of the head of the papillary muscle. **D:** Complete tear of the papillary muscle giving rise to gross valvular insufficiency **(E).**

The correct spatial relationships of parts of the mitral valve apparatus contribute to the integrity of the valve and ensure its normal function (Fig. 11-10). Ventricular dilation, resulting from infarction or ischemia, may interfere with this intricate mechanism and may be instrumental in the development of mitral insufficiency. For example, the papillary muscle may be necrotic, fibrosed, or, at times, normal and contract relatively well, but paradoxical movement of the adjacent left ventricular wall and impaired cardiac function can precipitate mitral insufficiency.

From the surgeon's point of view, mitral valve insufficiency may be the result of only annular dilation, a structural defect of the mitral valve apparatus such as ruptured or elongated chords, ventriculopapillary dysfunction such as an ischemic or infarcted papillary muscle, or various combinations of these defects.

The clinical presentation of a patient after myocardial infarction may be changed by the appearance of a new heart murmur that should be followed very closely in the coronary care unit. After a diagnosis of mitral regurgitation has been established, immediate surgery is recommended unless the degree of mitral insufficiency is slight and transitory, and the patient is otherwise in a stable condition. Often an intraaortic balloon pump and afterload reducing agents are used to optimize the patient's condition while preparing for surgery.

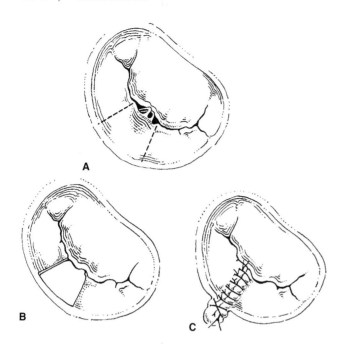

A

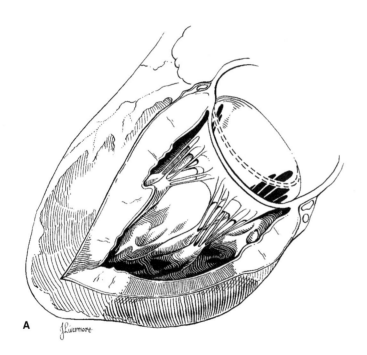

A

J. Livermore

B

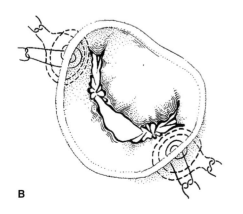

C

FIG. 11-11. A: Mitral insufficiency owing to rupture of chordae tendineae. The detached portion of the leaflet is excised **(B)**, and the defect is repaired with interrupted sutures **(C)**.

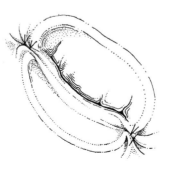

B

FIG. 11-12. A: Papillary muscle dysfunction and mitral annular dilatation owing to infarction of the inferior wall of the left ventricle. **B:** The mural annulus is reconstructed with a few figure-of-eight sutures at each commissure (modified after Kay).

Technique for Surgical Treatment of Ischemic Mitral Valve Disease

After cardioplegic arrest of the heart, the left atrium is incised longitudinally behind the interatrial groove, and the incision is extended behind the inferior vena cava for additional exposure. When the left atrium is small, the transverse transatrial incision from the right superior pulmonary vein across the right atrial wall and interatrial septum usually ensures excellent visualization of the mitral valve (see Chapter 7). At times, besides some minor annular dilation, the only significant lesion is the rupture of a few chordae tendineae that are attached to the mural leaflet of the mitral valve. On these occasions, conservative measures are preferred; the detached portion of mitral leaflet is excised and the defect is repaired (Fig. 11-11). The annulus is also appropriately reduced with a few figure-of-eight interrupted sutures (Fig. 11-12).

The role of annuloplasty is somewhat controversial. However, infarction of the left ventricular wall adjacent to the mural annulus, sometimes accompanied by papillary dysfunction, may stretch the mitral annulus and prevent the normal coaptation of the mitral leaflets. This leads to mitral insufficiency, which, in turn, may cause still more left ventricular dilation, thus compounding the already grave clinical picture (Fig. 11-12A). Therefore, some degree of mitral annular stretching may be present in all patients with left ventricular dilation and mitral insufficiency. When the mural annulus is considerably dilated and there are no lesions involving the mitral valve apparatus, a few interrupted sutures can incorporate parts of the mural annulus into both commissures without impinging on the anterior leaflet or anterior annulus of the mitral valve (Fig. 11-12B).

NB The use of an annuloplasty band or ring to reinforce the annular repair is an integral part of all mitral valve repair procedures (see Chapter 7).

Most commonly, conservative surgery will not be adequate because papillary muscles are friable and necrotic, chordae tendineae are slender and elongated, and there is marked left ventricular dilation with its consequent deformation of the mitral annulus. Occasionally, a ruptured papillary muscle can be reimplanted, but it may be hazardous if the reimplantation site is necrotic. Mitral valve replacement is indicated in the majority of patients and can be performed expeditiously with relative safety (see Chapter 7). Often, there are other associated lesions that require concomitant correction. Coronary artery bypass grafting to bypassable vessels is highly desirable to revascularize the viable myocardium as completely as possible. Resection of a ventricular aneurysm with endocardial resection may be indicated in selected patients.

INTRAAORTIC BALLOON PUMP

Occasionally, patients may require intraaortic balloon pump support after a cardiac surgical procedure. Depressed left ventricular function, ongoing myocardial ischemia, and ventricular arrhythmias are all indications for placement of the intraaortic balloon pump.

Technique for Placement of the Intraaortic Balloon Pump

If the patient has a palpable femoral pulse, the intraaortic balloon pump can be placed percutaneously using the Seldinger technique. After the common femoral artery is entered, the guidewire is passed through the needle, which is then removed. The dilator and finally the sheath are inserted over the wire. The deflated prewound balloon catheter is then introduced through the sheath and positioned in the descending thoracic aorta with the tip just distal to the takeoff of the left subclavian artery. Use of transesophageal echocardiography, if available, aids in proper positioning of the intraaortic balloon.

 BLEEDING IN HEPARINIZED PATIENTS
During or immediately after cardiopulmonary bypass, the patient is fully heparinized. Use of the percutaneous technique may lead to hematoma formation, retroperitoneal hemorrhage, or bleeding around the balloon sheath. This is especially likely to occur if it is difficult to palpate the femoral pulse, leading to inadvertent punctures of the femoral vein or back wall of the femoral artery.

 IMPROPER PLACEMENT OF THE BALLOON CATHETER
The balloon catheter should be placed via the common femoral artery. If it is inserted through the superficial femoral artery, lower extremity ischemia may result. The entry site of the balloon should be caudad to the inguinal ligament. Placement above this level may lead to bleeding, which is difficult to control by external pressure when the balloon catheter is removed.

NB *MANAGEMENT OF LOWER EXTREMITY ISCHEMIA*
If a patient develops evidence of leg ischemia after balloon pump placement, removing the sheath may allow improved distal blood flow. Alternatively, smaller diameter balloon catheters are available and should be used in patients with small femoral arteries.

In the operating room, when difficulties are encountered during weaning from cardiopulmonary bypass, placement of an intraaortic balloon may be helpful. In these patients, often no femoral pulse can be palpated.

Limited exposure of the common femoral artery is achieved through a small longitudinal incision with minimal dissection. A purse-string suture of 4-0 Prolene incorporating only adventitial tissue is placed on the anterior surface of the common femoral artery. The needle, wire, dilator, and balloon catheter are sequentially passed through this purse-string site. The suture is left long with the ends secured together by a Ligaclip and buried in the wound. The incision is closed in layers around the balloon catheter. Subsequently, the balloon may be removed under local anesthesia at the patient's bedside. The femoral arteriotomy is closed by simply tying the previously placed Prolene suture (Fig. 11-13).

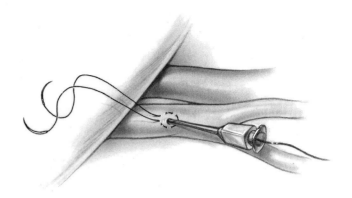

FIG. 11-13. Technique for placement of an intraaortic balloon catheter.

SECTION IV

Closed Procedures for Congenital Heart Defects

CHAPTER 12

Patent Ductus Arteriosus

INCISION

The ductus arteriosus can be adequately exposed through a small left anterior thoracotomy. A limited left posterolateral thoracotomy through the fourth intercostal space partially dividing the latissimus dorsi muscle and preserving the serratus anterior muscle provides good exposure and is more commonly used.

SURGICAL ANATOMY

The ductus arteriosus runs parallel to the aortic arch from the superior aspect of the origin of the left pulmonary artery and passes through the pericardium to join the medial margin of the aorta at an acute angle just opposite the origin of the left subclavian artery (Fig. 12-1). The left vagus trunk enters the thorax from the root of the neck in a groove between the left subclavian artery and the left common carotid artery, crosses the aortic arch and the ductus arteriosus, and continues downward. The recurrent laryngeal branch curves around the ductus arteriosus and extends back upward into the neck. The vagus nerve gives rise to many other small branches that are important tributaries to the pulmonary and cardiac plexuses. There are usually some lymph nodes buried in the hilum of the left lung that sometimes extend upward near the inferior margin of the ductus arteriosus. The left phrenic nerve enters the thorax medial to the vagus nerve and continues downward on the pericardium.

Technique for Exposing and Dissecting the Ductus Arteriosus

The left lung is pulled downward to bring into view the area of the ductus arteriosus. The parietal pleura is divided longitudinally behind the vagus nerve if the intention is to retract the vagus nerve medially. Alternatively, a pleural incision may be made between the vagus and phrenic nerves when the vagus nerve is to be retracted laterally (Fig. 12-1). The incision of choice is extended upward

along the left subclavian artery and downward into the left hilum. The pleural edges are then suspended.

In an infant, the ductus is exposed by sharp dissection with scissors both from above and below. A blunt right-angled clamp is then passed around the ductus to create a plane for its ligation or division. The ductus can also be occluded by the application of a metal clip.

 INJURY TO THE RECURRENT LARYNGEAL NERVE DURING DISSECTION OF THE DUCTUS ARTERIOSUS
If the ductus arteriosus is adherent posteriorly, the blunt technique for dissection may injure the ductus or the recurrent laryngeal nerve or both. Therefore, sharp dissection of the ductus, including its posterior wall, is recommended.

NB *RECURRENT LARYNGEAL NERVE LOCATION WITH MEDIAL RETRACTION*
To facilitate dissection and exposure of the posterior aspect of the ductus arteriosus, many surgeons prefer that the vagus nerve and its recurrent laryngeal branch be reflected medially on the pleural flap (Fig. 12-2). The surgeon should be aware that traction of the nerve toward the pulmonary artery causes the recurrent nerve to lie along a diagonal course behind the ductus arteriosus. Therefore, care must be taken to ensure that the recurrent nerve is not injured during dissection.

Alternatively, the vagus nerve and its branches can be isolated and retracted laterally to ensure its protection during the process of dissection of the posterior wall of the ductus. The aorta and the ductus are then mobilized by sharp dissection.

 COMPLETE EXPOSURE OF THE DUCTUS
Special care should be taken when dissecting near the angle between the pulmonary artery and the

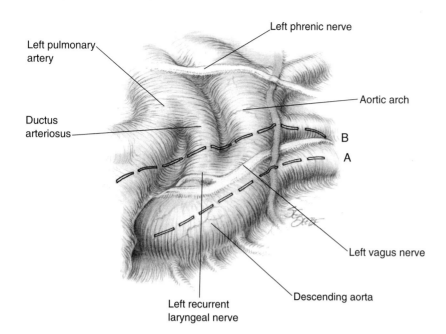

Left phrenic nerve

Left pulmonary artery

Ductus arteriosus

Aortic arch

B

A

Left vagus nerve

Descending aorta

Left recurrent laryngeal nerve

FIG. 12-1. Surgical anatomy of the ductus arteriosus. **A:** This incision line is used if the vagus nerve is to be retracted medially. **B:** This incision line is used if the vagus nerve is to be retracted laterally.

ductus arteriosus because the ductus is particularly susceptible to injury. A lappet of pericardium usually covers the ductus anteriorly. It should be dissected free to ensure complete exposure of the ductus (Fig. 12-3).

⊘ *DISSECTION OF THE AORTA*
The aorta is also dissected free, avoiding injury to the intercostal arteries. The posterior aspect of the ductus arteriosus is always adherent to the surrounding tissues and can be torn during the process of mobilization. Exposing the posterior aspect of the aorta and the ductus arteriosus can be facilitated

by retracting the aorta medially with two umbilical tapes or vessel loops passed around the aorta somewhat above and below the ductus (Fig. 12-4). This allows cautious dissection under direct vision.

Technique for Dividing and Ligating the Ductus Arteriosus

The vagus and recurrent laryngeal nerves are identified so that they are not divided inadvertently. Two heavy Ethibond sutures are individually passed behind the ductus, which is then securely ligated (Fig. 12-5). A finer suture material may cut through the friable ductus arte-

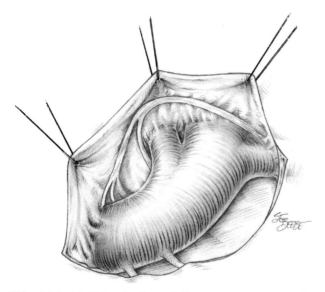

FIG. 12-2. Medial reflection of the vagus nerve on the pleural flap.

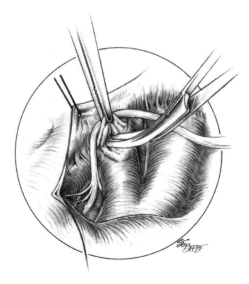

FIG. 12-3. Dissecting the lappet of pericardium to ensure complete exposure of the ductus.

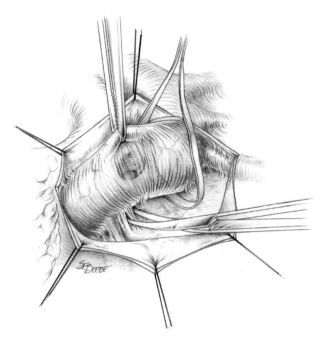

FIG. 12-4. Dissecting free the aorta.

riosus wall and result in hemorrhage. A purse-string suture of 4-0 Prolene may be placed between the ligatures to secure complete occlusion of the ductus (Fig. 12-5, inset). Alternatively, the ductus is divided between clamps and oversewn with fine, nonabsorbable sutures (Fig. 12-6). This technique is particularly useful when the ductus is exceptionally short and large. Another option is to occlude the ductus with one or two metal clips. This latter technique is especially applicable to premature infants.

DIFFICULTIES IN DISSECTION
Occasionally there may be some difficulty in dissecting near the posterior wall of the ductus arteriosus, particularly in older patients. Passage of suture material directly around the ductus may be somewhat hazardous. The vessel loops or umbilical tapes passed around the aorta can be manipulated to encircle and provide exposure and control of the ductus (Fig. 12-7).

INJURY TO THE RECURRENT LARYNGEAL NERVE DURING LIGATION OF THE DUCTUS ARTERIOSUS
The surgeon must always pay special attention to the recurrent laryngeal nerve. It can easily be divided during ductus mobilization. It can also be caught in the ligature, metal clip, or ductal clamp (Fig. 12-8).

A DUCTUS ARTERIOSUS TEAR
The ductus arteriosus is liable to be injured and torn any time during dissection, ligation, or division, resulting in massive hemorrhage. Mere digital pressure over the ductus usually controls the bleeding and provides adequate exposure in a dry field. The aorta can then be temporarily clamped above and below the ductus along the previously placed umbilical tapes while the torn ductus is oversewn with nonabsorbable sutures. The pulmonary artery end of the ductus can be similarly oversewn. Occasionally, this end of the ductus, if completely severed, may retract medially and its exposure may become impossible. Under these circumstances, while continuing digital control of bleeding, the surgeon must gain access to the pericardium by incising it longitudinally, anterior to the left phrenic nerve. Control of bleeding from the ductal end is

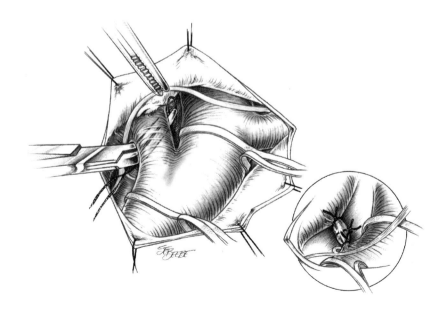

FIG. 12-5. Ligation of the ductus. **Inset:** Securing the occlusion with purse-string sutures.

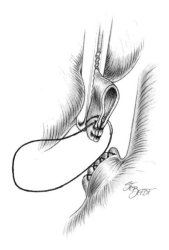

FIG. 12-6. Dividing the ductus arteriosus between clamps and oversewing it with fine, nonabsorbable sutures.

then achieved by temporarily occluding the left pulmonary artery from within the pericardium. The ductal opening is then oversewn under direct vision in a relatively dry field (Fig. 12-9).

 BACK CLAMPING OF THE AORTA AND PULMONARY ARTERY
Whenever the surgeon elects to divide the ductus arteriosus, it is essential that the clamps include the aorta and pulmonary artery walls proper and not

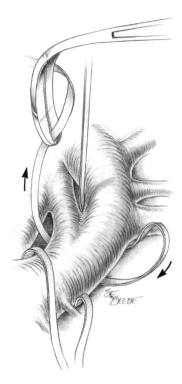

FIG. 12-7. Manipulating umbilical tape around the aorta to encircle the ductus arteriosus.

the ductal tissue alone, which is very friable and liable to be disrupted. By the same token, the ductus must never be directly gripped and pulled.

 INADVERTENT LIGATION OF THE AORTIC ARCH
The ductus arteriosus and aortic arch must both be identified. Occasionally, the ductus is very much larger than the arch, which may be underdeveloped and hypoplastic. This can be seen in infants and neonates. Inadvertent ligation of the arch instead of the ductus is a catastrophe that can be prevented by sequentially occluding the ductus and arch while looking for the disappearance of blood pressure as monitored in the left arm (Fig. 12-10).

 OCCLUDING THE DUCTUS ARTERIOSUS
It is a good practice always to occlude the ductus arteriosus with an atraumatic tissue forceps before its ligation or division. The occurrence of hypotension, bradycardia, and the like can then be noted, all of which suggest that the patient does not tolerate the ductal occlusion, possibly because of reversal of flow or some other complex congenital anomaly.

Closure of the Ductus Arteriosus in Premature Infants

The ductus arteriosus is visualized through a short, left lateral thoracotomy in the fourth intercostal interspace. The parietal pleura over the descending thoracic aorta is incised. Minimal scissor dissection is needed above and below the ductus. Occlusion of the ductus with a metal clip is the preferred method in premature infants. A small or medium metal clip is selected depending on the size of the ductus. The clip applier is positioned over the ductus arteriosus, directing the tips of the clip slightly inferiorly and away from the wall of the descending aorta. The ductus is then occluded with the metal clip. There is no need to pass an instrument around the ductus.

 EROSION OR CUTTING BY THE CLIP
If the ends of the clip are adjacent to the descending aorta or underside of the distal aortic arch, the clip may cut into these structures, resulting in immediate or delayed bleeding.

Completing the Operation

Rib blocks have been most effective in reducing postthoracotomy pain. A long-acting local anesthetic agent is injected near the neurovascular bundle at least two interspaces above and two below the level of the incision. The chest tube is brought through the skin and muscle opening and introduced through the fifth or sixth intercostal space. Heavy braided sutures are passed around the ribs above and below to reapproximate the opening. The mus-

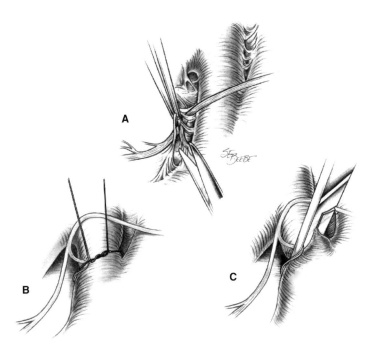

FIG. 12-8. Injury to the recurrent laryngeal nerve during ductal mobilization **(A)**, ligation **(B)**, and clamping **(C)**.

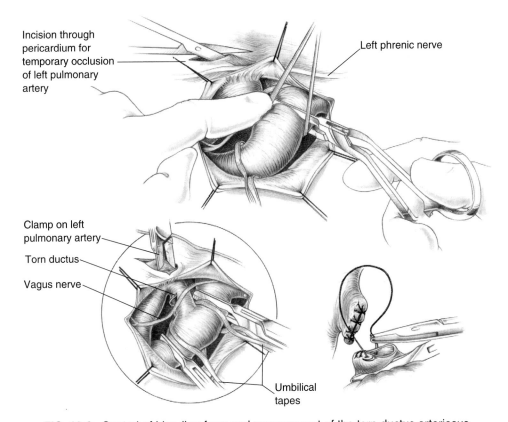

Incision through pericardium for temporary occlusion of left pulmonary artery

Left phrenic nerve

Clamp on left pulmonary artery

Torn ductus

Vagus nerve

Umbilical tapes

FIG. 12-9. Control of bleeding from and management of the torn ductus arteriosus.

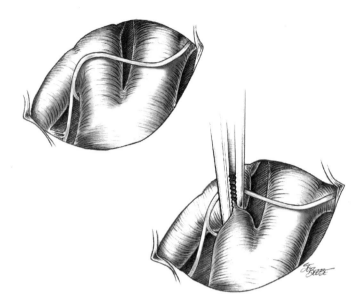

FIG. 12-10. Temporary occlusion of the ductus arteriosus to prevent the inadvertent ligation of the aortic arch.

cle layers, subcutaneous tissues, and skin are closed around the chest tube, which is connected to an underwater seal suction system. When the skin closure reaches the chest tube, several vigorous sustained ventilations are administered by the anesthesiologist. The chest tube is then withdrawn with the lungs inflated. A chest x-ray obtained in the operating room confirms reexpansion of the left lung and absence of pneumothorax.

 PLACEMENT OF PERICOSTAL SUTURES
The suture should hug the top of the rib to avoid injury to the intercostal artery or vein.

 INJURY TO THE LUNG
If injury to the lung is noted, the chest tube should be left in place on suction for 12 to 24 hours.

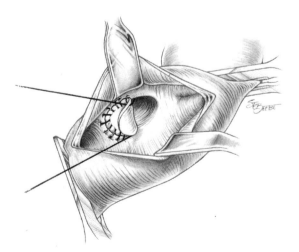

FIG. 12-11. Closure of the calcified ductus arteriosus through a left thoracotomy.

Thoracoscopic Closure of the Ductus Arteriosus

Some surgeons use thoracoscopic techniques for closure of the ductus arteriosus. The risk of recurrent laryngeal nerve injury is slightly higher with this approach; however, avoiding a thoracotomy incision may prevent future chest wall deformities.

Calcification of the Ductus Arteriosus

The ductus may be calcified and/or aneurysmal, and simple ligation or division may not be feasible. Under these circumstances, the aorta is clamped superiorly and inferiorly and the pulmonary artery is temporarily occluded from within the pericardium. The ductal opening is then closed through a longitudinal aortotomy with a Dacron, GORE-TEX, or pericardial patch (Fig. 12-11). However, it may be easier and safer to close the ductal opening through the left pulmonary artery under direct vision with the patient on cardiopulmonary bypass (see later).

 FRIABLE TISSUES
If the tissues are friable, the patch can be sewn into place with interrupted pledgeted sutures.

ANTERIOR APPROACH TO CLOSURE OF THE PATENT DUCTUS ARTERIOSUS

A median sternotomy incision is used for infants and children with a patent ductus arteriosus undergoing repair of other congenital heart defects. This approach is also useful in adults with both calcified and noncalcified and aneurysmal ducti.

Technique in Infants and Children

Before the initiation of cardiopulmonary bypass, the ascending aorta is retracted slightly to the right and the main pulmonary artery is retracted gently downward. The ductus is then dissected free of the left pulmonary artery and from the underside of the aortic arch. The ductus is encircled with a 2-0 braided suture and ligated or occluded with a metal clip at the onset of cardiopulmonary bypass (Fig. 12-12).

 FLOODING OF THE PULMONARY CIRCULATION
With the initiation of cardiopulmonary bypass, flooding of the pulmonary circulation and low systemic blood pressure are likely to occur unless the ductus is occluded. It is routine to look for a patent ductus arteriosus in every patient.

 TEARING OF DUCTAL TISSUE
The ductal tissue is friable, and care must be taken to prevent the suture or clip from cutting through the ductus. This results in bleeding that may be difficult to control, especially on the aortic side.

 STENOSIS OF THE LEFT PULMONARY ARTERY
The tie or clip should be placed sufficiently away from the origin of the left pulmonary artery to prevent narrowing of this vessel. This can result from external compression by the ligature or clip or from extrusion of ductal tissue into the lumen of the left pulmonary artery.

Technique in Adults

Closure of a patent ductus arteriosus in an adult can be safely accomplished through a median sternotomy on cardiopulmonary bypass. The patient is cooled systemically for 5 to 10 minutes to allow a brief period of very low perfusion. During low flow, the main pulmonary artery is opened longitudinally. The opening of the ductus is identified, and an appropriately sized Foley catheter is passed into the aorta (Fig. 12-13). After inflating the balloon with saline, the flow through the ductus is controlled by placing traction on the Foley catheter (the connector end of the catheter must be occluded to prevent the backflow of blood). Cardiopulmonary bypass flow can be increased while a patch of autologous pericardium treated with glutaraldehyde is sewn away from the edges of the ductal orifice using 5-0 monofilament suture (Fig. 12-14). Just before placing the last one or two stitches, the pump flow is turned very low while the Foley balloon is deflated, the catheter is removed, and the final stitches placed. Full flow is resumed, and the pulmonary arteriotomy is closed. The patient is weaned off cardiopulmonary bypass when systemic rewarming is completed.

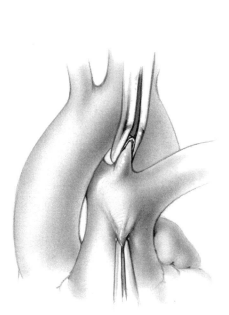

FIG. 12-12. Exposure and occlusion of the ductus arteriosus from the anterior approach.

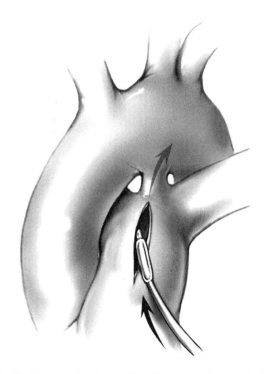

FIG. 12-13. Opening the main pulmonary artery and placing a Foley catheter in the ductus arteriosus.

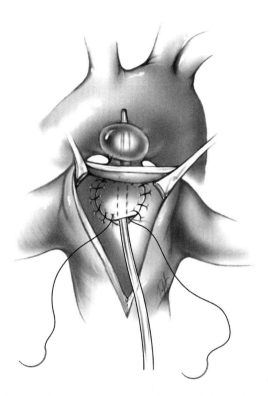

FIG. 12-14. Completing a patch closure of the pulmonary side of the ductus arteriosus with an inflated Foley balloon.

 FLOODING OF THE PULMONARY CIRCULATION
During cooling, the ductal flow must be occluded to prevent runoff of the aortic cannula flow into the pulmonary arterial bed. This is accomplished with forceful digital pressure on the distal main pulmonary artery.

 AIR EMBOLISM THROUGH THE DUCTUS ARTERIOSUS
When the pulmonary artery is opened, some flow must be maintained through the aortic cannula to prevent air embolism. In addition, the patient may be placed in Trendelenburg position to prevent this complication.

CHAPTER 13

Coarctation of the Aorta

More than 50% of infants with a coarctation of the aorta become symptomatic during the first month of life. Associated cardiac anomalies accompany this lesion in more than 75% of patients. In neonates, infusion of prostaglandin E_1 most often maintains or reopens the ductus. This improves lower body perfusion by allowing right-to-left shunting into the descending aorta and by partially relieving the obstruction of the coarctation by relaxing the aortic end of the ductus. Surgery can then be safely delayed until the left ventricular function, which is often poor, improves and any signs of low cardiac output syndrome, such as renal insufficiency, resolve. Older children may present with upper body hypertension and/or signs and symptoms of decreased lower extremity perfusion.

INCISION

In patients with an isolated aortic coarctation, the involved area can be adequately exposed through a fourth intercostal left posterolateral thoracotomy. Infants with associated lesions may be better served with a complete repair on cardiopulmonary bypass through a median sternotomy using a period of hypothermic arrest to resect or augment the coarcted segment (see Chapter 27). Even in infants with no other cardiac anomalies, the aortic arch may be hypoplastic. These patients should undergo patch augmentation of the entire arch and proximal descending aorta under hypothermic arrest (see Chapter 27).

Surgical Anatomy

A coarctation of the aorta in the thoracic cavity affects the junction of the aortic arch, descending aorta, and ductus arteriosus in more than 98% of patients. It can, however, occur anywhere along the course of the aorta.

The left vagus nerve enters the thoracic cavity from the root of the neck between the left subclavian and left common carotid arteries, crosses the aortic arch, and contin-

ues downward anteromedial to the descending aorta, traversing the ligamentum arteriosum. The recurrent laryngeal nerve has its origin in the vagus nerve, curves around the ligamentum arteriosum, and continues back upward into the neck (Fig. 13-1). There may be poststenotic dilation just distal to the coarctation. In older patients, the poststenotic dilation may be more pronounced and there may be extensive enlargement of collateral vessels about the shoulder and back muscles. This may include the intercostal arteries, whose walls may be paper thin and friable.

EXPOSURE TO THE COARCTATION

The left lung is retracted inferiorly and anteriorly. The parietal pleura is divided longitudinally over the left subclavian artery and descending thoracic aorta across the coarctation segment. The pleural edges are then suspended (Fig. 13-1). The left subclavian artery and the descending aorta are widely mobilized from the root of the neck to a distance well below the coarctation. Vessel loops may be passed around the aorta and the subclavian artery to facilitate exposure (Fig. 13-2).

 PROTECTION OF THE VAGUS AND RECURRENT LARYNGEAL NERVES
The left vagus nerve and its recurrent laryngeal branch may be injured during mobilization.

 ENLARGED INTERCOSTAL ARTERIES
The intercostal arteries are usually enlarged. They have extremely thin walls and can cause troublesome bleeding if traumatized.

 BLEEDING FROM AORTIC BRANCHES
Bronchial arteries may occasionally arise from the posterior surface of the aorta and the left subclavian artery. They can be inadvertently torn during mobilization and dissection, resulting in bleeding.

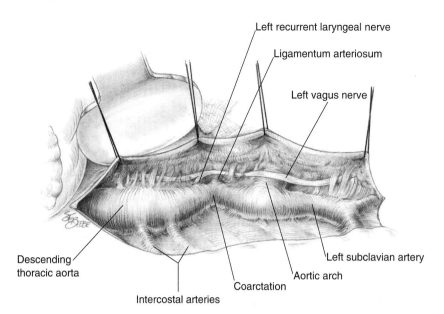

Left recurrent laryngeal nerve

Ligamentum arteriosum

Left vagus nerve

Descending thoracic aorta

Intercostal arteries

Coarctation

Aortic arch

Left subclavian artery

FIG. 13-1. Surgical anatomy of a coarctation of the aorta.

COARCTECTOMY

Whenever possible, a coarctectomy is the procedure of choice. It entails removal of stenosed or hypoplastic segments of the aorta and of abnormal ductal tissue in neonates. The ductus arteriosus (if present) or the ligamentum arteriosum is divided to give the aorta additional mobility. The coarcted segment is excised between clamps, and the aorta is sewn together with sutures of fine Prolene (5-0 in older children and 7-0 in neonates) to reestablish continuity (Fig. 13-3). A combination of straight and spoon-shaped atraumatic clamps with an approximator is most useful. This allows the clamps to remain immobile while the aortic ends are being sutured together without tension. The operative field is not obscured by the assistant's hands; this is an important point, particularly in neonates. Alternatively, the assistant surgeon has the critical responsibility of holding the two ends of the aorta together so that a satisfactory anastomosis can be completed.

 RESIDUAL COARCTATION
Inadequate resection of a coarctation may leave the patient with residual disease (Fig. 13-4).

 PRESERVING THE MAXIMAL DIAMETER OF THE LUMEN
The aortic anastomosis should incorporate the widest lumen of the aorta to prevent any local constriction. A clamp occluding the left subclavian artery and the aortic arch is placed obliquely across the upper segment of the aorta. This segment can be enlarged, if necessary, to conform with the poststenotic dilation of the lower aortic segment (Fig. 13-5).

 INTERRUPTED SUTURES IN NEONATES
Although continuous suturing provides better hemostasis and functions quite satisfactorily in most cases, interrupted suturing in the neonate is used by some surgeons to reduce the possibility of recurrent stenosis. Alternatively, the posterior layer is completed with a continuous technique, but the anterior layer is approximated with interrupted sutures. Although some surgeons have advocated using absorbable suture, such as polydioxanone (PDS), which theoretically should ensure better growth at the site of the anastomosis, no real difference between Prolene with PDS has been noted.

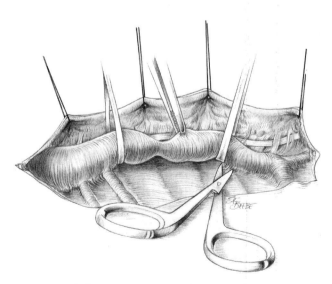

FIG. 13-2. Exposure of a coarctation.

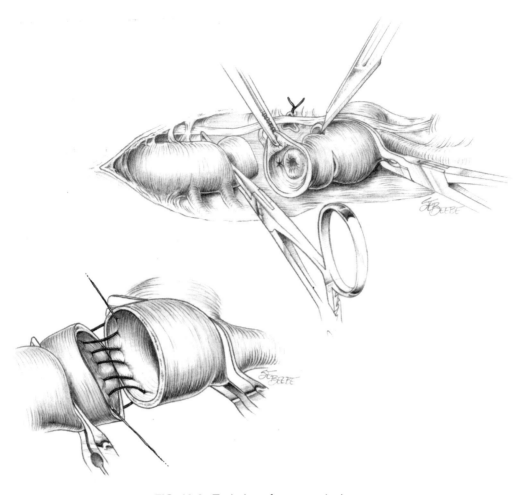

FIG. 13-3. Technique for a coarctectomy.

Ⓧ *SPINAL CORD ISCHEMIA*
There is always the possibility of ischemic spinal cord injury. Therefore, the operation must be performed expeditiously with a clamp time of less than 30 minutes.

In addition, the core body temperature should be allowed to drift down to 35°C by keeping the room cold

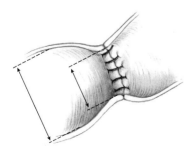

FIG. 13-4. Inadequate resection in a coarctectomy.

or using a cooling blanket to minimize the risk of spinal cord ischemia.

NB *DISTAL CIRCULATORY SUPPORT*
Femoral-femoral bypass or left atrial bypass, using a Gott shunt, can be used to provide distal perfusion in adults during the cross-clamp period (see Technique for Replacement of the Descending Thoracic Aorta section, Chapter 9).

NB *TUBE GRAFT INTERPOSITION IN OLDER CHILDREN AND ADULTS*
At times, the removed coarctation segment may be too long, and safe aortic reapproximation becomes hazardous. A tube graft may then be interposed to achieve aortic continuity in adults (Fig. 13-6).

Ⓧ *HEMOSTASIS*
There may be bleeding along the suture line, necessitating placement of additional sutures. The proximal clamp and occasionally the distal clamp are

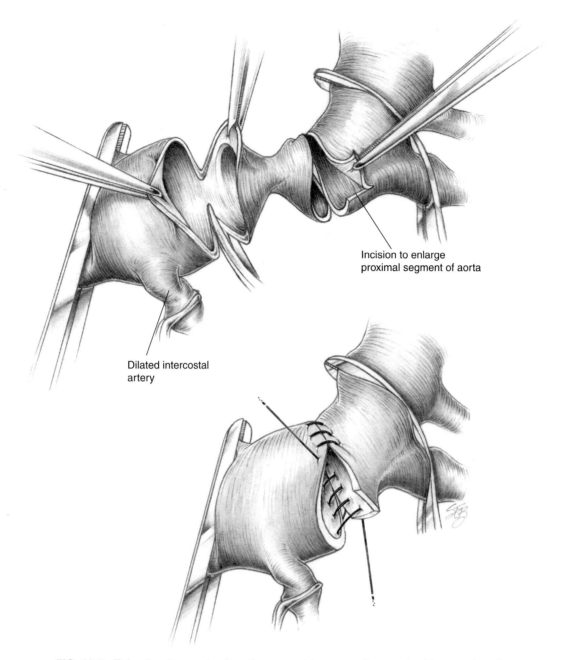

Incision to enlarge
proximal segment of aorta

Dilated intercostal
artery

FIG. 13-5. Enlarging the proximal aortic segment to ensure the maximal lumen diameter.

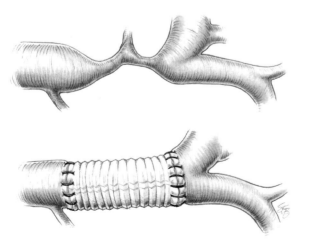

FIG. 13-6. Tube graft replacement when the coarctation segment removed is too long to allow safe aortic reapproximation.

then reapplied temporarily so that additional sutures can be placed without tension on the anastomosis.

 CLAMP PLACEMENT
The clamps should not be too far away from the cut edges of the aorta; the elastic aortic wall always retracts, thus increasing the distance between the ends of the aorta and the tension on the suture. Nevertheless, an aortic tissue cuff placed 1 to 1.5 cm distal to the clamps in older children and 0.5 cm in neonates is usually needed to secure a satisfactory anastomosis.

SUBCLAVIAN FLAP ANGIOPLASTY

The procedure is particularly suited for the neonate. The left subclavian artery is well mobilized up to the ori-

gin of its branches in the root of the neck; all the branches are ligated (Fig. 13-7). The proximal clamp is placed across the aortic arch just distal to the left carotid artery, and the descending aorta is clamped with a straight clamp (Fig. 13-8A). Alternatively, a single curved clamp can be used (Fig. 13-8C). The left subclavian artery is incised longitudinally downward along the aorta, well beyond the coarctation segment. Whenever a prominent coarctation ridge is present, it should be excised (Fig. 13-7C). The subclavian artery is then divided at the level of its branches, folded down, and sewn into the aortic incision as a patch using two continuous 7-0 PDS or Prolene sutures (Fig. 13-8B).

 SUBCLAVIAN STEAL SYNDROME
The vertebral artery must be identified and ligated separately to eliminate the possibility of the development of subclavian steal syndrome.

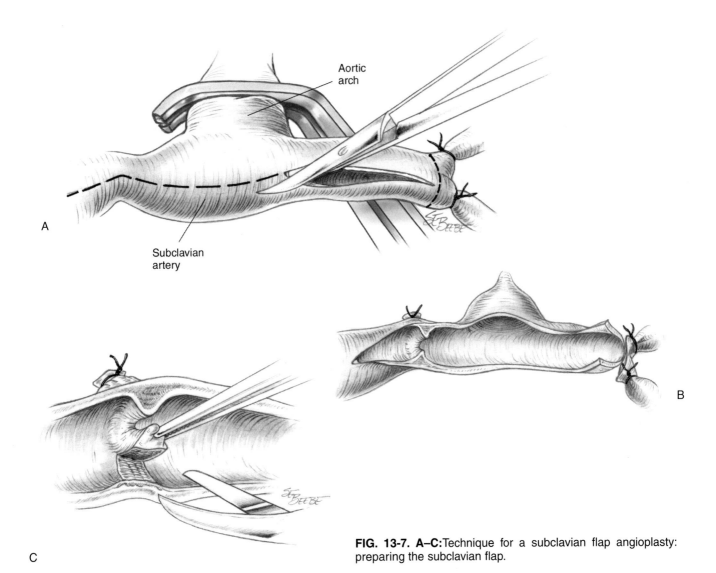

FIG. 13-7. A–C: Technique for a subclavian flap angioplasty: preparing the subclavian flap.

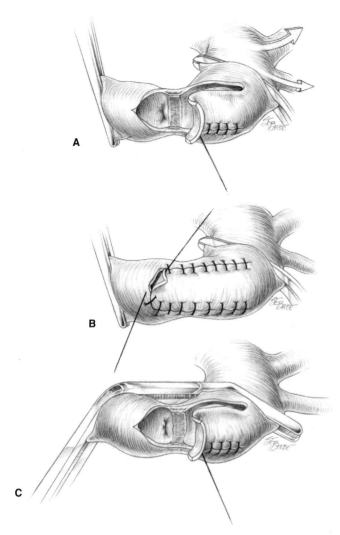

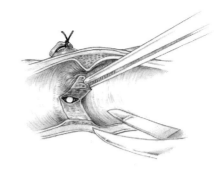

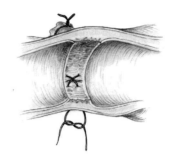

FIG. 13-9. Repairing a perforation in the posterior aortic wall.

FIG. 13-8. A and B: Technique for a subclavian flap angioplasty using two clamps. Note that the upper clamp is placed just distal to the left common carotid artery. **C:** Single-clamp technique.

⊘ *RESECTION OF THE COARCTATION RIDGE*
The coarctation ridge within the lumen of the aorta must be excised, but not so deeply as to weaken the posterior aortic wall. Any perforation must be sutured with fine Prolene and tied on the outside (Fig. 13-9).

⊘ *SHORT SUBCLAVIAN ARTERY*
Too short a subclavian artery will not reach beyond the coarcted segment and will leave residual stenosis (Fig. 13-10). A diamond-shaped prosthetic patch angioplasty (see later) must then be performed.

⊘ *DISTAL STENOSIS*
The toe of the anastomosis should be at least 8 to 10 mm distal to the site of coarctation. Otherwise, healing with its resulting fibrosis gives rise to recoarctation.

⊘ *POSITIONING THE SUBCLAVIAN ARTERY PATCH*
Ideally, the subclavian artery patch must balloon out evenly over the coarctation. A kink at the heel of the anastomosis suggests that excessive tension has been applied to the subclavian flap in an effort to bring it down far enough beyond the coarcted segment (Fig. 13-11).

⊘ *INCISION IN THE SUBCLAVIAN ARTERY AND THE AORTA*
The line of incision in the subclavian artery and the aorta should be straight. Any deviation interferes with a satisfactory anastomosis.

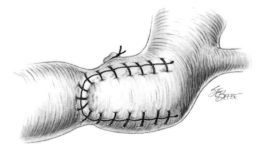

FIG. 13-10. Persistence of residual stenosis when the subclavian artery is too short to reach beyond the coarcted segment.

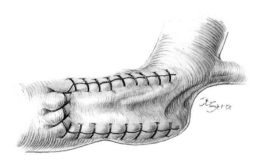

FIG. 13-11. A kink at the heel of the anastomosis, suggesting that excessive tension has been applied to the subclavian flap.

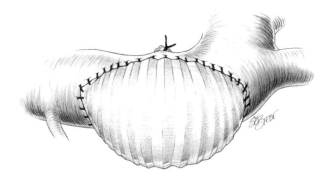

FIG. 13-13. Using an especially wide patch prevents recoarctation as the aorta grows.

DIAMOND-SHAPED PROSTHETIC PATCH ANGIOPLASTY

If the coarctation segment is too long, a coarctectomy with an end-to-end anastomosis or subclavian flap angioplasty may not be feasible. An alternative to graft interposition is to roof the defect with a prosthetic patch. This procedure is equally useful in cases of redo coarctation of the aorta.

The aorta is clamped above and below the coarctation segment as described previously. The aorta is then incised longitudinally across the lesion. The prominent coarctation ridge is then excised, taking the usual precautions. A

wide, diamond-shaped GORE-TEX or Hemashield prosthetic patch of appropriate size is sewn with fine continuous Prolene sutures to the aortic edges (Fig. 13-12).

 RECOARCTATION
Recoarctation can occur as the aorta grows. For this reason, the diamond-shaped prosthetic patch must be very wide, resulting in a redundant, patulous bulge over the coarctation (Fig. 13-13). An aesthetically satisfactory patch often results in recoarctation.

REVERSED SUBCLAVIAN ANGIOPLASTY

Hypoplasia of the aortic arch between the left carotid and left subclavian arteries can be treated by a reversed subclavian flap angioplasty. In patients with combined discrete coarctation and significant hypoplasia of the arch, this technique can be combined with a standard coarctectomy. The distal arch must be mobilized, as well as the take off of the left carotid artery and the portion of the arch just proximal to its origin. The left subclavian artery is ligated as in the standard subclavian flap angioplasty. One vascular clamp is placed across the left carotid artery and the aortic arch. The other clamp is placed on the descending aorta. The transected subclavian artery is opened medially onto the aortic arch, across the roof of the distal arch, and onto the base of the left carotid artery (Fig. 13-14A). The flap is then sutured in place with 7-0 PDS or Prolene sutures (Fig. 13-14B).

EXTENDED RESECTION AND ANASTOMOSIS

If the aortic arch is significantly hypoplastic, repair of the coarctation alone may result in an unacceptable gradient. In these cases, extended resection with an anastomosis of the distal aorta to the undersurface of the aortic arch can be carried out.

Extensive dissection and mobilization of aorta from the origin of the innominate artery along the descending thoracic aorta to the level of the third or even fourth intercostal artery are carried out. Ligation and division of the

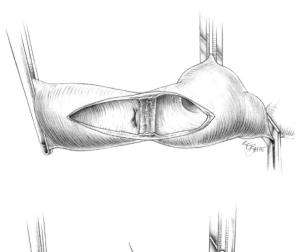

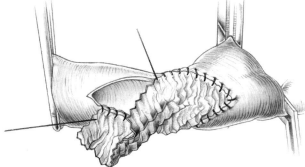

FIG. 13-12. Technique for a diamond-shaped prosthetic patch angioplasty.

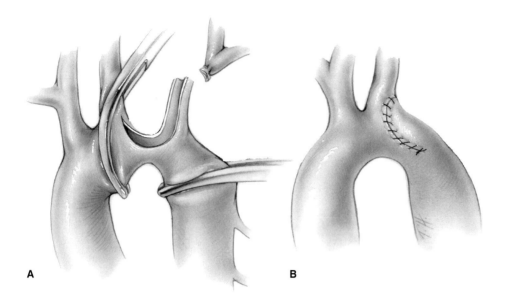

FIG. 13-14. A: The transected subclavian artery is opened medially across the roof of the aortic arch. **B:** The subclavian flap is sutured in place, augmenting the hypoplastic segment.

ductus arteriosus facilitate the dissection. A curved vascular clamp is placed across the origin of the subclavian and left carotid arteries as well as the proximal aortic arch just beyond the innominate artery. A straight clamp is also placed across the descending aorta. The coarcted segment and ductal tissue are resected. An incision is now made along the undersurface of the aortic arch while a second matching incision is made on the lateral aspect of the distal aorta (Fig. 13-15). The descending aorta is then anastomosed to the undersurface of the arch with fine continuous Prolene or PDS suture.

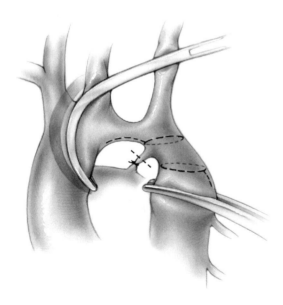

FIG. 13-15. Extended resection and anastomosis of the coarctation and hypoplastic arch. Note the improper placement of the clamp *(shaded)* on the innominate artery.

 OCCLUDING INNOMINATE ARTERY
In placing the curved clamp across the aortic arch, care must be taken to allow adequate flow into the innominate artery (Fig. 13-15).

 TENSION AT THE ANASTOMOSIS
Aggressive proximal and distal mobilization will avoid tension on the anastomosis; this will minimize the risk of suture line bleeding and the development of stenosis.

COMPLEX COARCTATIONS

Many recoarctations, which in the past may have required a bypass procedure or resection and interposition graft, can now be successfully treated with a balloon angioplasty with or without stenting. (Some institutions are balloon dilating native coarctations with good results.) Thus, the previously used left subclavian artery to descending aortic bypass graft and ascending-descending aortic bypasses are rarely, if ever, indicated.

Occasionally, when patients with previous tube grafts placed from the ascending to descending aorta to treat interrupted aortic arch or arch hypoplasia develop stenoses or outgrow the graft, an anterior bypass procedure may be the preferred approach.

Anterior Ascending-Descending Aortic Bypass Graft

A median sternotomy incision is made. The patient is placed on cardiopulmonary bypass. With the heart decompressed, the descending aorta is identified at the level of the diaphragm. The pericardium is incised, and the descending aorta is dissected free of surrounding tissues to allow placement of a large C-shaped or Satinsky clamp. The appropriately sized Hemashield tube graft is then anastomosed end to side with a side-biting clamp on the descending aorta. The graft is allowed to fill with blood and measured to the correct length to lie along side the right atrium and reach the right lateral aspect of the ascending aorta (Fig. 13-16). After trimming the graft obliquely, the proximal anastomosis is performed with a side-biting clamp on the ascending aorta. The graft is deaired before removing the clamp from the ascending aorta.

 ### KINKING OF THE GRAFT
Kinking of the graft will leave the patient with a persistent pressure gradient. The graft should course rightward between the diaphragm and heart, hugging the right atrium, and lie anterior to the superior vena cava to join the ascending aorta obliquely.

 ### DIFFICULTY WITH DISTAL ANASTOMOSIS
If exposure of the descending aorta is problematic, the heart can be arrested with cardioplegia and retracted upward toward the patient's head.

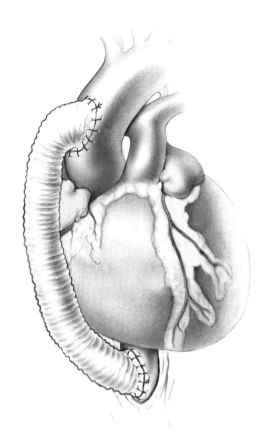

FIG. 13-16. Completed ascending-descending aortic bypass graft through a median sternotomy.

CHAPTER 14

Pulmonary Artery Banding

Because an increasing number of infants is undergoing total correction for congenital heart disease at an earlier age, banding of the pulmonary artery is only indicated for a specific subgroup of patients. This includes patients with multiple muscular ventriculoseptal defects or ventriculoseptal defects complicated by other noncardiac congenital anomalies as well as patients who present after 4 to 6 weeks of age with simple transposition of the great arteries (see Chapter 23) for whom a two-staged approach is used and some patients with univentricular hearts with excess pulmonary blood flow (see Chapter 29).

INCISION

Most surgeons use a median sternotomy because it allows the anatomy to be evaluated more accurately. A left thoracotomy incision is used in some patients, especially if the banding is performed in conjunction with the repair of a coarctation or ligation of a patent ductus arteriosus.

TECHNIQUE

Through a median sternotomy, the pericardium is opened longitudinally after resecting the thymus. (Removing the entire thymus in this operation makes dissection at reoperation easier.) A patent ductus arteriosus, if present, is first ligated (see Chapter 12). The main pulmonary artery is freed up from the aorta and the right pulmonary artery take off identified. A band of Silastic 3 to 4 mm wide is placed around the proximal pulmonary artery and tightened until the pressure distal to the band is approximately one-third systemic with an arterial oxygen saturation no less than 75% on 50% inspired oxygen (Fig. 14-1). The constriction site on the band is made permanent with stainless steel clips or interrupted sutures. The band is then secured to the adventitia of the pulmonary artery at various intervals with interrupted 6-0 or 5-0 Prolene sutures (Fig. 14-1, inset).

Through a left thoracotomy, a patent ductus arteriosus and/or coarctation of the aorta, if present, are first

corrected (see Chapters 12 and 13). The pericardium is then incised anterior and parallel to the phrenic nerve. The main pulmonary artery is isolated, and the Silastic band passed around it and narrowed as described previously.

⊘ **DAMAGE FROM THE BAND**
The pulmonary artery may be tense and its walls thin and friable. Regular suture material or a narrow band may cut through and produce hemorrhage that is difficult to control.

⊘ **DIFFICULTY PASSING THE BAND AROUND THE PULMONARY ARTERY**
It may be easier and safer to initially pass the tape around both the aorta and pulmonary artery through the transverse sinus and then between the aorta and pulmonary artery.

⊘ **TROUBLESOME BLEEDING**
Small vessels near the aorta and pulmonary artery may give rise to troublesome bleeding; they must be identified and cauterized.

⊘ **EXCESSIVE BANDING**
The degree of banding must not be too constrictive because this will result in unacceptable cyanosis and possible hemodynamic collapse.

⊘ **INADEQUATE BANDING**
Many times, the tightness of the band is limited by the hemodynamic response of the patient. Patients with subaortic narrowing may not tolerate adequate constriction of the band. If the band is loose, excess pulmonary blood flow will persist.

In this case, a complete correction or Damus-Kaye-Stansel anastomosis and shunt (see Chapter 28) may be indicated.

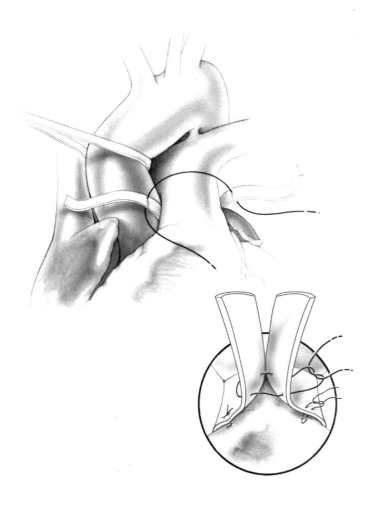

FIG. 14-1. Technique for placement of a pulmonary artery band. The band is tightened with interrupted sutures. Securing the band to the adventitia of the pulmonary artery **(inset)**.

⊘ *PLACING THE BAND TOO PROXIMALLY*

If the band is placed too low, the sinotubular ridge of the pulmonic valve will be distorted. To adequately relieve the gradient during the debanding procedure, the sinus portion(s) of the pulmonary root needs to be patched. This often results in an incompetent pulmonary valve. This is especially problematic when an arterial switch or Damus-Kay Stansel procedure is planned at the second stage.

⊘ *BAND MIGRATION*

The band should be *sewn to the adventitia of the proximal aspect* of the main pulmonary artery (see Fig. 14-1, inset). This precaution prevents the band from migrating upward, distorting and constricting the pulmonary artery at its bifurcation or branches.

After the optimal band constriction has been achieved, it is secured and the pericardium is approximated with multiple interrupted sutures. The median sternotomy or thoracotomy is then closed in the usual fashion.

PULMONARY ARTERY DEBANDING

When total correction of the congenital anomaly is initiated, the pulmonary artery band must be removed. It is usually necessary to reconstruct the pulmonary artery to eliminate any gradient across the constricted segment. With Silastic, if the band has been in place for a short time, simple removal of the band may result in no gradient.

Before the initiation of cardiopulmonary bypass, the band is dissected and removed (Fig. 14-2A). The pulmonary artery is then incised longitudinally across the constricted segment while on cardiopulmonary bypass. An appropriately sized patch of glutaraldehyde-treated autologous pericardium or GORE-TEX is then sewn onto the defect with continuous 5-0 Prolene sutures (Fig. 14-2B).

⊘ *PERSISTENCE OF THE GRADIENT*

Inadequate enlargement of the main pulmonary artery may be responsible for persistence of the gradient across the site of the band.

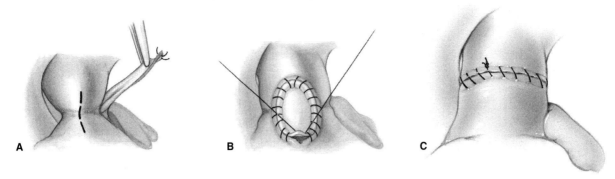

FIG. 14-2. Technique for pulmonary artery debanding. **A:** Removal of the band. **B:** Incision and patch enlargement of the pulmonary artery. **C:** Resection of the constricted segment and an end-to-end anastomosis of the pulmonary artery.

Alternatively, the portion of the main pulmonary artery involved in the banding can be resected and an end-to-end anastomosis performed between the proximal main pulmonary artery and the confluence of the right and left pulmonary arteries (Fig. 14-2C).

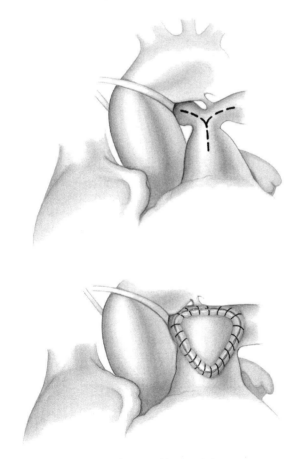

FIG. 14-3. Technique for patching pulmonary artery constriction at the bifurcation.

⊘ *CONSTRICTION OF AN ANASTOMOSIS*
All fibrotic tissue must be excised when the procedure is carried out. In addition, every fourth or fifth suture may be locked to prevent purse-stringing of the anastomosis.

⊘ *PULMONARY VALVE INSUFFICIENCY*
When the band has caused distortion of the sino-tubular ridge, patching anteriorly into one sinus only often causes valvular insufficiency. If the patient will not tolerate pulmonary valve incompetence, the pulmonary artery can be transected and all three sinuses patched as described for supravalvular aortic stenosis (see Chapter 22).

NB *INCORPORATION OF THE BAND INTO THE PULMONARY ARTERY*
With the passage of time, the band may burrow through the wall of the pulmonary artery to become subendothelial. The band can be divided anteriorly but left *in situ*, and the pulmonary artery enlarged with a patch angioplasty. Resection with an end-to-end anastomosis may also be used when this situation is encountered.

Occasionally, the band may migrate upward to the pulmonary artery bifurcation and cause distortion of its branches. The incision on the pulmonary artery is then extended distally onto the left or both the left and right pulmonary artery branches as needed. The defect is then closed with a pericardial patch (Fig. 14-3).

NB *SIZING THE PATCH*
The pericardial patch should be wide enough, particularly at its distal end, to prevent constriction.

CHAPTER 15

Vascular Ring and Pulmonary Artery Sling

Persistence of both the right and left embryonic dorsal aortic arches results in the development of a double aortic arch. The ascending aorta gives rise to right and left arches that encircle the trachea and esophagus and rejoin to form the descending thoracic aorta. This acts as a ring and compresses the trachea and esophagus, causing obstructive symptoms (Fig. 15-1). Each arch gives rise to a subclavian artery and a carotid artery. There is no innominate artery in this condition.

DOUBLE AORTIC ARCH

Incision

A left posterolateral thoracotomy in the fourth intercostal space is the approach most commonly preferred. A right thoracotomy is indicated if the left aortic arch is dominant, which occurs rarely.

Technique

The left lung is retracted anteriorly and downward toward the diaphragm to bring into view the area of the aortic arch and ductus arteriosus. The parietal pleura is incised longitudinally on the anterior surface of the descending aorta and left subclavian artery. The pleural flap containing the vagus nerve and its branches is retracted anteriorly; meticulous dissection is carried out to identify the local anatomy precisely. The surgeon should be aware that pulling the nerve toward the pulmonary artery causes the recurrent nerve to lie along a diagonal course behind the ductus arteriosus, thus increasing the risk of injury to the nerve. Alternatively, the vagus nerve and its branches can be isolated and retracted posterolaterally to ensure their protection during the process of dissection of the posterior wall of the ductus arteriosus.

The aorta and ductus arteriosus are then mobilized by sharp dissection. The ductus arteriosus is divided and oversewn (see Chapter 12).

🚫 ***INJURY TO THE DUCTUS ARTERIOSUS***
Special care should be taken when dissecting near the angle between the pulmonary artery and ductus arteriosus because this area is particularly susceptible to injury.

The smaller (usually left anterior) aortic arch is dissected free and divided between clamps. The ends are then oversewn with 5-0 Prolene suture in two layers (Figs. 15-2 and 15-3).

NB ***ADHESIONS OF THE ESOPHAGUS AND TRACHEA***
Both the trachea and the esophagus must be dissected free of any adhesions and fibrous bands to ensure that narrowing of these structures is relieved. This entails freeing up the divided ends of the arch from the surrounding tissues.

🚫 ***DIVISION OF A PATENT DUCTUS ARTERIOSUS***
The ductus arteriosus, whether patent or not, must always be doubly ligated and divided. Otherwise, continued compression of the trachea and esophagus may be caused by the aortic arch being pulled downward toward the pulmonary artery.

🚫 ***INJURY TO THE RECURRENT LARYNGEAL NERVE***
The vagus and recurrent laryngeal nerves are identified so that they are not inadvertently divided or traumatized.

🚫 ***DIVISION OF THE SMALLER ARCH***
The smaller of the two arches must always be divided; otherwise, a pseudocoarctation will sometimes develop. Therefore, both arches are dissected and the smaller one is identified and divided as described previously. As a precaution, blood pressure cuffs should be placed on one leg and both arms and a trial occlusion of the arch should be carried out to confirm the absence of a pressure gradient before dividing it.

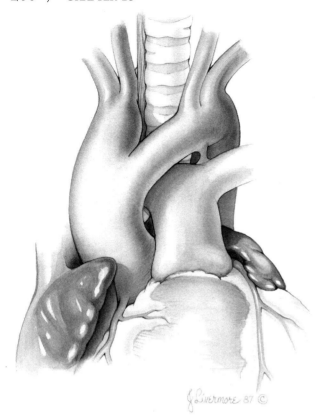

FIG. 15-1. Double aortic arch.

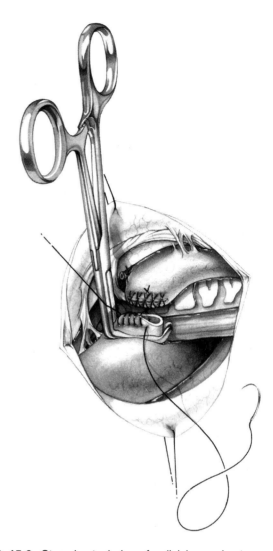

FIG. 15-3. Stepwise technique for division and suture occlusion of the left anterior arch.

PULMONARY ARTERY SLING

A pulmonary artery sling results when the left pulmonary artery arises from the right pulmonary artery and passes leftward between the trachea and esophagus to reach the hilum of the left lung. The ligamentum arteriosum extends from the superior aspect of the main pulmonary artery to the undersurface of the aortic arch. This creates a vascular ring that constricts the trachea but not the esophagus (Fig. 15-4). Hypoplasia of the distal trachea, with or without complete cartilaginous rings, is present in approximately 50% of these patients.

Incision

A left posterolateral thoracotomy in the fourth intercostal space is the traditional approach. If tracheal reconstruction is thought to be required, then a median sternotomy is performed and cardiopulmonary bypass is used.

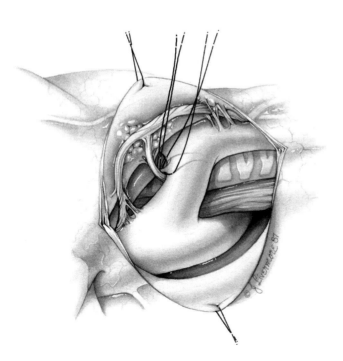

FIG. 15-2. Exposure of the left anterior arch.

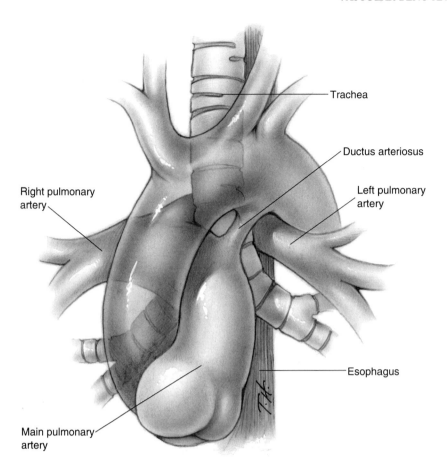

Trachea

Ductus arteriosus

Right pulmonary artery

Left pulmonary artery

Esophagus

Main pulmonary artery

FIG. 15-4. Pulmonary artery sling. Note the origin of the left pulmonary artery from the right pulmonary artery and its course behind the trachea.

Thoracotomy Technique

Through a left thoracotomy approach, the lung is retracted anteriorly and inferiorly to expose the descending thoracic aorta. The parietal pleura is opened longitudinally along the anterior surface of the descending aorta. The ligamentum arteriosum or patent ductus arteriosus is carefully dissected, using care not to injure the vagus or recurrent laryngeal nerves. This structure is doubly ligated with suture ligatures of 5-0 Prolene and divided. The left pulmonary artery is dissected as far medially as possible between the trachea and esophagus using sharp dissection. A straight vascular clamp is applied to the left pulmonary artery as close to its take off from the right pulmonary artery as feasible. A second straight vascular clamp is placed more distally on the left pulmonary artery, which is then divided close to the first clamp. The proximal portion of the left pulmonary artery is oversewn with a double layer of 6-0 Prolene suture. This clamp is then removed. A longitudinal incision in the pericardium anterior to the phrenic nerve is made. Traction sutures are placed on the pericardial edges to expose the main pulmonary artery. A second opening in the pericardium posterior to the phrenic nerve is then made, and the transected end of the left pulmonary artery is brought through this incision. The left pulmonary artery is trimmed in an oblique fashion to enlarge its opening. A C clamp is then placed on the supe-

rior aspect of the main pulmonary artery, and a generous incision is made to accommodate the opening of the left pulmonary artery. The two vessels are anastomosed together, using a running 6-0 or 7-0 Prolene suture. The two vascular clamps are then removed, and the suture line checked for hemostasis (Fig. 15-5).

 OBSTRUCTING THE TRACHEA
When applying the vascular clamp on the proximal take off of the left pulmonary artery, care must be taken to avoid compressing the trachea.

 OCCLUSION OF THE LEFT PULMONARY ARTERY
Occlusion of the left pulmonary artery after this procedure is not uncommon. Systemic heparinization with 1 mg per kilogram of body weight must be administered before clamping the left pulmonary artery. Adequate length on the left pulmonary artery must be obtained to prevent undue tension on the anastomosis to the main pulmonary artery, which could result in stenosis or occlusion of the left pulmonary artery.

 STENOSIS OF THE LEFT PULMONARY ARTERY
It is important to enlarge the opening of the left pulmonary artery with an oblique incision and to make a generous opening in the main pulmonary artery to

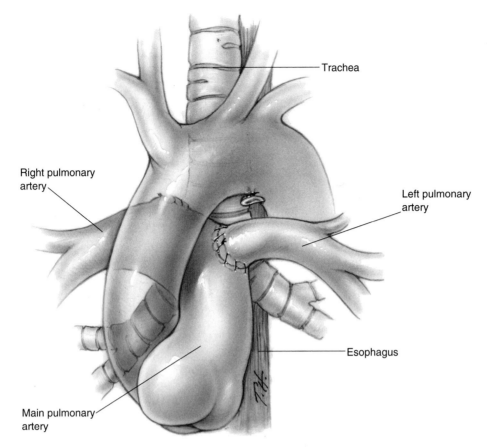

FIG. 15-5. Correction of a pulmonary artery sling. Note the division and reimplantation of the left pulmonary artery onto the main pulmonary artery in front of the trachea.

prevent narrowing of the anastomosis. In addition, it may be useful to lock every fourth to fifth stitch to prevent purse-stringing of the anastomosis.

Median Sternotomy Technique

A standard median sternotomy incision is performed, and cardiopulmonary bypass is instituted with an ascending aortic cannula and single straight venous cannula in the right atrium. The procedure is carried out on the beating heart.

The ductus or ligamentum arteriosus is doubly ligated and divided. The main right and left pulmonary arteries are extensively mobilized. With the aorta retracted leftward, the origin of the left pulmonary artery is identified and dissected free of the back of the trachea. The left pulmonary artery can now be detached from the main pulmonary artery and brought anterior to the trachea. The resultant opening in the distal main pulmonary artery is oversewn with a 6-0 Prolene running suture. The left pulmonary artery is reimplanted more proximally on the main pulmonary artery, using care not to twist or kink the left pulmonary artery (Fig. 15-5).

NB Because the median sternotomy approach allows complete mobilization of the right, left, and main

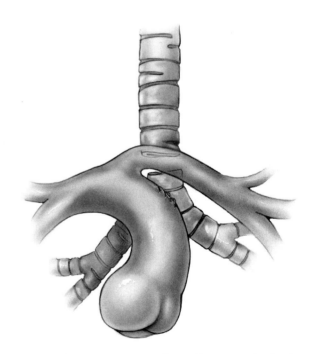

FIG. 15-6. Pulmonary artery sling with a stenotic distal trachea. The left pulmonary artery can be brought anteriorly between the divided ends of the trachea.

pulmonary arteries, tension on the anastomosis is minimized.

NB If a stenotic segment of the trachea is present, the trachea may be transected, allowing the left pulmonary artery to be brought anterior to the trachea through the space between the two divided ends of the trachea (Fig. 15-6). Subsequently, the stenotic portion of the trachea is resected and the two ends are reanastomosed. The lie of the left pulmonary artery must be assessed, and if kinking or stretching is noted, the left pulmonary artery should be detached and reanastomosed more proximally on the main pulmonary artery.

CHAPTER 16

Systemic Pulmonary Shunting

Increased experience with total correction of congenital heart defects in early infancy has considerably reduced the need for shunting procedures in recent years. Nevertheless, systemic to pulmonary artery shunts continue to offer excellent palliation in a select group of patients with anatomically complex cardiac anomalies. They are most beneficial when used as a bridging procedure in preparation for the definitive correction of the cardiac defects later in the patient's life or as part of a procedure in patients with single ventricles to provide controlled pulmonary blood flow. This multiple-stage approach is warranted in some specific clinical conditions.

Today, the most common application of the systemic to pulmonary artery shunt is in the neonate with a ductus-dependent pulmonary circulation. The ability to keep the ductus arteriosus patent with an infusion of prostaglandin E_1 has been instrumental in improving hypoxia and acidosis in these critically ill patients. Shunting procedures can therefore be performed on a semiurgent basis in an unhurried manner.

TYPES OF SHUNTS

The Blalock-Taussig shunt was introduced in 1945. Traditionally, it consists of anastomosing the subclavian artery to the pulmonary artery on the side opposite the aortic arch; however, with some technical modifications, the subclavian artery can also be anastomosed to the pulmonary artery on the same side as the aortic arch.

Other shunting procedures were subsequently introduced. They include Potts's shunt (descending aorta to the left pulmonary artery), Waterston shunt (ascending aorta to the right pulmonary artery), central shunt (interposing a graft between the ascending aorta and the main pulmonary artery), and the modified Blalock-Taussig shunt (interposing a GORE-TEX tube graft between the subclavian or innominate artery and the right or left pulmonary artery).

The Potts's shunt was abandoned because it is cumbersome to perform, difficult to close, and can cause high flow and early development of pulmonary vascular disease. Waterston shunt lost favor because of the high incidence of injury to the pulmonary artery and the difficulty in controlling the amount of flow through the shunt. The classical Blalock-Taussig shunt is rarely used. Today, most surgeons perform a central or modified Blalock-Taussig shunt through a median sternotomy. The relative disadvantage of this approach requiring a redo sternotomy and dissection of adhesions for the next procedure are outweighed by the superior exposure and ability to place the patient on cardiopulmonary bypass should hemodynamic instability occur. If the patient requires a second shunt procedure before definitive repair or as further palliation, a modified Blalock-Taussig shunt through a thoracotomy approach may be indicated.

MODIFIED BLALOCK-TAUSSIG SHUNT WITH GORE-TEX TUBE INTERPOSITION

Interposition of a GORE-TEX tube graft between the subclavian or innominate artery and the right or left pulmonary artery is the most commonly performed shunt procedure. Today, most shunts are performed through a median sternotomy as an isolated procedure or as part of a palliative operation for a single ventricle. Under some circumstances, a thoracotomy approach is indicated. With either approach, it should be remembered that the lumen of the subclavian or innominate artery is the limiting factor to the volume of flow. In neonates, a 3.5- or 4-mm graft is used; in older infants, a 5-mm graft is usually selected.

Median Sternotomy Approach

This approach has several advantages. The pulmonary end of the shunt can be placed more centrally, potentially allowing better and more uniform growth of both pulmonary arteries. The ductus arteriosus can be occluded at the conclusion of the procedure preventing excessive pulmonary circulation in the early postoperative period. The ductus arteriosus can be ligated when a left thoracotomy approach is used but rarely accomplished through a right thoracotomy. Finally, if the patient becomes unstable, cardiopulmonary bypass can be quickly initiated through a median sternotomy.

Incision

A standard median sternotomy with resection of the thymus is used.

Technique

After opening the pericardium, traction sutures are placed on the pericardial edges. The aorta and pulmonary artery are dissected free using scissors or an electrocautery on a low setting. Downward traction on the main pulmonary artery allows the ductus arteriosus to be identified and encircled with a tie or cleaned free of surrounding tissues in preparation for later Ligaclip closure. The innominate artery is dissected to allow application of a C clamp. The proximal right pulmonary artery is then dissected away from the underside of the ascending aorta and from the superior vena cava and mobilized circumferentially, identifying the right upper lobe branch.

NB *USE OF HEPARIN*

If the shunt is being performed without cardiopulmonary bypass, systemic heparinization (1 mg/kg) is initiated just before the clamp is applied to the innominate artery. The GORE-TEX graft is trimmed obliquely. A fine vascular C clamp is applied to the innominate artery so that the inferior aspect of the artery is centered in the excluded portion (Fig. 16-1). The handle of the clamp is then raised to position the inferior edge of the innominate artery anteriorly. A longitudinal incision is made in the artery, and a fine adventitial suture is placed on the superior edge of the arteriotomy to keep the lumen open. The anastomosis is started near the heel with 7-0 or 8-0 Prolene suture. With one end of the suture tagged, the other needle is passed from the inside to the outside of the graft at the heel. The suture is pulled through to the halfway point, then the same needle is passed from outside to inside the artery at the heel. The inferior suture line is completed using the same needle continuing one to two bites beyond the toe and tagging the suture line outside the graft (Fig. 16-2). The other needle is passed from inside the artery at the heel, and the suturing is continued until both suture lines meet. The sutures are tied together.

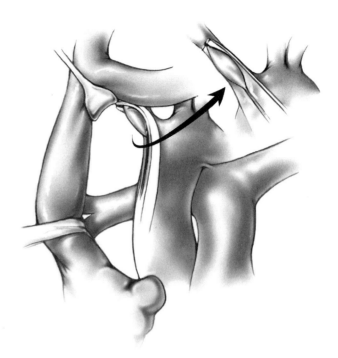

FIG. 16-1. Modified Blalock-Taussig shunt through a sternotomy. Placing a side-biting clamp on the innominate artery and rotating it to expose the inferior aspect of the artery. A vein retractor under the innominate vein improves exposure.

With the other end of the graft occluded, the vascular clamp on the innominate artery is carefully removed and the anastomosis is checked for leaks. The length of the GORE-TEX graft is measured to just reach the superior aspect of the proximal right pulmonary artery. The graft is divided transversely at this site after placing a fine straight vascular clamp on the graft just below the innominate anastomosis. Alternatively, the C clamp may be reapplied to the innominate artery to occlude inflow to the graft. The right pulmonary artery is grasped with a fine C clamp so that the superior aspect is in the middle of the clamp. The clamp is then rotated so that a longitudinal incision can be made on the superior edge of the pulmonary artery. The arterial opening should be approximately two-thirds of the diameter of the graft lumen as the pulmonary artery stretches. A double-armed, 7-0 or 8-0 Prolene suture is passed from inside to outside of the pulmonary arteriotomy at the 12-o'clock position. The other needle is tagged, leaving one-half of the suture pulled through. The first needle is then passed from outside to inside on the graft. The superior portion of the anastomosis is completed in this way, carrying the same needle two bites past the 6-o'clock position. The other needle is then passed from inside to outside on the graft, and the suturing is continued until the two sutures meet (Fig. 16-3). The C clamp on the pulmonary artery is now removed, and the sutures are tied together. The clamp on

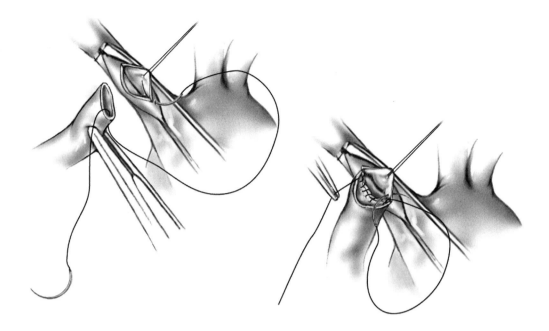

FIG. 16-2. Modified Blalock-Taussig shunt through a sternotomy. The end-to-side anastomosis of a GORE-TEX tube graft to the innominate artery. The inferior suture line is completed first.

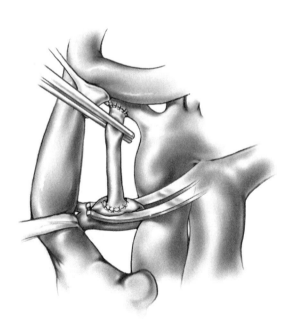

FIG. 16-3. Modified Blalock-Taussig shunt through a sternotomy: completing the pulmonary artery anastomosis. The side-biting clamp has been placed so that the superior edge of the right pulmonary artery is exposed.

the graft is removed, and a check for leaks is done. A thrill should be appreciated by palpating the graft.

NB *CENTRALLY LOCATED SHUNT*
The median sternotomy approach allows the pulmonary artery end of the shunt to be placed as centrally as possible. The aorta must be mobilized and retracted leftward with a traction suture on the right side of the aorta, a vein retractor, or the back of the C clamp itself (Fig. 16-3).

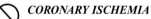 *CORONARY ISCHEMIA*
Care must be taken when applying traction to the aorta to prevent compression or kinking of the coronary arteries. If any electrocardiographic changes are noted or hemodynamic instability occurs, the traction suture, retractor, or clamp must be repositioned immediately.

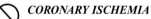 *PULMONARY FLOODING*
When the shunt is opened and flow through it confirmed, the ductus arteriosus, if present, should be occluded to prevent pulmonary overcirculation. Too much pulmonary blood flow may lead to systemic hypoperfusion and an inadequate diastolic blood pressure resulting in coronary ischemia.

HEMODYNAMIC INSTABILITY WITH RIGHT PULMONARY ARTERY CLAMPING
Before incising the pulmonary artery, hemodynamic stability and systemic oxygenation with the C clamp in place should be assessed. The clamp may interfere with ductal flow, and reapplying it more distally on the right pulmonary artery may rectify the problem. However, if desaturation or hemodynamic compromise persists after repositioning the clamp, the patient should be placed on cardiopulmonary bypass for support during this anastomosis.

 INCORRECT LENGTH OF THE TUBE GRAFT
Tension on the anastomosis owing to too short a tube graft may cause suture line bleeding and an upward pull on the pulmonary artery, which can lead to distortion or stenosis of the proximal right pulmonary artery. A graft that is too long may kink, thus compromising flow through the graft.

At the completion of the procedure, the pericardium is loosely reapproximated with three or four interrupted sutures. A small chest tube is placed in the anterior mediastinum before a standard sternotomy closure is performed.

NB **MODIFIED LEFT BLALOCK-TAUSSIG**
It may be preferable to place an interposition GORE-TEX tube graft between the subclavian and pulmonary arteries through a thoracotomy incision. This may apply when a child requires a second shunt procedure before definitive repair or palliation. In this case, a left thoracotomy approach is generally used. Some surgeons prefer a thoracotomy approach for the initial shunt. In this case, a right-sided shunt may be used because it is easier to take down. The technique is essentially the same for both sides. The following description pertains specifically to the left side.

Incision

A left thoracotomy through the fourth intercostal space provides satisfactory exposure.

Technique

The left lung is retracted downward and posteriorly, and the local anatomy is evaluated. The left pulmonary artery is identified. The parietal pleura overlying it is incised, and the artery is mobilized medially toward the pericardium and the hilum of the lung.

 IDENTIFICATION OF THE LEFT PULMONARY ARTERY
Sometimes the exact identity of the vessels within the hilum of the lung may not be clear. If there is any doubt as to the exact location of the pulmonary artery, it can be traced from within the pericardium through a short longitudinal incision of the pericardium, just anterior and parallel to the left phrenic nerve.

 COLLATERAL VESSELS
In older infants, many collateral vessels may have developed as a result of reduced pulmonary flow and marked cyanosis. They must be lightly coagulated to prevent troublesome blood oozing in the area of dissection.

 IDENTIFICATION OF THE LEFT UPPER LOBE BRANCH OF THE PULMONARY ARTERY
The division of the left pulmonary artery into its lobar branches within the hilum must be noted and its left upper lobe branch identified. This prevents anastomosis of the graft to the left upper lobe branch artery.

The left pulmonary artery, with its lobar branches having been clearly identified, is prepared for clamping or snaring with fine vascular elastic bands. The parietal pleura over the subclavian artery is incised, and the artery is mobilized and dissected free of its parietal sheath (Fig. 16-4).

A 5-mm GORE-TEX tube graft is most commonly used in older infants. A 3.5- or 4-mm tube graft is used for neonates, and a 6-mm graft is rarely used in older patients. Because the size of the lumen of the subclavian artery is the limiting factor to the flow of blood, grafts larger than the subclavian artery do not necessarily increase the flow to the lungs and therefore are not responsible for pulmonary flooding, if it occurs.

The distal end of the graft is trimmed obliquely. An appropriate segment of the subclavian artery is excluded within a delicate vascular clamp. A longitudinal incision is then made in the artery. A fine adventitial traction suture on the anterior edge of the arteriotomy will keep the lumen of the artery open.

The anastomosis is started near the toe with 7-0 Prolene suture with double-armed, swaged-on needles. The first stitch is passed from inside the graft to the outside at the toe, and the same needle is then passed from outside the subclavian artery to the inside at the distal part of the arteriotomy (Fig. 16-5A). The suture is pulled halfway through, and the other end is tagged. Suturing is continued with the same needle along the posterior edge of the arteriotomy passing the heel of the anastomosis; the needle is clamped when it is on the outside of the graft. The other needle is passed from the inside to the outside of the arterial lumen and then from the outside of the graft to the inside. The suturing is continued until both ends of the sutures meet. They are then tied together (Fig. 16-5B).

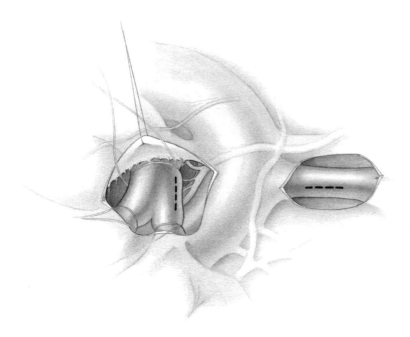

FIG. 16-4. Left modified Blalock-Taussig shunt: operative view of the hilum of the left lung and left subclavian artery.

With the other end of the graft temporarily occluded with fine, atraumatic forceps, the vascular clamp on the subclavian artery is loosened to detect a gross anastomotic leak that may require additional suture reinforcement. The clamp is then reapplied. The lung is now inflated to bring the pulmonary artery to its normal location. The length of the GORE-TEX tube graft is meticulously evaluated; it is divided transversely at the appropriate site so that when its divided end is in close apposition to the left pulmonary artery, it is under no tension and is not kinked.

The main left pulmonary artery is clamped down as proximally as possible. The pulmonary artery branches are snared down snugly. Alternatively, a fine vascular C clamp may be applied to the left pulmonary artery. A longitudinal incision is made on the superior surface of the left pulmonary. The arterial opening should be approximately two-thirds of the diameter of the graft lumen (Fig. 16-6A). A double-armed, 7-0 Prolene suture is introduced from the inside of the graft to the outside and from the outside of the artery to the inside at the 12-o'clock position of the anastomosis. Suturing is continued in an over-and-over fashion until the first needle exits the graft at the 7-o'clock position. This suture is then tagged, and the second needle is placed from inside to outside on the pulmonary artery. This suture is continued to meet the first suture. Before tying down the suture ends, the clamp on the subclavian artery is removed to flush the graft lumen of any blood clots that may have accumulated there. Occasionally, the graft is irrigated with dilute heparin solution. The clamp on the left pulmonary artery is also removed, and any snares around the upper and lower branches of the pulmonary artery are loosened. The sutures ends are now tied snugly. A good thrill should be felt (Fig. 16-6B).

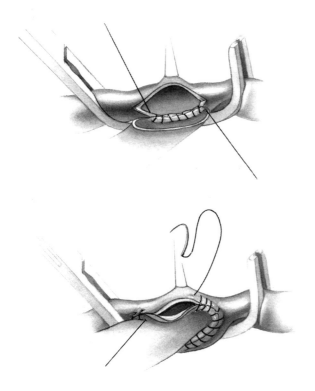

FIG. 16-5. Left modified Blalock-Taussig shunt: stepwise technique for anastomosing a GORE-TEX tube graft to the left subclavian artery.

NB *USE OF HEPARIN*
Systemic heparinization with 1 U per kilogram of body weight is initiated before clamping the subclavian artery. Although this may prolong bleeding

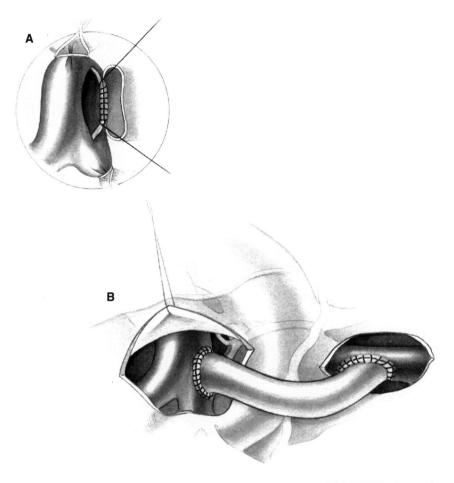

FIG. 16-6. Left modified Blalock-Taussig shunt. **A:** Anastomosing the GORE-TEX tube graft to the left pulmonary artery. **B:** Graft interposition between the left subclavian and left pulmonary arteries.

at the anastomotic site, it lessens the risk of early graft thrombosis. Additionally, systemic heparinization may be continued for the first 24 hours after surgery.

 TOO SHORT A TUBE GRAFT
Tension on the anastomosis owing to too short a tube graft not only causes suture line bleeding but also pulls upward on the pulmonary artery, narrowing the lumen for distal flow and bringing about early closure of the shunt. The inferior pulmonary ligament can be divided to allow the lung to move upward and to reduce some of the pull on the pulmonary artery in the hilum of the lung. If this maneuver does not rectify the problem satisfactorily, the shunting procedure must be repeated with a new tube graft of appropriate length.

 SUTURE LINE BLEEDING
Bleeding from the suture line is not uncommon. Packing the anastomotic site lightly with Surgicel or

Gelfoam and thrombin for approximately 5 minutes will achieve hemostasis in most cases. Additional sutures should be avoided, if possible, because they may jeopardize the lumen of the shunt.

 TRANSVERSE VERSUS LONGITUDINAL INCISION ON THE PULMONARY ARTERY
A transverse incision on the superior aspect of the pulmonary artery has been advocated by some surgeons. However, the risk of distortion and subsequent stenosis of the pulmonary artery appears to be greater with this incision as opposed to the longitudinal opening.

At the end of the procedure, a small chest tube is inserted and the thoracotomy is closed in the usual fashion.

CENTRAL SHUNT

This procedure entails interposing a tube graft between the main pulmonary artery and ascending aorta. It pro-

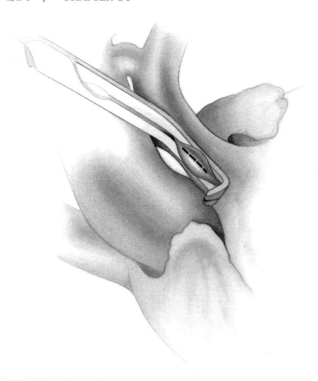

FIG. 16-7. Central shunt: isolation and incision of the pulmonary artery.

vides an alternative technique when other shunt techniques have failed or in cases in which the branch pulmonary arteries are very small. The approach is through a median sternotomy.

Technique

The ascending aorta and main pulmonary artery are dissected free of each other. A small side-biting clamp is placed on the main pulmonary artery. A vertical pulmonary arteriotomy is made (Fig. 16-7). A 3.5- or 4-mm GORE-TEX tube graft is cut transversely and anastomosed to the pulmonary artery with continuous 7-0 Prolene sutures. Similarly, another vascular clamp is applied to the ascending aorta and a small opening is made with a knife blade. This is enlarged to the appropriate size with an aortic punch. The other end of the GORE-TEX tube is cut obliquely and anastomosed to the aorta with 7-0 Prolene suture (Fig. 16-8). Air is removed by unclamping the pulmonary artery before tying down the suture on the aortic side of the anastomosis. The aortic clamp is removed as the last step. A good thrill should be felt.

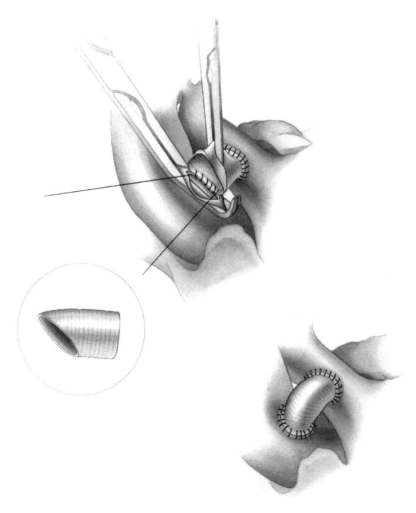

FIG. 16-8. Stepwise technique for creating a central shunt.

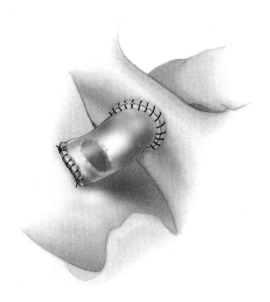

FIG. 16-9. Central shunt with a side-to-side aortic anastomosis and oversewing the end of the GORE-TEX tube graft.

 KINKING OF THE GRAFT

An inappropriate length of a GORE-TEX tube graft and too sharp an angle at its junction with either the aorta or pulmonary artery may contribute to kinking of the tube graft and subsequent shunt failure. Oblique division of the tube graft at the aortic end and a transverse cut at the pulmonary artery end usually prevent distortion of the graft. Alternatively, the GORE-TEX tube can be cut transversally and anastomosed end to side into the pulmonary artery. Then a 3.5- to 4-mm hole is created on the aortic side of the graft where it lies against the ascending aorta, and a side-to-side anastomosis is performed with a partial occlusion clamp on the ascending aorta. The distal end of the graft is then transected 4 to 5 mm distal to the aortic anastomosis, and the end is oversewn with 7-0 Prolene (Fig. 16-9).

PROSTHETIC ASCENDING AORTA–RIGHT PULMONARY ARTERY SHUNT

Occasionally, the aortic arch anatomy may make interposition from the innominate to the right pulmonary artery problematic. In these cases, a graft may be placed from the ascending aorta to the right pulmonary artery.

NB ***LIMITING FACTOR TO THE PULMONARY BLOOD FLOW***

In modified Blalock-Taussig shunt interposition with GORE-TEX tube graft, the size of the subclavian or innominate artery is the limiting factor to the flow of blood to the lungs. In an ascending

aorta–right pulmonary shunt, however, the diameter and length of the GORE-TEX tube graft are important factors regulating the pulmonary blood flow. Therefore, except on very rare occasions, a 3.5- or 4-mm tube graft should be used to prevent excessive blood flow, pulmonary edema, or premature development of pulmonary vascular disease.

Incision

A median sternotomy approach is used.

Technique

After removing the thymus, the pericardium is opened and traction sutures are placed. If the ductus arteriosus is patent, it is dissected free circumferentially for later closure after completion of the shunt. The right pulmonary artery is mobilized by gently retracting the aorta leftward and the superior vena cava rightward. The upper lobe branch of the right pulmonary artery is identified so that the shunt can replaced proximal to it. After systemic heparinization (1 mg/kg), a C clamp is placed on the proximal right pulmonary artery positioning the anterior portion of the artery in the center of the clamp. The appropriately sized GORE-TEX tube is cut transversely. A longitudinal arteriotomy is made in the pulmonary artery approximately two-thirds of the diameter of the graft. A traction suture is placed on the inferior edge of the arteriotomy. A double-armed, 7-0 Prolene suture is used, tagging one end and placing the needle from inside to outside the artery at the 12- o'clock position. The same needle is then passed from outside to inside on the graft, and suturing is continued to complete the superior edge of the anastomosis. The needle is brought outside the artery at the 5-o'clock position and tagged. The other needle is then passed from inside to outside the graft and used to complete the inferior suture line. The sutures are tied together. The graft is occluded, and the clamp on the pulmonary artery is removed. The suture line is inspected for leaks. Any traction on the ascending aorta is now released, and the location of the aortic anastomosis is carefully judged. The graft is marked as is the ascending aorta. The graft may be cut obliquely to meet the opening on the ascending aorta without distortion. However, it is often advisable to create an opening on the aortic side of the graft matching the aortic opening and perform a side-to-side anastomosis. This procedure is described.

After marking the graft, a fine vascular clamp is placed on the graft close to the pulmonary artery anastomosis. A small incision is made at the mark on the graft and enlarged to a size equal to the diameter of the graft with a 2.8-mm aortic punch. A side-biting clamp is now placed on the ascending aorta so that the marked area is centered in the clamp. A small incision is made and enlarged with the aortic punch. The side-to-side anastomosis is performed using a double-armed, 7-0 Prolene suture. One end is tagged, and the other needle is passed inside to outside on the graft and then outside to inside the aorta at the 8-o'clock position. Suturing is continued counterclockwise to the 4 o'clock position where the suture is tagged outside the graft. The other needle is now passed from inside to outside the aorta, and suturing is continued until the sutures meet. The sutures are tied together. The graft is now transected approximately 5 mm distal to the side-to-side anastomosis and oversewn with 7-0 Prolene suture, taking care not to distort the aortic anastomosis. Alternatively, the distal end of the GORE-TEX tube may be closed with a circular patch of GORE-TEX (Fig. 16-10). Before securing this suture line, both the aortic partial occluding clamp and the straight clamp on the graft are removed to deair the graft. If the ductus arteriosus is present, it is now occluded with a heavy tie or Ligaclip. The pericardium is loosely approximated with interrupted sutures, a small chest tube is placed in the anterior mediastinum, and standard sternotomy closure is performed.

 AORTIC PARTIAL OCCLUSION
The side-biting clamp must be placed carefully on the ascending aorta, especially in neonates and infants with small aortas to avoid hypotension or myocardial ischemia secondary to compromised coronary flow. Before incising the aorta, the position of the clamp should be tested to ensure that no hemodynamic changes are going to occur. Multiple reapplications of the clamp from different angles may be required before a satisfactory placement is found.

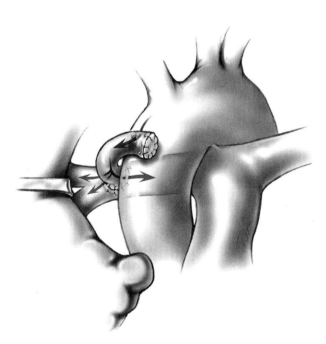

FIG. 16-10. Completed ascending aorta to the right pulmonary artery shunt. Note a circular patch closing the tube graft above the side-to-side aortic anastomosis.

 THROMBOSIS OR DISTORTION OF THE GRAFT ABOVE THE AORTIC ANASTOMOSIS
The length of graft beyond the side-to-side anastomosis is crucial with this technique. If too much graft extends above the aortic anastomosis, there will be an area of relatively stagnant flow that may predispose to graft thrombosis. If too little graft remains, the suture line may distort or compromise flow into the graft from the aorta. If the graft has been cut too short, the end can be closed with a circular piece of GORE-TEX cut from extra graft material (Fig. 16-10). This prevents distortion and minimizes dead space.

CLOSURE OF SYSTEMIC PULMONARY SHUNTS

All these shunts should be dissected free and exposed for complete occlusion just after initiation of cardiopulmonary bypass, when contemplating complete correction of the anomaly or further palliative procedures.

Right-Sided Modified Blalock-Taussig Shunts

The aorta and superior vena cava are retracted away from each other, and the posterior pericardium is incised above the superior margin of the right pulmonary artery. The GORE-TEX tube graft is identified and occluded with one or two medium or medium-large Ligaclips just after the initiation of cardiopulmonary bypass (Fig. 16-11).

 DISSECTION AROUND THE RIGHT PULMONARY ARTERY
There are many adhesions and collateral vessels in this area. A minimal dissection to isolate the shunt should suffice. It is usually unnecessary to pass a silk tie around the shunt.

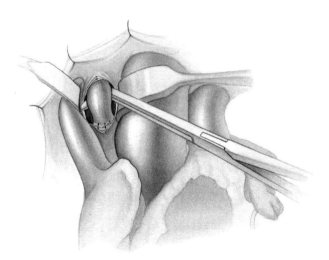

FIG. 16-11. Exposure of the right modified Blalock-Taussig shunt.

RIGHT PULMONARY ARTERY STENOSIS

If significant stenosis is present at the insertion site of the shunt into the right pulmonary artery, the tube graft should be divided after the initiation of cardiopulmonary bypass. The transected end should be secured with at least two adequately sized Ligaclips or oversewn with a 6-0 or 5-0 Prolene suture. The residual GORE-TEX material should then be removed from the right pulmonary artery and this area enlarged with an oval-shaped patch of autologous pericardium or pulmonary homograft wall.

DIVISION OF THE GORE-TEX SHUNT

Theoretically, as a child grows, an intact GORE-TEX tube graft may cause upward traction on the right pulmonary artery, which may lead to distortion and possible late development of pulmonary artery stenosis. If an adequate length of GORE-TEX tube graft can be dissected free without incurring excessive bleeding, the tube may be secured with two Ligaclips on each side and divided to prevent this potential late complication.

Left-Sided Modified Blalock-Taussig Shunts

Isolation of the left-sided shunt is somewhat more cumbersome and can be accomplished in many ways. Some surgeons prefer opening the left pleura. The GORE-TEX tube graft is then identified as it enters the left pulmonary artery (Fig. 16-12). It is minimally dissected free and doubly clipped, just before initiation of cardiopulmonary bypass. Less often, the left pulmonary artery is dissected free from within the pericardium, and

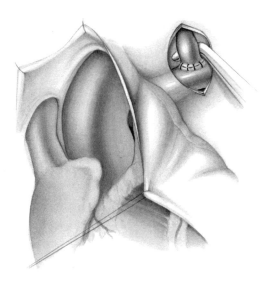

FIG. 16-12. Exposure of left modified Blalock-Taussig shunt.

the GORE-TEX tube graft is clipped, just above the junction with the pulmonary artery.

CLIP INJURY

Clips must be at least large enough to occlude the entire width of the graft. Smaller clips may pierce the graft and cause bleeding, in addition to closing it incompletely.

DIVISION OF A GORE-TEX SHUNT

With left-sided modified Blalock-Taussig shunts, the GORE-TEX is not divided. In this case, as the child grows, the left pulmonary artery is not pulled up, but rather the left subclavian artery is pulled down. Even if the left subclavian artery becomes occluded, no clinical consequences will result.

Central Shunt

With the initiation of cardiopulmonary bypass, the GORE-TEX tube is occluded with a metal hemoclip.

Prosthetic Ascending Aorta–Right Pulmonary Artery Shunt

The tube graft is dissected free on the lateral aspect of the ascending aorta and occluded with a metal hemoclip. Depending on the procedure to be performed, the shunt itself may need to be divided after commencing cardiopulmonary bypass and the aortic and pulmonary ends oversewn with a running 6-0 or 5-0 Prolene suture.

AORTIC INJURY

The GORE-TEX shunt is often very adherent to the side of the aorta. The correct plane for dissection must be identified, staying right on the GORE-TEX itself to avoid entry into the aorta. If the shunt cannot be safely dissected from the aorta, it should be occluded as much as possible with a vascular clamp or forceps when cardiopulmonary bypass is commenced and the dissection completed with the patient on a pump.

Waterston and Potts's Shunts

Waterston and Potts's shunts are no longer performed, but familiarity with the techniques of their closure is essential for the surgeon who operates on patients who have undergone these shunting procedures in the past.

Technique: Waterston Shunt

The easiest way to close a Waterston shunt is on cardiopulmonary bypass with the aorta cross-clamped. After administering cardioplegic solution, a small transverse aortotomy is made, and the shunt may be closed from within the aorta with a few interrupted sutures. The preferred method is to detach the right pulmonary artery from the aorta and oversew the defect in the ascending aorta with running 5-0 Prolene suture. The defect in the pulmonary artery can be closed transversely by direct suture or preferable patched with a piece of autologous pericardium or pulmonary homograft.

 PULMONARY ARTERY DISTORTION
If the shunt has created some stenosis or kinking of the right pulmonary artery, this should be reconstructed with an appropriate pericardial or homograft patch.

 FLOODING OF THE PULMONARY CIRCULATION
The site of the shunt must be occluded with the initiation of cardiopulmonary bypass, or flooding of the lungs will occur. If this cannot be achieved with a vascular forceps or clamp, the right and left pulmonary arteries should be dissected before beginning cardiopulmonary bypass and snared or clamped.

Technique: Potts's Shunt

Closure of Potts's shunt is performed on cardiopulmonary bypass with moderate hypothermia. The patient is placed in the Trendelenburg position, and with the heart decompressed, the perfusion pressure is temporarily reduced. A longitudinal incision is made on the main pulmonary artery and extended onto the left pulmonary artery. The site of a shunt orifice in the left pulmonary artery is identified and closed with a purse-string suture or patch.

 FLOODING OF THE PULMONARY CIRCULATION
Before instituting cardiopulmonary bypass, the site should be identified by palpating for a thrill along the left pulmonary artery. The shunt flow can be obliterated or markedly reduced by digital pressure on this site.

Open Procedures for Congenital Heart Defects

CHAPTER 17

Atrial Septal Defect

Defects in the atrial septum are relatively common developmental anomalies. They appear at various sites in the septum and are associated with other congenital abnormalities. Also, there is a real or potential slit-like opening, the foramen ovale, where the fossa ovalis flap disappears behind the superior septal limbus. Generally, the higher pressure in the left atrium keeps the fossa ovalis flap in apposition to the superior septal limbus, and thus the opening remains closed. In 20% of normal persons, however, it may remain open and allow minimal shunting. When pressure in the right atrium increases, as in right-sided heart failure, the septum becomes stretched and allows the foramen ovale to enlarge with significant shunting at the atrial level.

The sinus venosus atrial septal defect occurs high in the atrial septum and extends into the orifice of the superior vena cava, which becomes malpositioned slightly toward the left. There is usually anomalous drainage from the right superior pulmonary veins associated with these defects (Fig. 17-1).

The fossa ovalis type, also known as the ostium secundum defect, is the most common variety. This defect occurs in the mid-septum in the vicinity of the fossa ovalis and may be small or very large. Infrequently, the defect may occur low in the septum and extend into the orifice of the inferior vena cava, which also becomes malpositioned toward the left. This type of defect may occasionally be associated with anomalous pulmonary venous drainage. Rarely, the whole septum may be absent, giving rise to a single common atrium.

A defect low in the interatrial septum that extends down to the level of the atrioventricular valve orifices is part of the atrioventricular canal complex (see Chapter 20).

SURGICAL ANATOMY OF THE RIGHT ATRIUM

Although the right atrium is morphologically molded into a single chamber, it is formed by two components: the sinus venarum and the right atrial appendage (some-times referred to as the body of the atrium). Systemic venous return flows in from opposing directions through the superior and inferior venae cavae into the sinus venarum. This smooth-walled area is the most posterior portion of the right atrium and stretches between the orifices of the caval veins. From the viewpoint of the surgeon looking down into the right atrium, the sinus venarum is more or less horizontal with the superior vena cava entering from the left and the inferior vena cava entering (bounded by the eustachian valve) from the right (Fig. 17-2).

Just below and medial to the orifice of the superior vena cava arises a muscle bundle, the crista terminalis, which springs into prominence as it circles the orifice of the superior vena cava to the right lateral wall of the atrium and continues inferiorly toward the inferior vena cava, thus forming the boundary between the sinus venarum and the atrial appendage. This muscle bundle is evidenced on the outside of the atrium by a groove, the sulcus terminalis. Lying subepicardially in the sulcus terminalis, just below the entrance of the superior vena cava, is the sinoatrial node, which may be vulnerable to injury from the various surgical incisions and cannulations commonly performed on the right atrium. The remainder of the right atrium is made up of the atrial appendage, which begins at the crista terminalis and extends forward (upward from the surgeon's perspective) to surround the tricuspid valve and form an expanded chamber.

In contrast to the smooth-walled sinus venarum, the lateral wall of the atrial appendage is ridged with multiple narrow bands of muscle, the musculi pectinati. These bands arise from the crista terminalis and pass upward to the most anterior part of the atrium. Functionally, they supply the right atrium with enough pumping capacity to propel the venous inflow through the tricuspid valve into the right ventricle.

Just above the sinus venarum in the center of the medial wall is the fossa ovalis, a horseshoe- or elliptically shaped depression. The true interatrial septum consists of the

217

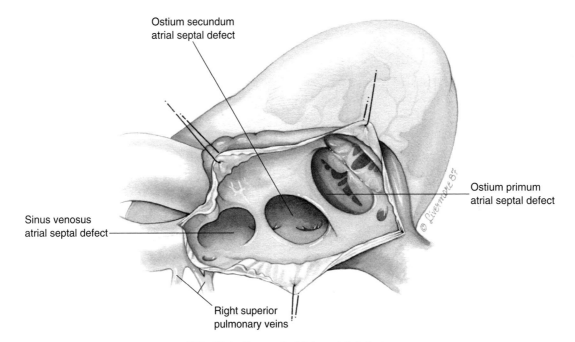

FIG. 17-1. Types of atrial septal defects.

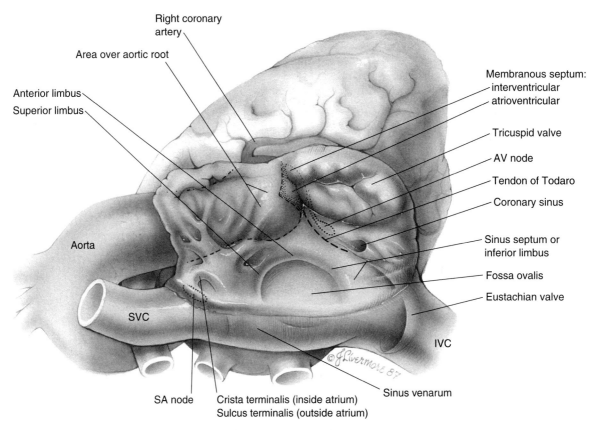

FIG. 17-2. Surgical anatomy of the right atrium.

fossa ovalis with variable contributions from the superior, anterior, and inferior limbic muscle bundles that surround it. The aortic root is hidden behind the anteromedial atrial wall between the fossa ovalis and the termination of the heavily trabeculated right atrial appendage. Segments of the noncoronary and right sinuses of Valsalva are in close apposition to the atrial wall in this area. Their location may be manifested by the aortic mound, which is a bulge above and slightly to the left of the fossa ovalis. The aortic valve here can be more clearly visualized if its continuity, through the central fibrous body, with the adjacent tricuspid valve annulus is taken into consideration.

Also invisible to the surgeon is the artery to the sinoatrial node, which can run through this same area. Although its origin and exact course are unpredictable, it takes a variable course toward the superior cavoatrial angle and the sinus node.

The tricuspid valve is located anteroinferiorly in the right atrium, where it opens widely into the right ventricle. The annulus of the tricuspid valve crosses over the membranous septum, dividing it into atrioventricular and interventricular segments. The membranous, or fibrous, septum is a continuation of the central fibrous body, through which the tricuspid, mitral, and aortic valves are connected. Immediately below the upper or atrioventricular section of the membranous septum lies the hidden atrioventricular node. It is situated at the apex of the triangle of Koch, the boundaries of which are the annulus of the septal leaflet of the tricuspid valve, Todaro's tendon (running intramyocardially from the central fibrous body to the eustachian valve of the inferior vena cava), and its base, the coronary sinus. Anderson describes Todaro's tendon as a fibrous extension of the commissure between the eustachian valve (of the inferior vena cava) and the thebesian valve (of the coronary sinus). Conduction tissue passes from the atrioventricular node as His's bundle, below the membranous septum, and down into the muscular interventricular septum. The coronary sinus, draining the cardiac veins, is situated alongside Todaro's tendon, between it and the tricuspid valve.

INCISION

All forms of atrial septal defect can be approached through a median sternotomy. Many surgeons now use a lower ministernotomy approach or submammary right thoracotomy for simple secundum atrial septal defects (see Figs. 1-16 through 1-20). Others prefer Brom's modification of the median sternotomy incision to allow full exposure of the pericardial space with acceptable cosmetic results in female patients (see Fig. 1-1).

CANNULATION

The ascending aorta is cannulated in the usual manner (see Chapter 2). The superior vena cava is usually cannulated directly, although it may be cannulated through the right atrial appendage. The inferior vena cava is cannulated through the atrial wall, just above the origin of the inferior vena cava. Tapes are then passed around both cavae.

NB *AORTIC CANNULATION WITH MINIMALLY INVASIVE APPROACHES*
The more distal ascending aorta is not easily accessible through a lower ministernotomy or submammary right thoracotomy. The aorta should be cannulated in its mid-portion where control of bleeding is relatively easy. Enough room should be left below the cannula to allow for deairing procedures.

NB *EXPOSURE OF THE SUPERIOR VENA CAVA*
A tie is placed on the right atrial appendage. Inferior traction on the appendage allows adequate visualization of the right superior vena cava for direct cannulation in most instances. If direct cannulation is not feasible, a straight venous cannula can be passed into the superior vena cava through a purse-string suture on the right atrial appendage.

⊘ *LEFT SUPERIOR VENA CAVA*
The left superior vena cava cannot be cannulated through minimally invasive incisions. Preoperative echocardiography must determine the presence or absence of the left superior vena cava.

MYOCARDIAL PRESERVATION

Cold cardioplegic arrest of the myocardium is achieved by infusion of cold blood cardioplegia into the aortic root (see Chapter 3).

Alternatively, closure of a simple septum secundum type defect can be accomplished safely without clamping the aorta. This approach is used when minimally invasive incisions are used because aortic cross-clamping in these cases is difficult or impossible. Before the atrium is opened, the heart is induced to fibrillate while the defect is being repaired. This prevents ventricular ejection and therefore any possibility of air embolism. If an extended period of time becomes necessary to deal with an unexpected anomaly, myocardial protection should be ensured with cold blood cardioplegic arrest of the heart.

SINUS VENOSUS ATRIAL SEPTAL DEFECT

Sinus venosus atrial septal defect usually occurs high on the septum close to the orifice of the superior vena cava and is associated with anomalous drainage of right upper lobe pulmonary veins into the superior vena cava and right atrium (Fig. 17-3). Approximately 10% of patients with this type of atrial septal defect also have a persistent left superior vena cava, which may be sus-

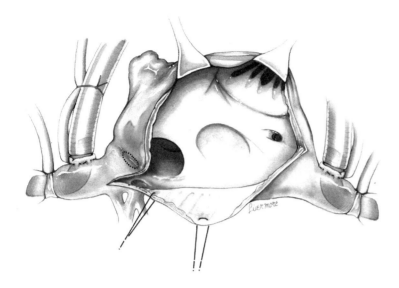

FIG. 17-3. Sinus venosus atrial septal defect and the superior extension of the atriotomy posterior to the sinoatrial node.

pected from a large coronary sinus on the preoperative echocardiogram.

Technique

The superior vena cava is cannulated directly above the entry site of the highest anomalous pulmonary vein.

The aorta is cross-clamped, and cardioplegic solution is administered into the aortic root (see Chapter 3). The vena caval snares are then snugged down. A longitudinal atriotomy is made starting at a point 0.5 to 1 cm posterior and parallel to the sulcus terminalis. The edges of the incision are then retracted to provide good exposure of the septal defect (Fig. 17-3). If additional exposure is required, the atriotomy is extended superiorly and posterolaterally across the superior vena caval–right atrial junction and onto the vena cava as far as necessary.

NB *DRAINAGE OF VENOUS RETURN FROM THE LEFT SUPERIOR VENA CAVA*
Although the venous return from a persistent left superior vena cava can be removed by pump suction, direct cannulation with a third venous cannula is the preferred approach. If an innominate vein is present and of adequate size, the left superior vena cava may be temporarily occluded with a snare.

🚫 *INJURY TO THE SINOATRIAL NODE*
The superior extent of the atriotomy may have to be retracted upward or, frequently, extended across the atriocaval junction onto the superior vena cava to provide adequate exposure. The sinoatrial node can be injured unless the atriotomy is extended well posterior to it.

🚫 *PERSISTENT LEFT-TO-RIGHT SHUNT*
It is important to ascertain that the tape around the superior vena cava is well above the level of the drainage of all the anomalous veins. Leaving a pulmonary vein draining into the superior vena cava results in a residual left-to-right shunt.

NB *DIFFICULT EXPOSURE*
The azygos vein, as it joins the superior vena cava, may at times obscure the surrounding structures. In this case, it may be divided to free up the superior vena cava and to provide better exposure of the anomalous pulmonary veins.

A patch of glutaraldehyde-treated autologous pericardium or GORE-TEX is cut to an appropriate size and shape after examining the extent of the defect. With a continuous suture of 5-0 or 6-0 Prolene, the patch is sewn around the lateral borders of the orifices of the anomalous veins and across to the anteromedial margin of the atrial septal defect (Fig. 17-4).

🚫 *PREVENTING OSTIAL STENOSIS OF ANOMALOUS VEINS*
It is preferable to place the sutures into the patch and the lateral margin of the defect before lowering the patch into position. Accurately placed sutures, well away from the anomalous vein orifices, will prevent subsequent stenosis. This technique facilitates complete drainage of all the pulmonary veins under the patch into the left atrium and prevents their late obstruction.

🚫 *OBSTRUCTION OF THE PULMONARY VENOUS RETURN*
If the atrial septal defect is relatively small, it should be enlarged to prevent obstruction of the

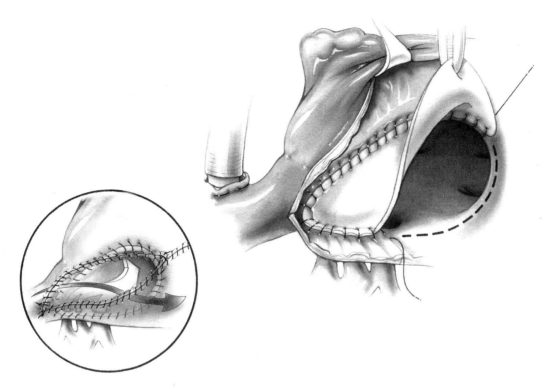

FIG. 17-4. First patch baffling anomalous pulmonary veins and closing the sinus venosus atrial septal defect. **Inset:** Second patch enlarging the superior vena caval–right atrial junction.

pulmonary venous return. The direction of septal incision for enlarging the septal defect should be caudal (usually to the fossa ovalis) rather than cranial so as not to sever the sinus node artery. In addition, the patch should be generous, creating a hood when the heart fills with blood and allowing unobstructed flow under the patch into the left atrium.

The atriotomy is then closed. Occasionally, this can be done primarily with a continuous suture of 5-0 Prolene. Most often, a second patch of pericardium is required to prevent narrowing of the superior vena cava–right atrial junction (Fig. 17-4, inset).

NB *AIR REMOVAL*
By having the anesthesiologist inflate the lungs before securing the patch, the left side of the heart is flooded with blood to displace any loculated air bubbles from within the pulmonary circulation and left atrium. The patch is kept partially open until all air has been removed; only then should the suture ends be snugly tied together, closing the defect completely. Venting through the aortic root is also used to remove air from the left heart (see Chapter 4).

 PREVENTING OBSTRUCTION OF THE SUPERIOR VENA CAVA
Often the atriotomy has been extended onto the superior vena cava for some distance for precise

exposure of the anomalous pulmonary veins. Direct closure may cause narrowing of the superior vena cava and give rise to subsequent obstruction. Unless the superior vena cava is unusually large, it should be enlarged with a patch of pericardium (Fig. 17-4, inset). Alternatively, a V-Y atrioplasty can be performed if the right atrium is very large.

 SINOATRIAL NODE INJURY
As mentioned previously, the atrial and superior vena caval closure line is in close proximity to the sinoatrial node. The edges of the atriotomy should be handled with care to prevent conduction abnormalities from sinoatrial node injury.

 CYANOSIS AFTER CARDIOPULMONARY BYPASS
If decreased systemic oxygen saturations are noted after completion of cardiopulmonary bypass, consideration should be given to the existence of a right-to-left shunt. This may occur if the azygos vein is included in the baffle of pulmonary veins to the sinus venosus atrial septal defect. *Ligating the azygos vein will rectify this situation.*

OSTIUM SECUNDUM ATRIAL SEPTAL DEFECT

Ostium secundum defects are the most common form of atrial septal defect. They are usually large and include the entire fossa ovalis (Fig. 17-5A).

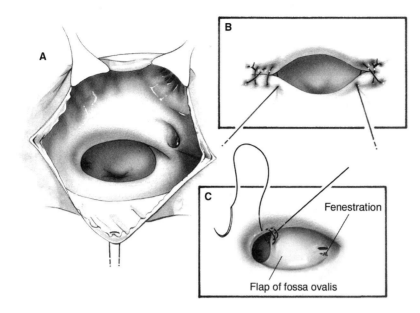

FIG. 17-5. **A:** Secundum atrial septal defect. **B:** Direct suture closure of a secundum atrial septal defect. **C:** Using the fossa ovalis flap to close the defect. Very small fenestrations of the flap can be primarily sutured.

Technique

The aorta is cross-clamped, and cardioplegic solution is administered into the aortic root (see Chapter 3). Alternatively, if a minimally invasive approach has been used, two pacing wires are secured on the anterior right ventricle and connected to a fibrillator to induce ventricular fibrillation. The venae caval snares are then snugged down. An oblique atriotomy is made and is extended toward the orifice of the inferior vena cava. The edges of the incision are then retracted to provide good exposure of the septal defect.

Some smaller secundum defects can be closed directly. Sutures are placed at the superior and inferior ends of the defect and continued toward each other, incorporating the margins of the defect (Fig. 17-5B).

 DEPTH OF SUTURES
The sutures must incorporate the thickened endocardium on both sides of the interatrial septum. The tissue of the fossa ovalis is usually too weak and friable to provide secure closure. Deep sutures should be avoided along the superior aspect of the defect because this area overlies the aortic root (Fig. 17-2).

NB *USING THE FOSSA OVALIS FLAP TO CLOSE A DEFECT*
Occasionally, the fossa ovalis flap is of sufficient size and quality to allow a tension-free primary suture closure, approximating the superior edge of the flap to the superior limbus (Fig. 17-5C). This is often the case in infants with a stretched patent foramen ovale. One must always check for fenestrations in the inferior aspect of the flap that could

result in residual atrial septal defects. If fenestrations are present or the flap is thin and friable, patch closure should be undertaken.

Unless the size of the defect is small and the rim of the opening is quite strong, a patch of glutaraldehyde-treated autologous pericardium or GORE-TEX is used to close a secundum defect to eliminate any tension along suture lines. An appropriately sized patch is prepared and sewn into position with continuous sutures of 5-0 or 6-0 Prolene (Fig. 17-6).

 EXTENSION OF THE DEFECT INTO THE INFERIOR VENA CAVA
Occasionally, the defect may extend into the orifice of the inferior vena cava, making its exposure difficult. The inferior vena caval cannula should be retracted to allow closure of this margin under direct vision, with a continuous suture of 5-0 Prolene incorporating the patch.

 CREATING A RIGHT-TO-LEFT SHUNT
The inferior free margin of the defect must be identified and distinguished from the eustachian valve. Inadvertent approximation of the edge of the eustachian valve to the anterior margin of the defect will create a tunnel, diverting the drainage from the inferior vena cava into the left atrium.

 DEPTH OF SUTURES
As with direct closure, the suture must incorporate the thickened endocardium on both sides of the septum and not the fossa ovalis tissue, which is often very thin and friable.

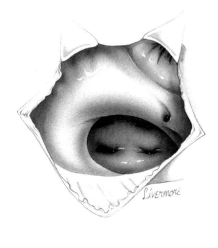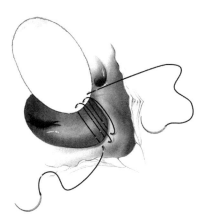

FIG. 17-6. Patch closure of a secundum atrial septal defect.

 AIR REMOVAL
The best way to prevent air embolism is to avoid introducing air into the left side of the heart. Whether the operation is performed under cardioplegic arrest or with the heart fibrillating, care should be taken to not place the sucker through the atrial septal defect.

By having the anesthesiologist inflate the lungs, the left side of the heart is flooded with blood to displace any loculated air bubbles from within the pulmonary circulation and left atrium. The patch is kept partially open until all air has been removed; only then should the suture ends be snugly tied together, closing the defect completely. Venting through the aortic root is also used to remove air from the left heart (see Chapter 4). When fibrillation has been used, the ascending aorta is aspirated with a large bore needle and syringe as the heart is defibrillated.

RIGHT PULMONARY VEIN DRAINAGE INTO THE RIGHT ATRIUM
The posterior margin of the defect may be so deficient as to allow the drainage of the right pulmonary veins directly into the right atrium. The patch must then be sewn to the atrial wall, anterior to the pulmonary vein orifices, to allow diversion of their drainage behind the patch into the left atrium (Fig. 17-7). The atriotomy is then closed with a continuous suture of 5-0 or 6-0 Prolene.

NB **MINIMALLY INVASIVE APPROACHES**
When limited incisions are used, the aorta is generally not clamped. Two pacing wires are attached to the right ventricle and connected to a fibrillator after cardiopulmonary bypass is initiated. The caval tapes are tightened, and with the ventricle fibrillating, the right atrium is opened. A concerted effort is made not to place a sucker through the atrial septal defect, thereby preventing air from entering the left atrium. The lungs are inflated before tying the suture line of the patch. A large needle on a syringe is used to aspirate the ascending aorta when fibrillation is discontinued, and this needle hole is allowed to bleed for 1 or 2 minutes after the heart is full and ejecting.

INADVERTENT DISCONTINUANCE OF FIBRILLATION
The failure to continue ventricular fibrillation when the heart is open may result in ejection of air into the ascending aorta with disastrous consequences. The pacing wires must be sewn securely to the right ventricle. The cable connections must be protected from contact with metal, which can short circuit causing loss of fibrillating current.

DEFIBRILLATION
Some patients will spontaneously regain sinus rhythm when the fibrillator is turned off. Many will require defibrillation. With limited incisions, small paddles must be used and oftentimes higher settings are required for successful defibrillation.

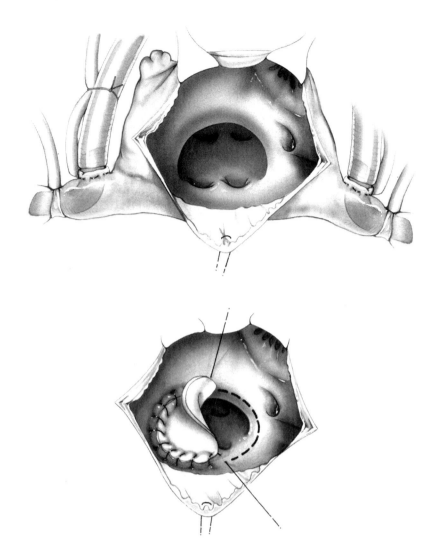

FIG. 17-7. Patch closure of an ostium secundum defect with malpositioned right pulmonary veins opening into the right atrium. The posterior edge of the patch is sutured in front of the orifices of the veins to reroute drainage into the left atrium.

COMMON ATRIUM

On rare occasions, the atrial septum may be absent, giving rise to a single common atrial chamber. Other lesions, such as anomalous systemic venous drainage with or without left superior vena cava and endocardial cushion defects, may also coexist. Each anomaly should be managed individually with subsequent septation of the common atrium.

A patient with complete absence of the atrial septum, absence of the right superior vena cava, persistent left superior vena cava, and a cleft mitral valve (Fig. 17-8) underwent complete correction, taking into consideration the following guidelines.

Aortic cannulation is carried out in the usual fashion. Tapes are passed around the left superior vena cava and inferior vena cava. Both inferior vena cava and left superior vena cava are cannulated directly. Alternatively, when exposure of the left superior vena cava is difficult, only the infe-

rior vena cava is cannulated and partial cardiopulmonary bypass is initiated. The snare around the inferior vena cava is snugged down, and the traditional atriotomy (above and parallel to the sulcus terminalis) is then made. The left superior vena cava is cannulated from within the right atrium, and the snare around it is now snugged down. In this manner, complete cardiopulmonary bypass is achieved.

The aorta is cross-clamped, and cold blood cardioplegia is administered into the aortic root. The cleft mitral valve is repaired with multiple interrupted sutures (see Chapter 20). A large patch of pericardium or GORE-TEX is then sewn to the posterior wall (Fig. 17-9).

The septation should start in the region of the annulus between the atrioventricular valves. Suturing should include the annulus and a small amount of tricuspid valve tissue (Fig. 17-9C). The mitral valve leaflet should be spared to avoid producing mitral insufficiency. The suturing is continued in a clockwise direction around the orifice of the coronary sinus (which may be absent) so that

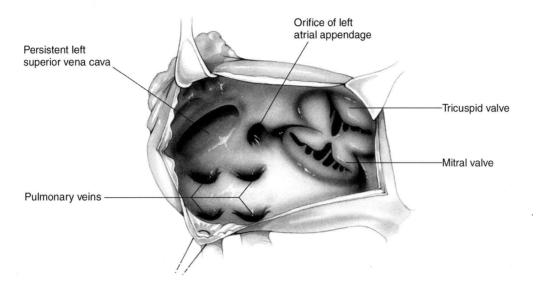

FIG. 17-8. Operative view of a single atrium with the absence of the right superior vena cava, persistent left superior vena cava, and cleft mitral valve.

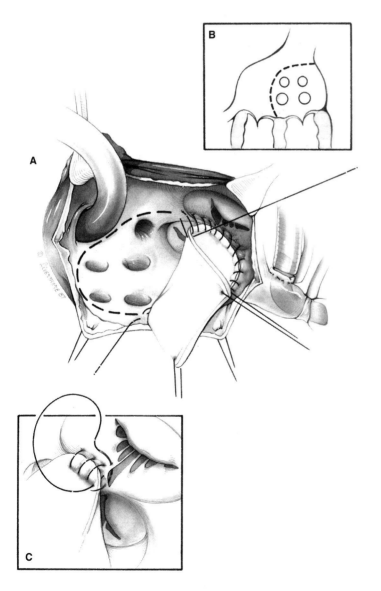

FIG. 17-9. A: Technique for repair of the defect shown in Fig. 17-8. **B:** Schematic illustration of repair. **C:** Suturing patch to tricuspid valve tissue (see text).

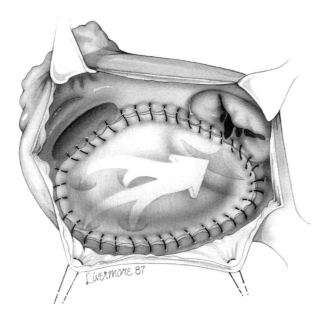

FIG. 17-10. Completed repair of the defect shown in Fig. 17-8.

it drains into the pulmonary venous atrium. The same suture is continued farther along the posterior atrial wall around the orifices of the right pulmonary veins. The other end of the suture is continued in a counterclockwise direction below and behind the orifice of the left superior vena cava until the patch takes on the configuration of a septum (Fig. 17-10). The patch should always be generous in size; if excess patch is present, it can be trimmed before suturing is completed. Otherwise, it may need to be augmented by sewing another patch to it.

PARTIAL ANOMALOUS PULMONARY VENOUS RETURN

The most common type of partial anomalous pulmonary venous return is seen in association with a sinus venosus atrial septal defect (see previously). Rarely, the right superior pulmonary vein enters the superior vena cava directly without an associated atrial septal defect. Repair of this anomaly requires creation of an adequately sized atrial septal defect and tunnel closure of the anomalous pulmonary vein to the left atrium (Fig. 17-4).

Scimitar syndrome consists of a large anomalous pulmonary vein draining the entire right lung or the right middle and lower lobes, passing inferiorly to enter the inferior vena cava just above or below the diaphragm. An interatrial baffle technique can be used to tunnel the flow from the anomalous pulmonary vein orifice within the inferior vena cava up to an existing or surgically created atrial septal defect. Alternatively, the anomalous vein may be ligated at its entrance into the inferior vena cava, transected, and anastomosed directly to the left atrium.

Anomalous drainage from the left lung into the innominate vein as an isolated lesion is rare. If only left upper lobe pulmonary venous drainage is involved, the defect may be left uncorrected. However, the left lung pulmonary veins drain through a vertical vein into the innominate vein, it must be dealt with. The vertical vein is ligated at its junction with the innominate vein and transected. The end of the vertical vein is opened obliquely and anastomosed to the left atrium at the base of the left atrial appendage.

CHAPTER 18

Total Anomalous Pulmonary Venous Connection

In a total anomalous pulmonary venous connection, there is no direct continuity between the pulmonary veins and left atrium. For the neonate to survive, there must be some mixing of circulation through a small atrial septal defect or a patent foramen ovale. The pulmonary veins converge to form a common pulmonary venous sinus that in turn connects to the systemic venous system and right atrium. The common pulmonary vein lies posterior to the pericardial sac behind the heart. The common pulmonary vein may rarely be atretic, a condition that results in death after a short time. Anomalous pulmonary venous connection may also be partial, as in the sinus venosus type of atrial septal defect, in which venous return from segments of the right lung drain into the junction of the right atrium and superior vena cava (see Sinus Venosus Atrial Septal Defect section in Chapter 17). The same kind of defect is seen less commonly near the orifice of the inferior vena cava.

In 45% of patients with total anomalous pulmonary venous drainage, a common pulmonary venous channel drains into an anomalous vertical vein joining the innominate vein or vena cava and reaches the right atrium in a supracardiac fashion. In approximately 25% of such patients, the drainage is directly into the right atrium or coronary sinus. The drainage in these cases is thus exclusively intracardiac. In another 25% of patients, the drainage is through infracardiac connections, i.e., the hepatic and portal veins. In approximately 5% of cases, the drainage can be into all or any combination of supracardiac, intracardiac, and infracardiac connections. Very rarely, in common pulmonary vein atresia (a condition in which life cannot be sustained for any great length of time), there is no connection to either atrium except through some collateral vessels.

Given the diversity of drainage connection, it is obviously essential to obtain an accurate diagnosis. Two-dimensional echocardiography can usually delineate the anatomy and demonstrate any associated anomalies. Rarely is cardiac catheterization or magnetic resonance imaging necessary.

TECHNIQUE

Most patients are neonates with unstable cardiorespiratory status. Those who present with pulmonary venous obstruction are true surgical emergencies. In neonates, the procedure is usually carried out during a period of deep hypothermic circulatory arrest. Continuous cardiopulmonary bypass using bicaval cannulation with aortic cross-clamping and moderate systemic hypothermia is used in older elective patients.

A median sternotomy is performed. The pericardium is opened, and the distal ascending aorta is cannulated. If hypothermic arrest is to be used, a single cannula is introduced into the right atrium through the right atrial appendage. Cardiopulmonary bypass is initiated, and the patient is cooled for 10 to 15 minutes. The aorta is cross-clamped, and cardioplegic solution is administered into the aortic root. Pump flow is discontinued, and after draining blood from the infant, the venous cannula is clamped and removed.

NB *LIGATION OF THE DUCTUS*
  The ductus must be dissected and occluded with a tie or Ligaclip before the initiation of cardiopulmonary bypass.

Intracardiac Type

A generous right atriotomy is made, somewhat below and parallel to the atrioventricular groove. The edges are retracted with fine sutures to provide maximal exposure. The inside of the right atrium is assessed carefully to delineate the precise anatomy. A patent foramen ovale or an atrial septal defect is always present. There may be a common pulmonary vein orifice opening into the right atrium, or the pulmonary veins may drain directly into the coronary sinus. In the latter case, the orifice of the coronary sinus is somewhat enlarged. The pulmonary venous return is rerouted into the left atrium by enlarging the atrial septal defect and using a pericardial patch to baffle the anomalous veins through the atrial septal defect.

⊘ SIZE OF THE ATRIAL SEPTAL DEFECT
The defect in the septum must be large enough to allow an unobstructed flow of pulmonary venous return. Most commonly, it is enlarged by extending its inferior margin toward the inferior caval or common pulmonary vein orifice.

NB DRAINAGE INTO THE CORONARY SINUS
Whenever the common pulmonary vein returns to the coronary sinus, its orifice is extended superiorly to reach the atrial septal defect. This incision must be well away from the anterior margin of the coronary sinus to prevent damage to the atrioventricular node and the conduction system (Fig. 18-1). In addition, the incision in the roof of the coro-

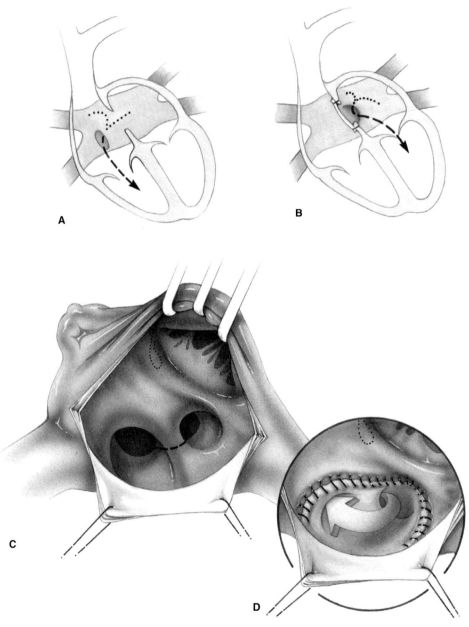

FIG 18-1. Intracardiac type of total anomalous pulmonary venous drainage. **A:** Schematic illustration of the defect. **B:** Schematic illustration of the correction of the defect. **C:** Operative view of the extension of the atrial septal defect to incorporate the coronary sinus orifice. **D:** Correction of the anomaly by roofing the septal defect and rerouting the pulmonary venous drainage into the left atrium.

nary sinus should be extended to the posterior wall of the heart. The resulting defect in the atrial septum is closed with an autologous pericardial patch using 6-0 Prolene suture.

 SUTURING INSIDE THE CORONARY SINUS
The continuous suturing of the patch must incorporate the wall of the coronary sinus well below its anterior rim to avoid the conduction system. Alternatively, very shallow bites of endocardium only are taken along the anterior rim of the coronary sinus.

When the patch is satisfactorily sewn in place, the atriotomy is closed with a continuous 6-0 Prolene suture. The heart is filled with saline, the venous cannula is replaced, cardiopulmonary bypass is recommenced, and the patient is warmed. The aortic cross-clamp is removed, and the cardioplegic site is allowed to bleed freely.

Infracardiac Type

This type is usually associated with obstruction and represents a true surgical emergency. During the cooling phase on cardiopulmonary bypass, the heart is elevated upward and to the right to expose the anomalous descending vertical vein. A 5-0 Prolene suture is placed at the apex of the left ventricle to simplify retraction of the heart. The posterior pericardium is opened, and a vertical incision is made in the anomalous vein to decompress the pulmonary veins (Fig. 18-2). The heart is replaced in the pericardial well until full cooling is achieved. The aorta is cross-clamped, and cardioplegia is given. After emptying the circulating volume into the pump, the venous cannula is removed. The heart is again lifted out of the pericardial well, and the previous incision on the anomalous vertical vein is extended longitudinally along the length of the pulmonary confluence.

A matching incision is made on the posterior left atrial wall and is extended onto the left atrial appendage. A tie placed on the left atrial appendage helps to expose and position the left atrium for the anastomosis. It is of paramount importance for the atriotomy to fall directly on the common pulmonary vein opening when the heart is allowed to resume its normal position.

NB *ENLARGEMENT OF THE COMMON PULMONARY VEIN OPENING*
The vertical incision on the common pulmonary vein channel may be extended slightly onto the left upper pulmonary vein tributaries, thus enlarging the opening.

The superior (rightward) aspect of the anastomosis is completed first with a continuous 7-0 Prolene suture. The inferior (leftward) aspect is similarly completed (Fig. 18-2C).

A small right atriotomy is now performed to close the atrial septal defect, usually a patent foramen ovale. If primary suture closure appears to compromise left atrial size, an autologous pericardial patch should be used (see Chapter 17). Cardiopulmonary bypass is started again, and the patient is warmed. Generally, the descending vein is not ligated because the systemic venous connections become obliterated quite quickly.

 HIGH PULMONARY ARTERY PRESSURE
It is often useful to insert a catheter through a purse-string suture on the right ventricular outflow tract into the pulmonary artery before weaning off cardiopulmonary bypass. Nearly all these patients have elevated pulmonary vascular resistance secondary to preoperative pulmonary venous obstruction. In addition, most patients have a relatively hypoplastic left atrium and left ventricle and may require fairly high left atrial pressures in the early postoperative period. The use of nitric oxide routinely in these patients is helpful in managing the pulmonary hypertension in addition to 100% oxygen and hyperventilation. Continued elevation of pulmonary artery pressures to near systemic should raise concerns about an obstructed anastomosis. Intraoperative transesophageal echocardiography can confirm an unobstructed flow from the pulmonary venous confluence into the left atrium.

 ANASTOMOTIC LEAK
A secure, leakproof anastomosis must be ensured. Suture reinforcement in this area is most difficult and may disrupt or distort the anastomosis.

Supracardiac Type: Biatrial Incision

After achieving deep hypothermic arrest, a transverse incision is started near the base of the right atrial appendage just posterior to the right atrioventricular groove and is extended toward the interatrial groove. The incision is then continued into the left atrium across the interatrial septum and foramen ovale (Fig. 18-3).

 OVEREXTENSION OF THE SEPTAL INCISION
The septal incision is not extended much farther than the anterior limbus of the fossa ovalis so that it does not end outside the heart.

The posterior wall of the left atrium is now incised transversely toward, but not reaching, the left appendage. The common pulmonary vein, which lies behind the parietal pericardium, is identified and the pericardium overlying it incised. Similarly, the common pulmonary vein is generously incised along a line as similar as possible to the incision of the posterior left atrial wall; 7-0 Prolene is then used to anastomose the

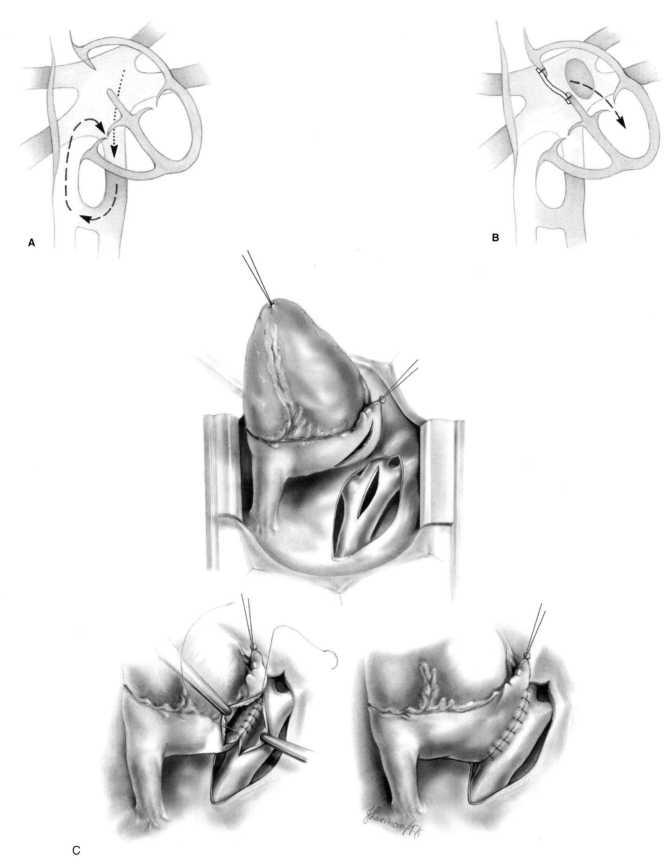

FIG. 18-2. Infracardiac type of total anomalous pulmonary venous drainage. **A:** Schematic illustration of the defect. **B:** Schematic illustration of the correction of the defect. **C:** Operative technique for the correction of the defect.

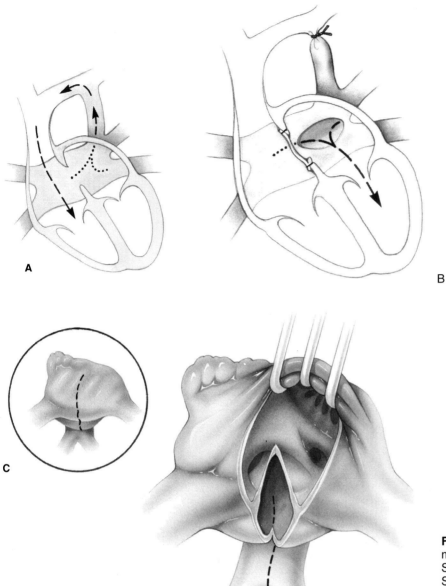

FIG. 18-3. Supracardiac type of pulmonary venous drainage. **A:** Schematic illustration of the defect. **B:** Schematic illustration of the correction of the defect. **C:** Biatrial incision for the total correction of the defect.

posterior atrial wall to the common pulmonary vein (Fig. 18-4A).

 SUTURE LINE BLEEDING
The sutures must be very close together, incorporating a good margin of tissue, to ensure a watertight anastomosis. Bleeding from this posterior suture line may be very difficult to control.

The atrial septum and right atrial wall are now sutured together to approximate the posterior edge of the right atriotomy. A patch of pericardium of appropriate size should be used to enlarge the interatrial septum to ensure an unobstructed flow of pulmonary venous return (Fig. 18-4B). The right atriotomy is then closed (Fig. 18-4C).

Supracardiac Type: Superior Approach

Another technique for dealing with the supracardiac type is the superior approach. The aorta is retracted leftward, and the dome of the left atrium is exposed. A tie is placed on the left atrial appendage. The posterior pericardium just superior to the dome of the left atrium is incised, and the pulmonary venous confluence is identified. A longitudinal incision is made along the entire length of the confluence and extended into a pulmonary vein orifice, if necessary, to create a patulous opening. A matching incision is made on the posterior aspect of the top of the left atrium, placing gentle traction leftward on the left atrial appendage (Fig. 18-5). The suture line is started at the leftward extent and carried along the supe-

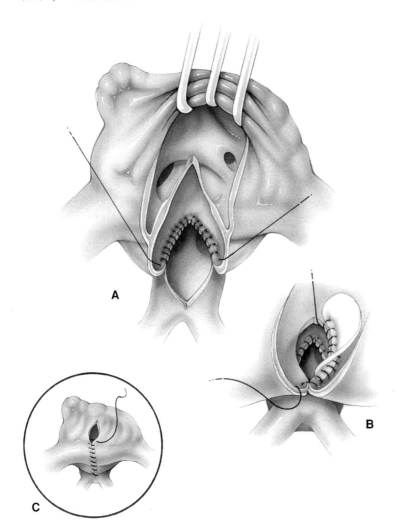

FIG. 18-4. Biatrial incision and technique for the total correction of the supracardiac type of anomalous pulmonary venous drainage. **A:** Anastomosing the left atrial wall to the pulmonary venous confluence. **B:** Patch enlargement of the opening of the atrial septum. **C:** Closure of the right atrium.

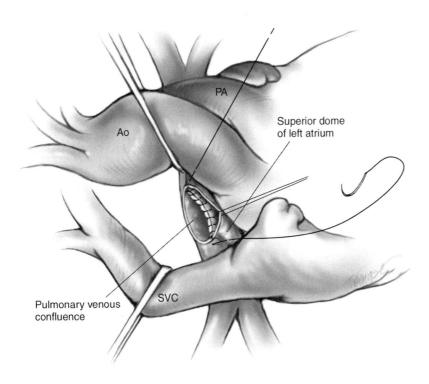

FIG. 18-5. Superior approach to the supracardiac type anastomosing the posterior aspect of the dome of the left atrium to the pulmonary venous confluence.

rior edge of the atriotomy and the inferior edge of the venous confluence. It is completed by joining the two remaining edges.

NB *CLOSURE OF THE ATRIAL SEPTAL DEFECT*
A patent foramen ovale or a small atrial septal defect, which is invariably present, must be closed in the usual fashion through a right atrial incision.

 LIGATION OF THE ASCENDING VERTICAL VEIN
The ascending vertical vein is encircled with a heavy tie during cooling. After rewarming, this vein may be kept open as cardiopulmonary bypass is discontinued. This can serve as a pop off if left atrial pressures are too high. After stable hemodynamics are achieved, the vein is ligated as far away from the venous confluence as possible.

ANASTOMOTIC LEAK
Every precaution must be taken to ensure a watertight anastomosis. Control of an anastomotic leak in this area may be somewhat difficult and hazardous.

COR TRIATRIATUM

Cor triatriatum is a rare defect in which the pulmonary veins drain into a common atrial chamber, usually located behind and above the true left atrium. This chamber is separated from the left atrium by a diaphragm. The upper chamber may or may not communicate with the right atrium through an atrial septal defect or foramen ovale.

Surgical Technique

Complete correction can be performed either on continuous cardiopulmonary bypass using bicaval cannulation or on cardiopulmonary bypass using a single atrial cannula with a period of deep hypothermic circulatory arrest. Transatrial incision beginning on the right superior pulmonary vein provides excellent exposure. The incision is extended across the right atrium and then across the atrial septum to the fossa ovalis (see Transatrial Oblique Approach section in Chapter 7). Retractors are placed beneath the edge of the atrial septum to inspect the left atrium. The entrance of all four pulmonary veins must be noted as well as the left atrial appendage and mitral valve. At this point, the membrane is resected, taking care not to extend the incision outside the heart.

The incision on the atrial septum can then be closed primarily or more often with a patch of autologous pericardium prepared with glutaraldehyde using a running 5-0 or 6-0 Prolene suture. The incisions on the right superior pulmonary vein and right atrium are then closed with a running 5-0 or 6-0 Prolene suture. The patient is rewarmed, the aortic cross-clamp is removed, and deairing is carried out in the usual fashion.

CHAPTER 19

Ventriculoseptal Defect

A ventriculoseptal defect can occur as an isolated lesion or in combination with other anomalies.

SURGICAL ANATOMY

The embryologic development of ventriculoseptal defects is indeed interesting and has been the basis for many complex classifications. Nevertheless, an increasing number of clinicians prefer a classification proposed by Anderson, which is simple and has many clinical implications, particularly from the surgeon's point of view. Anderson divides ventriculoseptal defects into perimembranous, subarterial-infundibular, and muscular types.

The perimembranous variety of ventriculoseptal defects encompasses subgroups of defects that occur near the membranous segment of the interventricular septum and includes those septal defects commonly seen in tetralogy of Fallot and the atrioventricular canal (Fig. 19-1). Because the path of the conduction tissue is intimately related to the inferior rim of these defects, an accurate knowledge of the surgical anatomy of this region is most helpful.

The atrioventricular node is situated in its usual position in the apex of Koch's triangle, whose boundaries consist of the septal attachment of the tricuspid valve, Todaro's tendon, and the coronary sinus as its base (Fig. 19-2). The conduction tissue passes from the atrioventricular node as His's bundle through the central fibrous body and the tricuspid annulus into the ventricular septum, following a course along the inferior rim of the defect toward the left ventricular side of the septum.

Surgical Approach

All forms of ventriculoseptal defects are approached through a median sternotomy.

CANNULATION

Cardiopulmonary bypass with moderate systemic hypothermia is used in most patients. In very small infants (<2 kg), deep hypothermic arrest using a single venous cannula through the right atrial appendage for cooling and warming may be preferred. In all others, the superior vena cava is cannulated directly; similarly, the inferior vena cava is cannulated through the atrial wall just above the origin of the inferior vena cava (see Chapter 2). Tapes are then passed around both cavae.

MYOCARDIAL PRESERVATION

Cardioplegic arrest of the myocardium is maintained by intermittent infusion of cold blood cardioplegia into the aortic root (see Chapter 3).

TRANSATRIAL APPROACH TO A VENTRICULOSEPTAL DEFECT

Almost all the perimembranous and atrioventricular canal types of ventriculoseptal defects and many of the muscular variety can be exposed and closed through the right atrium. The subarterial-infundibular type is best approached through a limited right ventriculotomy or preferably a pulmonary arteriotomy.

The aorta is cross-clamped, and cardioplegic solution is administered into the aortic root. The venae caval snares are then snugged down. A longitudinal or oblique atriotomy is made, starting at a point 0.5 to 1 cm anterior and parallel to the sulcus terminalis, and is extended toward the orifice of the inferior vena cava. The edges of the incision are then retracted to provide a good exposure of the tricuspid valve and Koch's triangle (Fig. 19-3).

 COEXISTING PATENT DUCTUS ARTERIOSUS
If a patent ductus arteriosus is present, it should be occluded with a metal clip before the initiation of

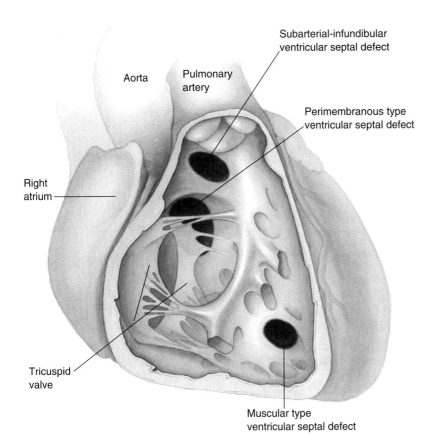

Subarterial-infundibular
ventricular septal defect

Perimembranous type
ventricular septal defect

Aorta   Pulmonary
artery

Right
atrium

Tricuspid
valve

Muscular type
ventricular septal defect

FIG. 19-1. Types of ventricular septal defects.

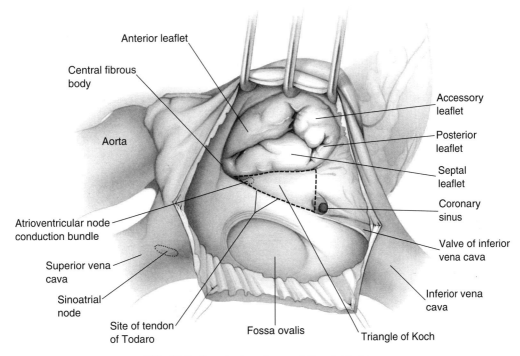

Anterior leaflet

Central fibrous
body

Aorta

Accessory
leaflet

Posterior
leaflet

Septal
leaflet

Coronary
sinus

Valve of inferior
vena cava

Atrioventricular node
conduction bundle

Superior vena
cava

Sinoatrial
node

Inferior vena
cava

Site of tendon
of Todaro   Fossa ovalis   Triangle of Koch

FIG. 19-2. Surgical anatomy of the right atrium.

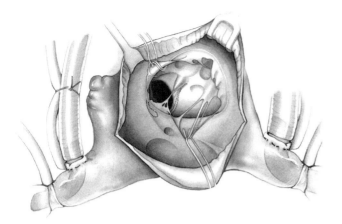

FIG. 19-3. Exposure of a ventricular septal defect by retracting the tricuspid valve leaflets.

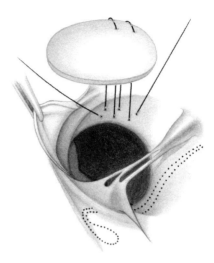

FIG. 19-4. Patch closure of a ventricular septal defect using a continuous suture technique.

cardiopulmonary bypass to prevent further overcirculation in the already overburdened plethoric lungs (see Chapter 12).

 SINOFATRIAL NODE INJURY
The sinoatrial node is vulnerable to injury from the snare around the superior vena cava. It can also be injured if the atriotomy is extended too far superiorly.

Technique for Closure

The anterior leaflet of the tricuspid valve is retracted with a 6-0 Prolene suture or small vein retractor to expose the defect and its margins for identification (Fig. 19-3). The defect can be closed with a continuous suture technique using 5-0 Prolene or multiple interrupted sutures of 4-0 or 5-0 braided sutures buttressed with Teflon felt pledgets or a combination thereof.

Continuous Suture Technique

With a double-armed, half-circle needle of 5-0 Prolene, the suturing is started at the 12-o'clock position along the muscular rim. The needle is then passed through a patch of Dacron velour slightly larger in size than the defect, again through the muscular rim, and then again through the patch, which is subsequently lowered into position (Fig. 19-4).

The suturing is continued in a counterclockwise direction along the superior rim, which overlies the aortic valve, until the central fibrous junction of the septum, aortic root, and tricuspid annulus is reached. The needle is passed through the septal leaflet of the tricuspid valve. During the procedure, the placement of each stitch is

facilitated by the assistant applying slight traction on the Prolene suture.

 BUTTRESSING THE SUTURES
Occasionally, the muscular rim of the ventriculoseptal defect may be very friable, allowing the fine Prolene to cut through. This is more likely to happen when there is associated long-standing muscular hypertrophy, as in tetralogy of Fallot. Multiple interrupted sutures buttressed with pledgets are then substituted for the continuous suture technique (Fig. 19-5).

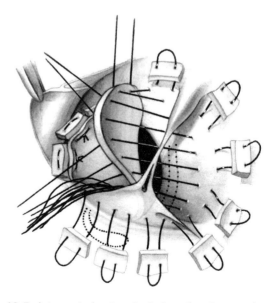

FIG. 19-5. Interrupted suture technique for closure of a ventricular septal defect.

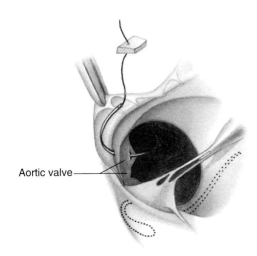

Aortic valve

FIG. 19-6. Proximity of an aortic valve leaflet to the rim of the septal defect.

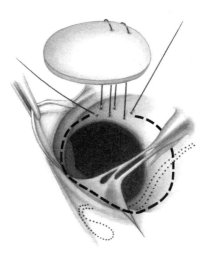

FIG. 19-8. Sutures are placed 3 to 5 mm from the rim of the defect inferiorly to avoid the conduction tract.

 INJURY TO THE AORTIC VALVE
The aortic valve leaflets are immediately below the superior margin of the defect and can be punctured during suturing if deep needle bites are taken in this area (Fig. 19-6).

 TRANSITIONAL SUTURES
The junction of the tricuspid annulus, aortic root, and septum is a vulnerable area where a residual defect may occur. A transitional stitch incorporating the tricuspid leaflet, the rim of the defect, and the patch (in that order) will ensure a more secure closure. This can be satisfactorily accomplished with either an interrupted or a continuous suturing technique.

The other arm of the Prolene suture is then continued in a clockwise direction; superficial bites that include only endocardium are taken just along the inferior rim of the defect, before piercing the tricuspid leaflet (Fig. 19-7). Alternatively, the other arm of the suture is continued, moving outward to a distance of 3 to 5 mm from the rim of the defect to avoid the underlying conduction tissue before again penetrating the septal leaflet of the tricuspid valve (Fig. 19-8).

 PREVENTION OF HEART BLOCK
As already described, His's bundle pierces the central fibrous body and the tricuspid annulus before penetrating the ventricular septum, where it follows a course along the inferior margin of the defect toward the left ventricular side of the septum. Because suturing along this course can be hazardous and culminate in heart block (Fig. 19-9A), shallow superficial bites are taken that include only the whitish endocardium close to the rim of the defect. In fact, the needle should be visible through the translucent endocardium (Fig. 19-9B). A more conservative and safer approach is to place sutures 3 to 5 mm from the inferior rim of the defect (Fig. 19-8).

 INTERFERENCE BY CHORDAE TENDINEAE AND PAPILLARY MUSCLES
If the view of the ventriculoseptal defect is obscured by chordae tendineae or papillary muscles, the septal leaflet and a portion of the anterior leaflet of the tricuspid valve may be detached, leaving a 2- to 3-mm rim of tissue along the annulus (Fig. 19-10A). Retraction of these leaflets pro-

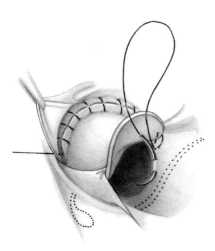

FIG. 19-7. Continuous suture technique for closure of a ventricular septal defect.

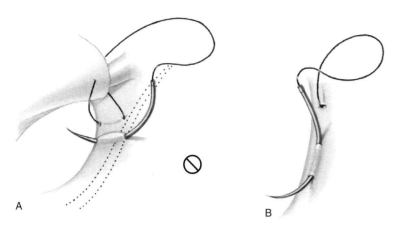

A

B

FIG. 19-9. A, B: Shallow bites of endocardium prevent the occurrence of heart block.

vides an unobstructed view of the ventriculoseptal defect (Fig. 19-10B). After patch closure of the defect, the leaflets are resutured to the rim of leaflet tissue along the annulus with a 6-0 Prolene suture.

The needle is now passed through the tricuspid leaflet approximately 2 mm from the annulus in a horizontal mattress fashion back into the right ventricle, taking a bite of the patch before penetrating the leaflet once again. This maneuver is continued in a clockwise direction until the other arm of the Prolene suture is met, so that both arms of the suture can be snugly tied to each other (Fig. 19-10C).

 BUTTRESSING THE SUTURES
The Prolene suture may cut through the thin, tricuspid leaflet tissue. The suture line can be buttressed with multiple pledgets or a strip of autolo-

gous pericardium. With the interrupted suture technique, pledgeted sutures are used.

 PREVENTION OF TRICUSPID INSUFFICIENCY
Incorporation of excessive leaflet tissue in the suture line results in tricuspid insufficiency (Fig. 19-11). The suture line along the tricuspid leaflet should not exceed a distance of 2 mm from the tricuspid annulus.

NB *TRICUSPID VALVE REPAIR*
After securing the patch, the anterior and septal leaflet tissue is carefully teased back over the patch with a nerve hook or fine forceps. Often one or two interrupted 6-0 Prolene sutures are used to approximate the anterior and septal leaflets and/or septal and posterior leaflets to ensure a competent tricuspid valve. The valve may be tested by injecting saline into the right ventricle.

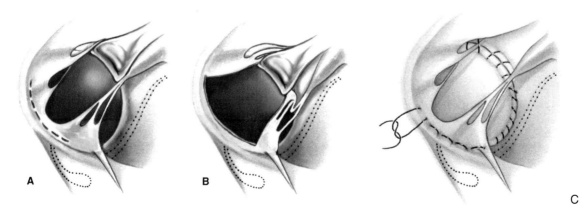

A

B

C

FIG. 19-10. A: Line of detachment of a septal leaflet to provide improved exposure. **B:** Retraction of a detached septal leaflet. **C:** Completed closure of a ventricular septal defect.

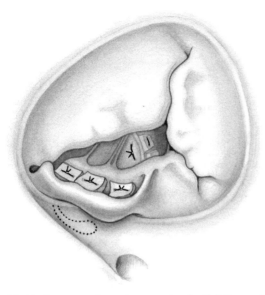

FIG. 19-11. Incorporation of excessive leaflet tissue in the suture line producing tricuspid valve insufficiency.

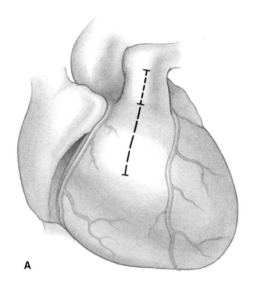

A

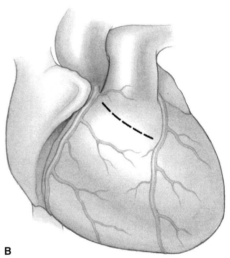

B

FIG. 19-12. A, B: Types of ventriculotomy.

When the repair is completed, the atriotomy is then closed with continuous suture of 5-0 or 6-0 Prolene.

TRANSVENTRICULAR APPROACH TO A VENTRICULOSEPTAL DEFECT

All septal defects, except those occurring near the left ventricular apex, can be closed through a right ventriculotomy. When there are associated lesions, such as infundibular or pulmonary valvular stenosis (as in tetralogy of Fallot), a vertical ventriculotomy becomes the approach of choice because it can be extended along the right ventricular outflow tract, thus providing excellent exposure. A transverse ventriculotomy has some theoretical advantages, especially when an aberrant coronary artery crosses the anterior wall of the right ventricle (Fig. 19-12).

 AVOIDING THE CORONARY ARTERIES
Every precaution should be taken to avoid dividing an aberrant coronary artery (Fig. 19-13). When the left anterior descending coronary artery originates in the right coronary artery, it courses across the anterior wall of the right ventricle. Its accidental division may result in severe myocardial dysfunction.

NB *INFUNDIBULAR HYPERTROPHY OBSCURING THE LOCATION OF THE DEFECT*
Infundibular hypertrophy may obscure the location of the perimembranous type of defect. The excess hypertrophied muscle mass, which may also be responsible for some right ventricular outflow obstruction, must be cautiously incised and/or

excised to expose the margins of the defect and relieve the obstruction (see Chapter 21).

Interrupted Suture Technique

The technique for transventricular closure of the perimembranous ventriculoseptal defect is essentially the same as that described for the transatrial approach. The edges of the ventriculotomy incision are retracted with fine pledgeted sutures or vein retractors. The margins of the defect are inspected, and interrupted, fine pledgeted sutures of double-armed 4-0 Tevdek are started at the 12-o'clock position, along the muscular rim in an everting fashion. Both needles are then passed through a patch of Dacron velour slightly larger than the defect (Fig. 19-14). Slight traction on this stitch by the assistant improves exposure and facilitates the placement of the next stitch (Fig. 19-15).

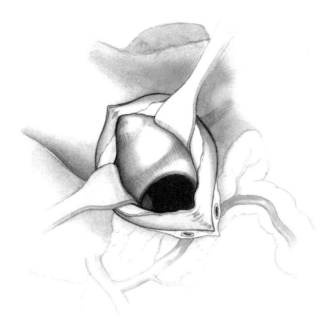

FIG. 19-13. Division of an aberrant coronary artery by a ventriculotomy.

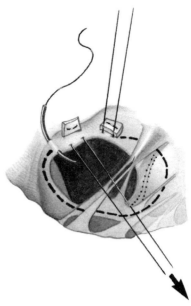

FIG. 19-15. Exposure is improved by gentle traction on the previously placed stitch.

Suturing is continued in this fashion in a counterclockwise direction along the superior rim (which overlies the aortic valve) until the central fibrous junction of the septum, aortic root, and tricuspid annulus is reached. Both needles of the next pledgeted interrupted suture incorporate the muscular rim of the defect, the patch, and the tricuspid leaflet (in that order). Depending on the consistency of the tricuspid leaflet, the needles may be passed through another pledget before tying on the atrial aspect of the tricuspid valve. Alternatively, the needle close to the previous

stitch is passed through the tricuspid tissue close to the annulus, the muscular rim of the defect, and the patch. The other arm of the needle is now passed through the tricuspid tissue and the patch. This is a true transitional stitch.

Suturing is then continued from the starting point in a clockwise direction, moving outward to a distance of 3 to 5 mm from the rim of the defect to avoid the underlying conduction tissue. (The alternative technique of taking very shallow bites that include only endocardium in the region of the inferior rim can also be used; see Transatrial Approach to a Ventriculoseptal Defect section.)

Where the tricuspid annulus becomes part of the inferior rim of the defect, the needle following the previous suture is passed through the tricuspid leaflet, the muscular septum 6 to 8 mm from the rim of the defect, and the patch. The other arm of the needle is now passed through the tricuspid valve and the patch. Alternatively, both needles of the pledgeted interrupted suture take shallow bites of the thickened endocardium, the patch, the tricuspid valve, and another pledget (in that order). The remaining sutures are passed from the right atrium through the tricuspid leaflet approximately 2 mm from the annulus before they are passed through the patch. When all the sutures are satisfactorily placed, the patch is lowered into position and the sutures are snugly tied (Fig. 19-16). It may be preferable to place all the sutures first, tagging each one separately, and then bring each suture through the patch held by the assistant.

Alternatively, a continuous 5-0 Prolene suture can be used in the same fashion as already described (see Transatrial Approach to a Ventriculoseptal Defect section). When the septal defect has been satisfactorily repaired, the ventriculotomy is closed with two layers of continuous or 5-0 Prolene sutures (Fig. 19-17).

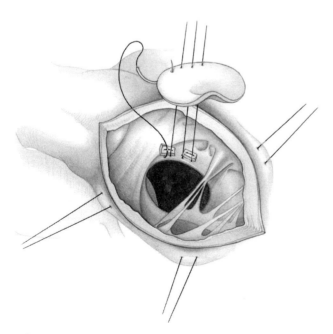

FIG. 19-14. Stepwise technique for closure of a ventricular septal defect by interrupted sutures (see text).

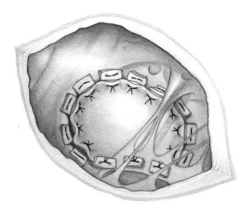

FIG. 19-16. Completion of a patch closure of a ventricular septal defect using the interrupted suture technique.

⊘ *INJURY TO THE AORTIC VALVE*
The aortic valve leaflets are immediately below the superior margin of the defect and can be punctured during suturing if deep needle bites are taken in this area. Suturing in this area should therefore incorporate the crista marginalis, which holds sutures well.

⊘ *PREVENTION OF HEART BLOCK*
As already described, the His's bundle pierces the central fibrous body and the tricuspid annulus before crossing into the ventricular septum and following a course along the inferior margin of the defect toward the left ventricular side of the septum. Because suturing along this course can be somewhat hazardous and culminate in heart block, shallow bites including only the whitish endocardium close to the rim of the defect are taken (Fig. 19-9). A more conservative and safer technique is to place sutures 6 to 8 mm from the inferior rim of the defect.

⊘ *TRANSITIONAL SUTURES*
The junction where the tricuspid annulus forms the margin of the defect is also most vulnerable to a

residual septal defect. Again, a transitional stitch incorporating the tricuspid leaflet, the muscular septum well away from the rim of the defect, and the patch (in that order) ensures a more secure closure.

SUBARTERIAL TYPE VENTRICULOSEPTAL DEFECT

These defects may be associated with progressive aortic insufficiency. Even if small, these defects should probably be closed to prevent progression of aortic insufficiency and aortic valve leaflet damage.

Technique for Closure

A right ventriculotomy may be used; however, the transpulmonary approach is preferred. If there is significant aortic insufficiency, the aortic valve should be repaired before the ventriculoseptal defect is closed.

Standard cannulation is performed with a single venous cannula. Cardiopulmonary bypass is commenced, and moderate systemic cooling is begun. The aorta is cross-clamped, and cold blood potassium cardioplegic solution is infused directly into the aortic root. If aortic regurgitation is significant, an oblique aortotomy is performed and direct infusion of cardioplegic solution is made into the left and right coronary ostia (see Chapter 3). A small vein retractor is placed in the aortotomy to expose the aortic valve. The midpoints of the three aortic cusps are brought together with a Frater stitch of 6-0 Prolene suture (Fig. 19-18). Usually one leaflet is prolapsed

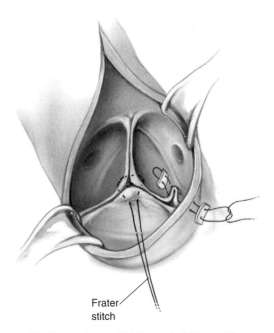

FIG. 19-18. Excessive leaflet tissue is folded at the commissure.

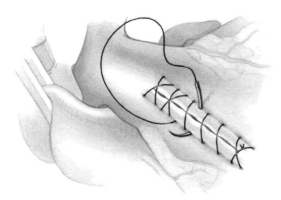

FIG. 19-17. Closure of a ventriculotomy.

and has excessive length along the free edge. The excess leaflet tissue is folded at the commissure and sewn to the aortic wall with one or two mattress sutures of 6-0 Prolene reinforced with a pericardial pledget (Fig. 19-18). Alternatively, a V-shaped wedge of leaflet tissue is resected from the middle of the involved leaflet and the leaflet reapproximated with interrupted sutures of 6-0 or 7-0 Prolene to correct the length of the free edge. The valve can now be tested with saline to ensure competence before cutting the temporary 6-0 Prolene suture through the midpoints of the commissures.

The aortotomy is closed with a running 6-0 or 5-0 Prolene suture. At this point, an additional dose of cardioplegic solution can be infused into the aortic root, allowing additional assessment of aortic valve competence.

The main pulmonary artery is opened transversely just above the commissures. A small vein retractor is then placed through the pulmonary valve to expose the ventriculoseptal defect. To further assess the degree of the aortic valve prolapse and insufficiency, blood cardioplegic solution is administered into the aortic root. All the aortic cusps can be well visualized through the septal defect if it is at least moderate in size. In fact, one of the aortic valve leaflets may be prolapsing through and partially closing the defect. An autologous pericardial patch fixed with glutaraldehyde is cut slightly larger than the defect and attached to the right ventricular aspect of the defect using 6-0 or 5-0 Prolene continuous suture. Superiorly, the patch must be secured to the base of the posterior cusp of the pulmonic valve. In this area, the needle is brought through the patch and then passed through the base of the valve leaflet. The needle is then placed back through the leaflet and again through the patch. This weaving suture line is continued until the edge of the defect is seen apart from the pulmonary annulus. If the leaflet tissue is friable, the pulmonary artery side of the suture line can be reinforced with a thin strip of pericardium. When the suture line is completed, the sutures are tied snugly (Fig. 19-19).

The pulmonary arteriotomy is then closed with a running 5-0 or 6-0 Prolene suture. The aortic cross-clamp is removed after filling the heart, and deairing is carried out through the cardioplegic site. Transesophageal echo evaluation should confirm adequate aortic valve repair and complete closure of the ventriculoseptal defect.

 INJURY TO THE AORTIC VALVE
Because there is often a close association between the aortic and pulmonary valve annulus with this anomaly, care must be taken in placing these sutures along the superior aspect of the ventriculoseptal defect. A too deeply placed needle may incorporate the aortic leaflet tissue and result in significant aortic insufficiency. In addition, if one of the aortic leaflets is prolapsing through the defect, care must be taken to not incorporate or injure the leaflet during closure of the defect.

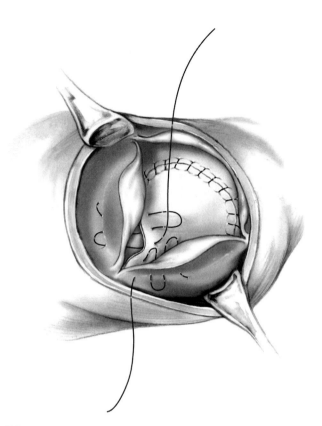

FIG. 19-19. Closure of a subarterial ventricular septal defect through the pulmonary artery.

 INJURY TO THE PULMONARY VALVE
The superior rim of the septal defect is adjacent to the pulmonary annulus. Closure of the defect entails placing sutures from within the pulmonary artery at the annulus. The leaflets of the pulmonary valve can be traumatized or perforated in the process. Use of a pericardial strip on the pulmonic side to buttress the suture line may be required.

LEFT VENTRICULOTOMY APPROACH

Depending on their location, muscular defects can be approached through both the right atrium and a right ventriculotomy. In the past, a limited left ventriculotomy near the apex was used to close muscular defects in the more distal portion of the septum. However, because there has been significant operative mortality and postoperative morbidity owing to left ventricular dysfunction and the late formation of aneurysms after left ventriculotomy, this approach should probably no longer be used. Many muscular ventriculoseptal defects can be located and closed through a right atriotomy using a small right-angled clamp or coronary artery probe passed through the foramen ovale into the left ventricle to demonstrate the defect. Apical muscular ventriculoseptal defects can be closed in the cardiac catheterization laboratory using transcatheter closure devices.

CHAPTER 20

Atrioventricular Septal Defects

There has been much discussion in recent years about the definition and embryogenesis of what has been called the atrioventricular canal complex. It is appropriate to refer to this anatomic complex as atrioventricular septal defects because, after all, that is what is actually seen clinically. The defect usually includes the inferior segment of the atrial septum and the superior segment or the inflow portion of the interventricular septum. The atrioventricular valves are also developed in an abnormal but varied fashion.

In all but the mildest forms, there is a common atrioventricular valve that can be said to consist of six leaflets of variable size and shape attached to normally or abnormally located papillary muscles by chordae tendineae. This common atrioventricular valve can be subdivided into mitral and tricuspid components or segments, each with three leaflets. The leaflets constituting the tricuspid valve are designated right superior, right inferior, and right lateral, and those comprising the mitral valve are designated left superior, left inferior, and left lateral (Fig. 20-1).

It is of clinical and anatomic significance that in normal hearts, the anterior mitral leaflet contributes to only one-third and the posterior leaflet contributes to two-thirds of the annulus of the mitral valve. In an atrioventricular defect, this ratio is reversed; the posterior (left lateral) leaflet contributes to one-third and the bileaflet anterior cusp (the left superior and inferior leaflets together) contributes to two-thirds of the mitral valve annulus (Fig. 20-2).

From the clinical point of view, however, there are partial, intermediate, and complete forms of atrioventricular septal defects. In the partial form, there exists an ostium primum type of interatrial septal defect. Here the atrioventricular valves are attached to the crest of the interventricular septum, and there is usually no interventricular communication below the valves. The anterior leaflet of the mitral valve, which has a cleft of varying degree, is considered to form part of a trileaflet mitral valve. Most commonly, this mitral valve is competent, although on occasion it may have some degree of incompetence (Fig. 20-1B).

The intermediate form is essentially similar to the partial form of atrioventricular septal defect. The main distinguishing feature is the incomplete attachment of the atrioventricular valves to the ventricular septum. In fact, some gaps may exist, and various degrees of underdevelopment of the leaflet tissues may also be present.

The complete form of atrioventricular septal defect, as its name implies, is a defect in both the lower atrial and upper ventricular septum. The configuration and details of the attachment of the atrioventricular leaflets to the ventricular septum are quite variable.

Rastelli reviewed atrioventricular canal specimens obtained at autopsy at the Mayo Clinic and proposed a classification of atrioventricular septal defects that essentially focuses on the shape, size, location, and details of the attachments of the left superior leaflet. In type A, which is very often seen, the left superior leaflet is over the left ventricle and its chordal attachment is to the crest of the ventricular septal defect (Fig. 20-3A).

In type B, which is rarely seen, the chordal attachment of the left superior leaflet is to an abnormally located papillary muscle on the right ventricular aspect of the interventricular septum (Fig. 20-3B). In type C, which is seen quite often, the left superior leaflet is large and bridges the ventricular septal defect and right ventricle. Its chordal attachments are variable (Fig. 20-3C). It is a matter of degree of the overriding of the left superior leaflet on the ventricular septum that determines the type of defect.

OSTIUM PRIMUM ATRIAL SEPTAL DEFECT

The ostium primum type of atrial septal defect is, in fact, part of the atrioventricular defect complex, sometimes referred to as a partial form of the atrioventricular canal. Clinically, a large ostium primum that is usually

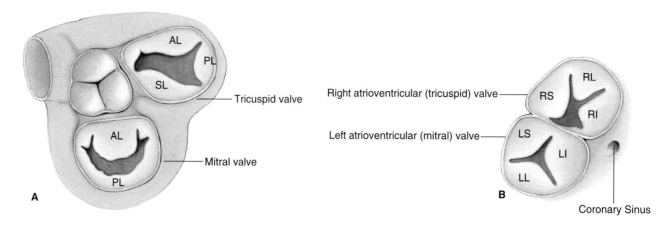

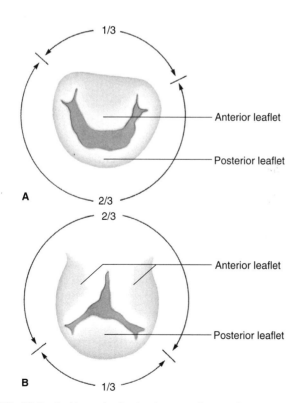

FIG. 20-1. Mitral-tricuspid valve relationship. **A:** In the normal heart, the mitral and tricuspid valve annuli are not in direct contact with each other. They are connected only by the fibrous skeleton of the heart as it encircles the aortic annuli. **B:** Partial atrioventricular septal defect (ostium primum atrial septal defect). The mitral and tricuspid valve annuli are fused, but there is no interventricular communication between the left and right sides of the heart. **C:** Complete atrioventricular septal defect. AL, anterior leaflet; LI, left inferior; LL, left lateral; LS, left superior; PL, posterior leaflet; RI, right inferior; RL, right lateral; RS, right superior; SL, septal leaflet.

nonrestrictive is detected, but there is always a cleft of varying degree in the anterior leaflet of the mitral valve (see Chapter 17) (Fig. 20-4). As already pointed out, the mitral valve in these cases should be considered a trileaflet structure; this should be borne in mind whenever a repair is attempted.

Incision

This form of atrial septal defect is usually approached through a median sternotomy. A right submammary thoracotomy incision can be used (see Chapter 1).

Cannulation

The ascending aorta is cannulated in the usual manner (see Chapter 2). The superior vena cava is cannulated directly, and the inferior vena cava is cannulated through the atrial wall just above the origin of the inferior vena cava. Tapes are then passed around both cavae. A vent is placed through the right superior pulmonary vein and positioned in the left atrium proximal to the mitral valve. (The correct position can be obtained after the heart is opened.)

Myocardial Preservation

Cold cardioplegic arrest of the heart is achieved and maintained by intermittent infusion of cold blood cardioplegic solution into the aortic root (see Chapter 3).

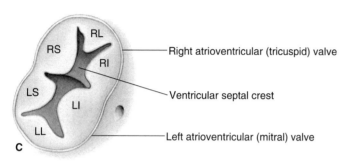

FIG. 20-2. A: Normal mitral valve annular configuration. **B:** Mitral valve annular configuration in an atrioventricular defect.

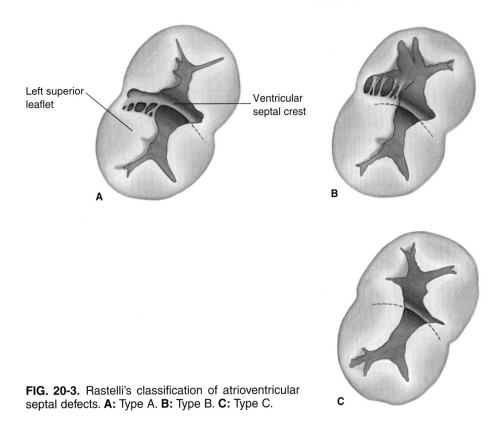

Left superior leaflet

Ventricular septal crest

FIG. 20-3. Rastelli's classification of atrioventricular septal defects. **A:** Type A. **B:** Type B. **C:** Type C.

Technique

A generous atriotomy is made from the base of the atrial appendage to near the site of the inferior vena cava cannulation, parallel with the atrioventricular groove. The atriotomy edges are retracted with fine sutures that are sometimes pledgeted (Fig. 20-5A). The presence and severity of the mitral regurgitation must be carefully assessed. This may be carried out by simply injecting saline forcefully through the mitral valve. The cleft on the anterior leaflet of the mitral valve should probably always

be closed even if there is no valve incompetence at the time of surgery because these valves often become insufficient over time. This can be accomplished by approximating the "kissing" edges of the cleft starting at the annulus with three or four interrupted 6-0 Prolene sutures.

 CLOSURE OF THE CLEFT
Care must be taken to approximate only the kissing edges of the leaflet tissue, which are not the same

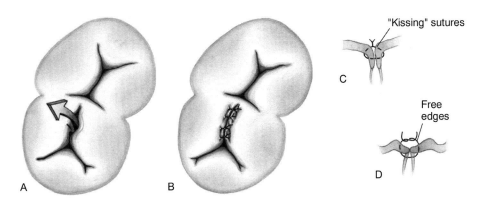

"Kissing" sutures

Free edges

FIG. 20-4. Insufficient anterior mitral leaflet. **A:** Regurgitation through the cleft. **B:** Repair of the cleft. **C:** "Kissing" edges of the cleft. **D:** Free edges of the cleft.

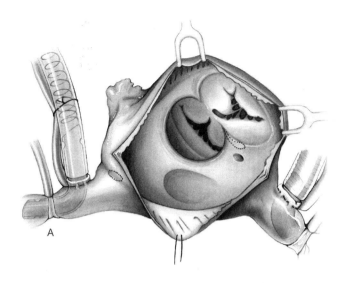

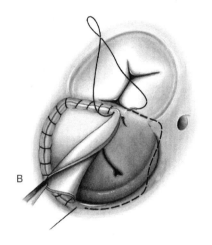

FIG. 20-5. A: Exposure of an ostium primum atrial septal defect. **B:** Suturing technique for repair.

as the free edges of the cleft (Fig. 20-4). Incorporation of an additional extent of the leaflet to secure a better repair usually results in severe valvular insufficiency. The edges of the cleft are strong and quite fibrotic in older patients and consequently hold sutures well. In infants, the valve tissue may be somewhat friable. In these cases, horizontal mattress sutures reinforced with pericardial pledgets can be used to close the cleft.

It is rare (10% of patients) to have significant valvular incompetence in the ostium primum type of defect. Occasionally, it does occur, however, and aggressive reconstruction should be undertaken (Nitral Valve Reconstruction). If the ostium primum defect is small and does not allow full visualization of the mitral valve, the atrial septal defect should be enlarged toward or into the fossa ovalis.

 OVERCORRECTION OF THE ANTERIOR LEAFLET REPAIR
Overzealous attempts to achieve perfection may produce mitral stenosis. In most patients, it is not necessary to close the cleft completely. In fact, the last one or two sutures may distort the anterior leaflet, pulling it down into the left ventricle, causing mitral valve insufficiency.

When all the maneuvers to evaluate the adequacy of mitral valve repair have been completed, the atrial septal defect is closed with a patch of autologous pericardium. A double-armed 5-0 or 6-0 Prolene suture is started at the cleft of the anterior mitral leaflet, taking small bites of tricuspid leaflet tissue where it is attached to the annulus (Fig. 20-5B). The suturing is continued in both clockwise and counterclockwise directions, taking small bites of the septal tricuspid leaflet tissue until the superior and inferior annuli are met.

 INCORPORATION OF THE TRICUSPID LEAFLET
To prevent the possibility of developing or aggravating mitral incompetence, the suturing should not extend onto the mitral leaflet. The bites should include tricuspid tissue just where it is adherent to the underlying ventricular septum.

After completing the suture line along the septal crest, the height of the pericardial patch is carefully measured. Too short a patch will pull up on the annulus and can cause mitral insufficiency. The patch is trimmed appropriately, and suturing is continued in both directions until all the edges of the primum defect are incorporated and the defect is closed by the patch (Fig 20-5B). The suture ends are tied. The atriotomy is then closed with a continuous suture of 5-0 or 6-0 Prolene. The process of air removal is meticulously followed, and finally the aortic clamp is removed. The aortic root vent is kept open in the field or connected to suction until good ejection of the ventricles takes place.

 RISK TO THE CONDUCTION TISSUE
Deep suturing in the area between the tricuspid annulus and the coronary sinus may injure the conduction tissue and produce heart block. Every precaution should be taken to avoid such a catastrophic event when suturing by taking superficial bites of endocardium only (you should be able to see the needle through the tissue) in this region. The first several bites are near the mitral valve annulus (Fig. 20-5B). Alternatively, the right-hand side of the patch should be left a little longer and sutured around the orifice of the coronary sinus so that it drains under the patch into the left atrium to prevent heart block (Fig. 20-6).

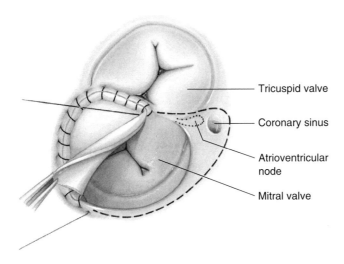

FIG. 20-6. Alternative suture technique for repair of an ostium primum atrial septal defect.

PREVENTING HEMOLYSIS

A patch of autologous pericardium fixed in glutaraldehyde should be used. The use of Dacron or GORE-TEX may result in hemolysis if a small amount of residual mitral regurgitation is present.

AIR EMBOLISM

Recommendations for air removal (see Chapter 4) must be followed to prevent the possible development of air embolism either systemically or into the orifice of the right coronary artery.

COMPLETE ATRIOVENTRICULAR DEFECT

The most crucial factor to consider in making repairs is competence of the mitral valve. A two-patch or single-patch technique can be used.

Cannulation

In small infants weighing less than 3 kg, hypothermic circulatory arrest allows optimal exposure. In most patients, however, direct cannulation of the superior vena cava and the inferior vena cava at its junction with the right atrium is carried out. Placement of the venous cannulae must not cause undue tension on the valvular apparatus. Aortic cannulation is performed as usual. When hypothermic arrest is used, a single venous cannula is placed through the right atrial appendage for cooling and rewarming and removed during the period of circulatory arrest. When continuous flow cardiopulmonary bypass is used, a vent is placed through the right superior pulmonary vein and positioned proximal to the mitral valve after the heart is opened.

Two-Patch Technique

A generous atriotomy is performed from just below the atrial appendage down toward the inferior vena cava parallel with the atrioventricular groove. The edges of the atriotomy are retracted with fine sutures, sometimes buttressed with pledgets. Small leaflet retractors are used to provide additional exposure. The precise functional and pathologic anatomy is assessed. Saline is injected into the ventricles to assess the coaptation relationships between the inferior and superior leaflets.

A 6-0 Prolene stay suture is used to approximate the left superior and left inferior leaflets just at the level of the ventricular septum, which should be a landmark for the establishment of the future common annulus (Fig. 20-7). It is often necessary to divide the left superior and/or left inferior leaflets for better exposure and a more secure closure of the ventricular septal defect. Any secondary chordal attachments to the ventricular septum that may interfere with closure of the defect are divided, although usually these attachments can be preserved and the patch secured on the right ventricular side of the crest below them. An appropriately sized, semicircular Dacron velour patch is sutured with double-armed 5-0 Prolene to the right ventricular aspect of the ventricular septum (usually starting in the middle). This first bite may be buttressed with a pledget (Fig. 20-7).

PREVENTION OF HEART BLOCK

The course of the atrioventricular node and His's bundle are described in the Surgical Anatomy of the Tricuspid Valve and the Right Ventricle section in Chapter 8. Suturing of the patch to the ventricular septum

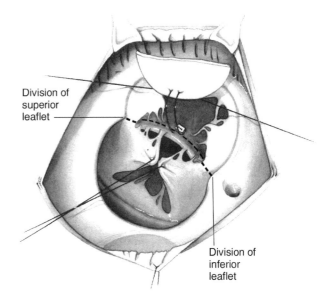

FIG. 20-7. Repair of a ventricular septal defect in a complete atrioventricular defect. Dotted line shows proposed division of the inferior and superior leaflets.

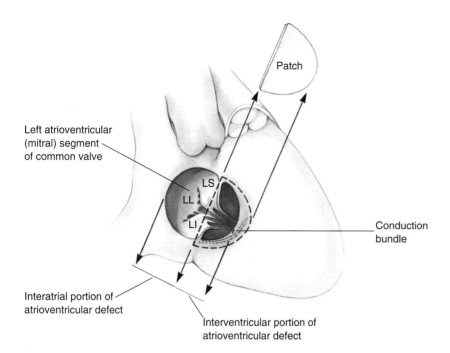

Left atrioventricular (mitral) segment of common valve

LS
LL
LI

Patch

Conduction bundle

Interatrial portion of atrioventricular defect

Interventricular portion of atrioventricular defect

FIG. 20-8. Diagrammatic view of a complete atrioventricular defect from the right. The tricuspid or right half of the common valve and the remainder of the right side of the heart have been removed to show the dimensions for sizing the interventricular patch. The upper edge of the patch suspends the leaflets at the level of their annuli, and the lower edge extends below the muscular crest on the right side of the interventricular defect so that suturing will not injure the conducting bundle. LS, left superior; LL, left lateral; LI, left inferior.

should be well beyond the rim of the ventricular septal defect so as not to produce any conduction injury.

Gentle traction on the suture facilitates suturing in both directions until the superior and inferior annuli are reached. The needles are then brought out through the leaflets superiorly and inferiorly, and both ends of the suture tagged.

 HEIGHT OF THE INTERVENTRICULAR SEPTAL PATCH
Resuspension of the valve leaflets at the appropriate level is critical. Therefore, the height of the ventricular septal defect patch is of paramount importance (Fig. 20-8).

A large patch of pericardium is then appropriately tailored to cover the atrial septal defect. The suture line that crosses the common atrioventricular valve incorporates leaflet tissue as well as the Dacron velour patch used to close the ventricular septal defect. A continuous over-and-over suture is used if the leaflet has not been divided. If the leaflet tissue has been divided, particular care must be taken to incorporate both sides of the leaflet tissue, i.e., left and right atrioventricular valve tissue, as well as the interventricular Dacron velour patch and the interatrial pericardial patch. This is best accomplished with several horizontal mattress sutures of 6-0 Prolene passed first through the tricuspid leaflet component, then through the upper edge of the Dacron patch, then through the mitral leaflet tissue, and finally through the bottom edge of the pericardial patch. All the sutures are placed and tagged separately, then the pericardial patch is lowered into place and the sutures tied.

 DEFORMATION OF THE LEAFLET ANATOMY
Overzealous incorporation of the atrioventricular leaflet tissue in suturing may shorten the height of the leaflet and produce valvular incompetence.

Once continuity of the ventricular and atrial patches has been established, the atrial patch is drawn into the right atrial cavity, and the cleft between the left superior and inferior leaflets is approximated with interrupted sutures bringing the kissing edges together. The left atrioventricular valve is again tested for competence by injecting saline into the left ventricle (Fig. 20-9A). Leakage at the inferolateral or superolateral commissure may be controlled with pericardial pledgeted sutures placed at the corresponding commissure to accomplish a mitral annuloplasty (Fig. 20-9B). Trivial central regurgitant flow can be accepted, but every effort should be made to achieve most competent valve possible. Sometimes a suture annuloplasty using a double-armed 5-0 Prolene suture along the mitral annulus from commissure to commissure achieves the best results. A pericardial pledget is placed at both ends of the double suture line, and the suture is tied over a Hegar's dilator, which is the Z-zero mitral diameter for the patient's size (Fig. 20-9C).

The correct height of the pericardial patch is then carefully gauged, and the patch is trimmed accordingly. The pericardial patch is then sewn to the edges of the atrial septal defect, leaving the coronary sinus on either its left or right side, as described for repair of an ostium primum defect (Figs. 20-5B and 20-6). This is achieved by a continuous suture of 5-0 or 6-0 Prolene. Should the coronary sinus be left in the right atrium, care must be taken to take superficial bites near the conduction tissue.

HIGH LEFT ATRIAL PRESSURE

After separation from cardiopulmonary bypass, the left atrial pressure may be elevated secondary to mitral valve incompetence or left ventricular dysfunction. If the coronary sinus has been placed on the left atrial side of the patch, this high pressure may interfere with coronary arterial perfusion.

NB *VALVULAR COMPETENCE*

Residual severe valvular incompetence is most deleterious. It is sometimes better to overcorrect and produce mild stenosis than to accept even mild mitral valve insufficiency.

 INCORRECT HEIGHT OF PATCHES

A perfect valvular repair can be distorted, leading to mitral valve incompetence if either the ventricular or atrial septal patch is too tall or too short.

One-Patch Technique

Before cannulation, a large piece of pericardium is harvested, placed in glutaraldehyde, and rinsed in saline. After the right atrium is opened, the leaflets are assessed by filling the ventricles with saline. Coaptation of the superior and inferior leaflets overlying the ventricular septum is evaluated. A 6-0 Prolene suture is placed at the leading edges of the inferior and superior leaflets to determine the point of partition of the common atrioventricular valve into left- and right-sided valves.

The distance between the two points on opposite sides of the annulus where the ventricular septal crest meets the atrioventricular groove is measured. This determines the width of the patch at the annular level. If the patch is too wide, the left atrioventricular valve annulus will be increased, and this may lead to mitral regurgitation. If the left atrioventricular valve tissue is believed to be insufficient, then the width of the patch should be less than the measured distance between the two points on the annulus. This will reduce the size of the left atrioventricular valve annulus and, it is hoped, create a competent valve.

Leaflet incisions are nearly always required in the superior and inferior leaflets to allow placement of the pericardial patch. The leaflets should be incised in a line parallel with and overlying the ventricular septal crest, with the incision extending to the level of the annulus (Fig. 20-10).

 INADEQUATE LEFT-SIDED VALVE TISSUE

The superior and inferior leaflets should be divided somewhat on the right ventricular side to ensure

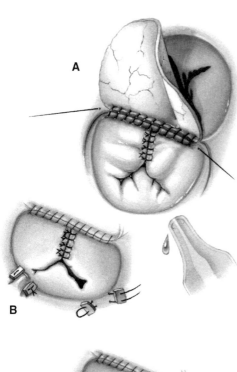

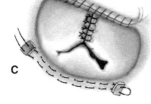

FIG. 20-9. A: Atrial patch with the completed suture line across the common atrioventricular valve. **B:** Mitral annuloplasty with pledgeted sutures at the commissures. **C:** Suture annuloplasty tied over appropriately sized Hegar's dilator.

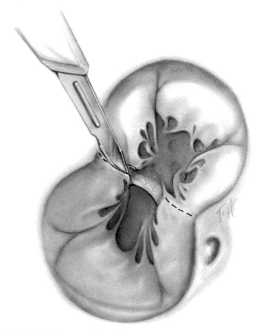

FIG. 20-10. Division of leaflets overlying the ventricular septal crest.

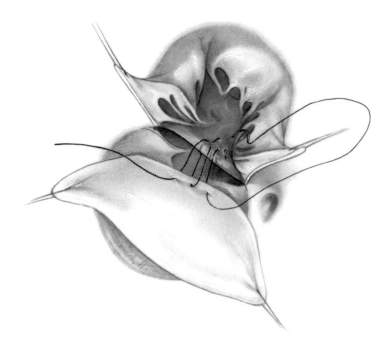

FIG. 20-11. Attaching a pericardial patch to the right ventricular aspect of the defect.

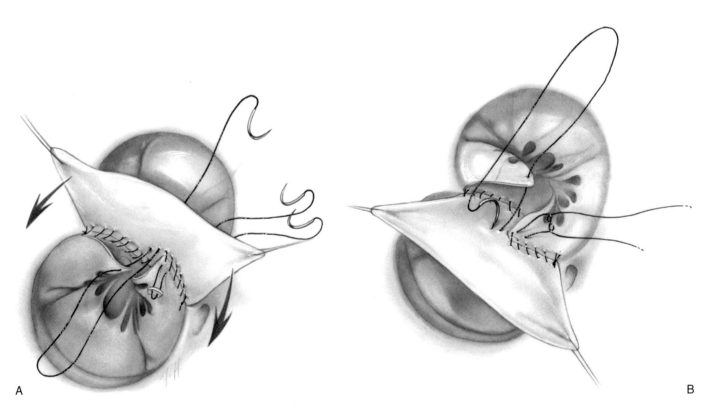

A

B

FIG. 20-12. Attaching mitral and tricuspid valve components to the pericardial patch. Running suture is completed inferiorly and interrupted reinforcing mattress sutures are placed from the left side through the mitral component, patch, and then tricuspid component and tied on the right side. **A:** Left-sided view. **B:** Right-sided view.

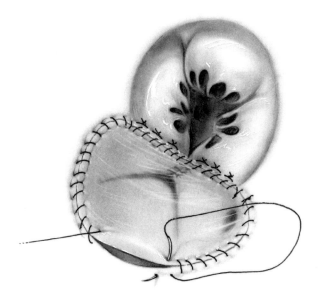

FIG. 20-13. The remainder of the pericardial patch is used to close the atrial septal defect.

adequate left-sided leaflet tissue for a competent mitral valve.

The pericardial patch is attached to the right ventricular aspect of the defect beginning in the midportion and continuing the suture line in a running fashion, weaving in and out of the chordal attachments. The suture line is continued along the septal crest until the annulus of the atrioventricular valve is reached (Fig. 20-11). This suture line is accomplished with a running 5-0 Prolene suture. With the two ends of this running suture on tension, the pericardial patch is held up within the atrium and the leaflets are suspended from the patch at an appropriate level so that valve competence is preserved. This should correspond with the leaflet level when the chordal structures are under slight tension. The left- (mitral) and right- (tricuspid) sided valve components are reattached to the pericardial patch initially with a running 6-0 Prolene suture that is secured on both ends of the patch by tying it to the previously placed 5-0 Prolene stitch. The leaflet attachment to the pericardium is then reinforced with multiple pericardial pledgeted horizontal mattress sutures of 5-0 or 6-0 Prolene (Fig. 20-12A, B). Traction sutures on the upper edges of the pericardial patch allow the surgeon to deflect the patch back and forth to visualize the left and then the right side of the repair.

The cleft between the superior and inferior leaflet components of the left atrioventricular valve is approximated with interrupted sutures as described above. The left atrioventricular valve is again tested with saline, and any areas of regurgitation are noted and repaired as discussed in the Two-Patch Technique section. The remainder of the pericardial patch is then secured to the atrial septal defect as described previously (Fig. 20-13).

COMPLETION OF THE OPERATION

The right atriotomy is closed with a running 6-0 or 5-0 Prolene suture. If the operation has been performed on cardiopulmonary bypass, rewarming is begun during closure of the atrial septal defect component; after closing the right atrium, the heart is filled, the aortic cross-clamp is removed, and deairing procedures are performed. If the operation has been accomplished under circulatory arrest, the heart is filled with saline after closing the right atriotomy, cardiopulmonary bypass is recommenced, the aortic cross-clamp is removed while deairing through the ascending aorta, and rewarming is carried out in the usual fashion.

CHAPTER 21

Right Ventricular Outflow Tract Obstruction

The right ventricular outflow tract includes the right ventricular outlet chamber (or the infundibulum); the pulmonary valve; the main, right, and left pulmonary arteries; and the peripheral pulmonary arterial branches. Obstruction can occur at any specific site or involve many segments of the right ventricular outflow tract. Obstruction of the right ventricular outflow tract is commonly associated with other cardiac anomalies.

DOUBLE-CHAMBERED RIGHT VENTRICLE

This consists of an hypertrophied muscle band creating obstruction between the inlet and infundibular portion of the right ventricle. A prominent, acute marginal branch of the right coronary artery often overlies the area of obstruction. Most often, a double-chambered right ventricle is associated with the perimembranous type ventriculoseptal defect.

Technique for Repair

Cardiopulmonary bypass with bicaval cannulation is used. After aortic cross-clamping and cardioplegia delivery, a transverse right ventriculotomy is made just superior to the suspected obstructing muscle band (Fig. 21-1A). This can most often be identified by the associated enlarged coronary branch, external palpation of the right ventricle, or careful pressure measurements before beginning cardiopulmonary bypass. By retracting the inferior margin of the ventriculotomy, a circular opening can be seen, often covered with fibrous tissue. This obstruction is incised anteriorly initially. After identifying the papillary muscles of the tricuspid valve, the remainder of the obstructing muscle is resected. The accompanying ventriculoseptal defect should now be apparent. This ventriculoseptal defect may be closed through the right ventriculotomy or through a separate right atrial incision, working through the tricuspid valve (see Chapter 19). The right ventriculotomy is then closed with a running 5-0 Prolene suture.

 MISIDENTIFYING THE VENTRICULOSEPTAL DEFECT
The circular opening visualized through the right ventriculotomy may, on first examination, appear to be the ventriculoseptal defect. Care must be taken to identify the location of the tricuspid valve to avoid this mistake.

TETRALOGY OF FALLOT

An anatomic anomaly consisting of a ventriculoseptal defect, right ventricular outflow tract obstruction with resultant right ventricular hypertrophy, and dextroposition of the aorta was described by Fallot in 1888. These children usually present with mild to moderate cyanosis and may have intermittent hypoxic spells.

The anatomy must be accurately defined to plan the management of these patients. Echocardiography can demonstrate the presence of additional ventriculoseptal defects, can usually delineate the initial course of the right and left coronary arteries, and can size the main and proximal right and left pulmonary arteries. Cardiac catheterization is reserved for those patients in whom the echocardiographic diagnosis is incomplete, when aortopulmonary collateral vessels are suspected, or for patients with previous palliative procedures.

Staged Approach

Although several centers have reported satisfactory results with complete repair of tetralogy of Fallot in neonates, the general approach has been to perform a shunt procedure initially in patients who become symptomatic within the first month of life. These patients often have small pulmonary arteries and may be ductal dependent. Three percent to 5% of patients with tetralogy of Fallot have an anomalous left anterior descending coronary artery arising from the right coronary artery. The course of the left anterior descending coronary artery

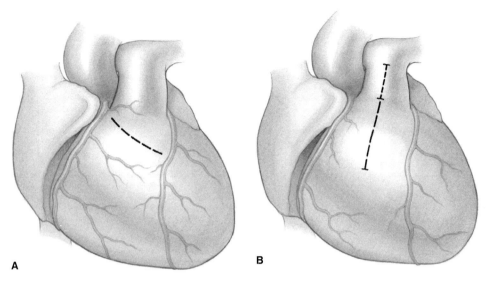

FIG. 21-1. A, B: Types of ventriculotomy.

across the right ventricular outflow tract interferes with an appropriate ventriculotomy to relieve the obstruction. These patients probably should undergo an initial shunt procedure because they will ultimately require a right ventricular to pulmonary artery conduit as part of their repair, which is ideally delayed until age 1 or 2 years (see Chapter 16).

Technique for Complete Repair

A median sternotomy provides excellent exposure. A generous patch of autologous pericardium is harvested, attached with Ligaclips to a cardboard from a suture pack, placed in 0.6% glutaraldehyde solution for 6 to 8 minutes, and then rinsed in saline. Such treatment fixes the pericardium and thereby lessens the chances of aneurysmal dilation of the patch. Except in very small infants in whom deep hypothermic arrest may be used, standard bicaval and aortic cannulation is used to initiate cardiopulmonary bypass. A vent is placed through the right superior pulmonary vein into the left ventricle. Systemic cooling to 28°C is achieved, the aorta is clamped, and cold blood cardioplegic solution is infused into the aortic root (see Chapter 3). If it is believed that a right ventricular outflow tract patch will not be required, the ventriculoseptal defect and infundibulum of the right ventricle as well as the pulmonary valve annulus can be explored through the right atrium. Tapes around the venae cavae are snugged down, and an oblique right atriotomy is made. The ventriculoseptal defect and right ventricular outflow tract are evaluated through the tricuspid valve. If the pulmonary annulus is of adequate size, the ventriculoseptal defect and hypertrophied infundibular muscle may be resected through the right atrium. Otherwise, a

right ventriculotomy provides excellent exposure and is the approach of choice. A vertical right ventriculotomy is made, and the edges are retracted with pledgeted sutures (Fig. 21-1B). The hypertrophied infundibular muscle bundles are carefully but aggressively excised (Fig. 21-2). The large malalignment type of ventriculoseptal defect now comes into view.

The margins of the defect are inspected, and an interrupted, fine, pledgeted, double-armed 5-0 braided suture is started at the 12-o'clock position along the muscular rim in an everting fashion. Both needles are then passed through a patch of Dacron velour that is slightly larger than the defect (Fig. 21-3). Slight traction on this stitch by the assistant improves exposure and facilitates the placement of the next stitch (Fig. 21-4).

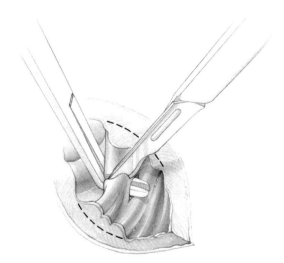

FIG. 21-2. Resection of infundibular muscle bands.

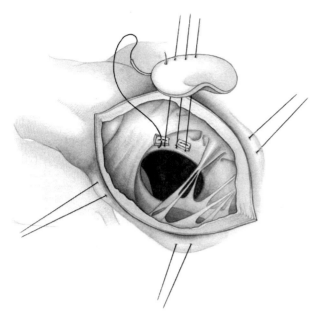

FIG. 21-3. Stepwise technique for the closure of a ventricular septal defect by interrupted sutures (see text).

Suturing is continued in this fashion in a counterclockwise direction along the superior rim, which overlies the aortic valve, until the central fibrous junction of the septum, aortic root, and tricuspid annulus is reached. Both needles of the next pledgeted, interrupted suture incorporate the muscular rim of the defect, the patch, and the tricuspid leaflet (in that order). Depending on the consistency of the tricuspid leaflet, the needles may be passed through another pledget before they are tied. The suturing process is then continued from the starting point in a clockwise direction, moving outward to a distance of 3 to 5 mm from the rim of the defect to avoid the underlying conduction tissue.

The alternative technique of taking very shallow bites that include only endocardium in the region of the inferior rim may also be used. Where the tricuspid annulus becomes part of the inferior rim of the defect, both needles of the pledgeted, interrupted suture take shallow bites of the thickened endocardium, the patch, the tricuspid valve, and another pledget (in that order). The remaining sutures are passed from the right atrium through the tricuspid leaflet approximately 2 mm from the annulus before passing through the patch. When all the sutures are satisfactorily placed, the patch is lowered into position and the sutures are snugly tied (Fig. 21-5). Alternatively, the Dacron velour patch is anchored with a continuous suture of 5-0 Prolene. The continuous suture technique takes less time and is the preferred technique as long as the exposure of the defect is satisfactory. With this technique, traction on the patch by the assistant facilitates placement of the next stitch. Suturing begins at the 1-o'clock position and continues clockwise around the tricuspid annulus where shallow bites of thickened endocardium are taken up to the aortic annulus where the suture is tagged at the 8-o'clock position (Fig. 21-6). The other needle is then used to complete the suture line.

Another option is to close the ventriculoseptal defect through the right atrial approach before opening the right ventricle. In some cases with marked overriding of the aorta, the inferior portion of the ventriculoseptal defect can be approached through the right atrium and the superior sutures placed through the right ventriculotomy.

 RESIDUAL VENTRICULOSEPTAL DEFECT
The edges of the patch are carefully checked for a residual ventriculoseptal defect. Additional sutures buttressed with pledgets are used to close any small residual defects.

 INJURY TO THE AORTIC VALVE
The aortic valve leaflets are immediately below the superior margin of the defect and can be punctured

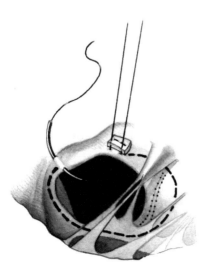

FIG. 21-4. Exposure is improved by gentle traction on the previously placed stitch.

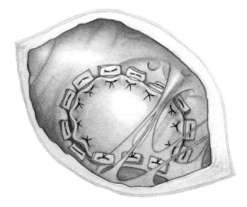

FIG. 21-5. Completion of a patch closure of a ventricular septal defect using the interrupted suture technique.

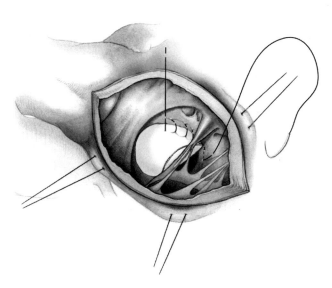

FIG. 21-6. Continuous suture technique for the closure of a ventricular septal defect through a right ventriculotomy.

during suturing if deep needle bites are taken in this area (Fig. 21-7). Suturing in this area should therefore incorporate the crista marginalis, which holds sutures well.

🚫 PREVENTION OF HEART BLOCK

As already described, His's bundle pierces the central fibrous body and the tricuspid annulus before crossing into the ventricular septum and follows a course along the inferior margin of the defect toward the left ventricular side of the septum. Because suturing along this course can be somewhat hazardous and culminate in heart block, shallow superficial bites including only the whitish endocardium 3 to 5 mm from the rim of the defect are taken.

NB *TRANSITIONAL SUTURES*

The junction where the tricuspid annulus forms the margin of the defect is also most vulnerable to residual septal defect. A transitional stitch incorporating a shallow bite of the thickened endocardium, the patch, and the tricuspid leaflet (in that order) ensures a more secure closure.

🚫 *BUTTRESSING THE SUTURES*

The Prolene suture may cut through the thin and friable tricuspid leaflet tissue. The suture line can be buttressed with multiple pledgets or a strip of Teflon felt or autologous pericardium.

The pulmonary valve and annulus are evaluated with Hegar's dilators. Pulmonary valvotomy is carried out by bringing the pulmonary valve leaflets downward into the ventriculotomy. Alternatively, a separate vertical incision is made in the main pulmonary artery and the valvotomy performed from above.

The orifices of the right and left pulmonary arteries are then evaluated. If stenosis of the takeoff of the left pulmonary artery is noted, the pulmonary arteriotomy can be carried out onto the left pulmonary artery as far as necessary to adequately relieve the stenosis. If narrowing of the right pulmonary artery is noted, this may be best handled by extending the pulmonary arteriotomy onto the anterior surface of the right pulmonary artery behind the aorta. In this case, a separate rectangular patch is used to enlarge the opening of the right and left pulmonary arteries (Fig. 21-8).

If the annulus is of adequate size, the pulmonary arteriotomy may be closed primarily with running 6-0 Prolene suture or closed with an appropriately sized patch of autologous pericardium to enlarge the main or left pulmonary arteries, as indicated. When used to enlarge the left pulmonary artery, the patch should be tailored with a

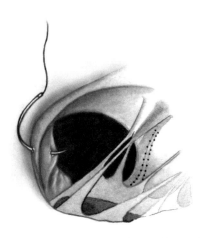

FIG. 21-7. Proximity of an aortic valve leaflet to the rim of a septal defect.

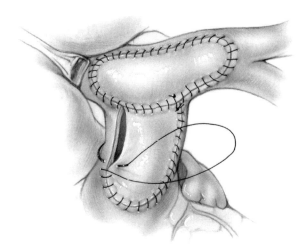

FIG. 21-8. Two-patch technique to enlarge the proximal right and left pulmonary arteries.

squared-off end to provide optimal enlargement. A double-armed 5-0 or 6-0 Prolene suture is placed through the patch and the left pulmonary artery at the toe of the anastomosis several times before lowering the patch into position. The right ventriculotomy is then closed with an oval patch of autologous pericardium or GORE-TEX, using running 5-0 Prolene sutures.

 ### COMPRESSION OF RIGHT PULMONARY ARTERY AUGMENTATION

The separate patch used to enlarge the opening of the right pulmonary artery may be compressed by the ascending aorta. Reinforced GORE-TEX patch material tailored from a large reinforced GORE-TEX tube graft has been used in such cases but may erode into the ascending aorta and therefore should probably not be used.

If the size of the annulus is not adequate, a transannular patch is required. Many surgeons use a patch with a monocusp valve made from pericardium, GORE-TEX, or excised from a large pulmonary homograft (Fig. 21-9A). The patch may extend only onto the proximal main pulmonary artery if the right and left pulmonary arteries are of adequate size (Fig. 21-9B). Often, however, the distal main artery and the origin of the left pulmonary artery are small and the transannular incision is extended out onto the left pulmonary artery (Fig. 21-10A). The patch should be tailored in such a way that the new pulmonary artery dimension is equal to or slightly larger than the Z-zero value for the pulmonary valve based on the patient's body surface area. When a monocusp is used, the patch is tailored so that the position of the valve leaflet is at the level of the patients annulus (Fig. 21-9A). The patch is sewn into place starting at the distal pulmonary arterial opening, using running 6-0 or 5-0 Prolene suture. If a standard pericardial patch is used, it may be useful to place the correct size of a Hegar's dilator into the new main pulmonary artery as the patch reaches the level of the pulmonary valve annulus. The patch can then be trimmed to fit snugly over the Hegar's dilator at this level as it is being sewn into place (Fig. 21-10B).

At this point, systemic rewarming is begun. If an atrial septal defect or patent foramen ovale is present, it is now closed, and if the right atrium has been opened, it is also closed. Venting of the ascending aorta is carried out as the aortic cross-clamp is removed. If the surgery has been performed under hypothermic arrest, the circulation may be resumed after closure of the ventriculoseptal defect, and the right ventricular outflow tract reconstruction can be performed while rewarming is proceeding.

NB SURGERY IN NEONATES

In neonates, the patent foramen ovale is generally left open. If pulmonary hypertension and/or right ventricular dysfunction occur in the postoperative period, right-to-left shunting at the atrial level can maintain left-sided filling pressures and adequate systemic cardiac output. The consequent desaturation is usually well tolerated. Because neonates have no secondary right ventricular hypertrophy, resection of muscle mass from the right ventricular outflow tract should be minimal.

At the end of cardiopulmonary bypass, pressures in the right ventricle, pulmonary artery, and left ventricle are measured directly or estimated by transesophageal echocardiography. The right ventricular pressure should be less than 70% of left ventricular pressure. If the right ventricular pressure is greater than this and a transannu-

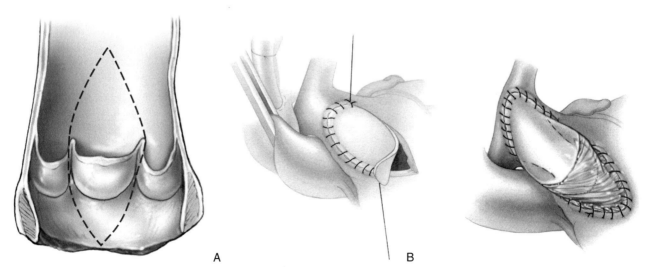

FIG. 21-9. Enlargement of a pulmonary valve annulus. **A and C:** With a monocusp patch. **B:** With a pericardial patch.

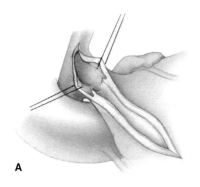

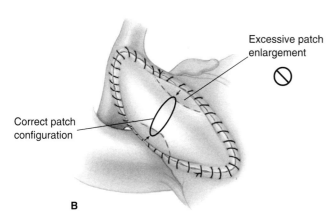

FIG. 21-10. Patch enlargement of the right ventricular outflow tract (see text). **A:** Extension of a pulmonary arteriotomy onto the left pulmonary artery. **B:** Correct patch configuration.

lar patch has not been placed, cardiopulmonary bypass should be recommenced and a transannular patch placed. If a transannular patch has been used, the site of obstruction should be localized by echocardiography or multiple pressure measurements proximal to, along the length of the patch, and distal to the right ventricular outflow tract patch. If a correctable obstruction is identified, cardiopulmonary bypass should be recommenced and the right ventricular outflow reconstruction should be revised. If the right ventricular pressure remains high despite these interventions and the patient is unstable, consideration should be given to creating a small atrial septal defect or a hole in the ventriculoseptal defect patch. This can be done on cardiopulmonary bypass during a brief period of aortic cross-clamping.

POOR EXPOSURE OF THE BRANCH PULMONARY ARTERIES

Before placing the patient on cardiopulmonary bypass, the main and right pulmonary arteries must be dissected completely free from the aorta. This allows the aortic cross-clamp to be applied in such a way as to not limit exposure or distort the distal main pulmonary artery and right pulmonary artery takeoff.

WIDTH OF THE OUTFLOW TRACT PATCH

The width of the patch across the pulmonary annulus must be generous enough to eliminate most of the gradient between the right ventricle and pulmonary artery. It is better to accept a mild to moderate gradient than to create wide open pulmonic insufficiency. The new annulus diameter should not be much greater than the Z-zero pulmonary annulus size for the patient.

STENOSIS OF THE DISTAL PATCH

The toe of the patch must be oval or square to minimize the risk of subsequent anastomotic stenosis.

PULMONARY ATRESIA AND VENTRICULOSEPTAL DEFECT

The intracardiac anatomy of pulmonary atresia and a ventriculoseptal defect resembles that of tetralogy of Fallot, except that there is no connection between the right ventricular outflow tract and pulmonary artery. There is a wide range of anatomic subtypes, ranging from those patients with well-developed pulmonary arteries connected to all bronchopulmonary segments, to those with hypoplastic pulmonary arteries in whom aortopulmonary collateral arteries are important sources of pulmonary blood flow, to the group of patients in whom no true mediastinal pulmonary arteries are present. In this last group of patients, all bronchopulmonary segments are supplied exclusively by aortopulmonary collateral arteries.

To plan the surgical approach in these patients, it is important to identify all aortopulmonary collateral arteries at the time of cardiac catheterization. Smaller aortopulmonary collateral arteries may be embolized in the cardiac catheterization laboratory. Larger collateral vessels that supply a significant area of lung parenchyma must be detached from the aorta and anastomosed to a branch of the pulmonary artery, so-called unifocalization. This process may require one or more thoracotomies to incorporate as many aortopulmonary collateral arteries as possible before complete repair. Alternatively, unifocalization of collaterals to both lungs can be performed at one setting through a clamshell incision with the option of connecting the unifocalized pulmonary arteries to the right ventricle with a homograft conduit with or without closure of the ventricular septal defect.

Patients with well-developed pulmonary arteries are usually dependent on a patent ductus arteriosus for adequate pulmonary blood flow. These infants require treatment with prostaglandin E_1 and a shunt procedure as a neonate (see Chapter 16). Complete repair can then be performed at 1 to 2 years of age.

Patients with hypoplastic, confluent pulmonary arteries may undergo an initial modified Blalock-Taussig shunt procedure (see Chapter 16). Better pulmonary artery growth may be achieved by early establishment of forward pulmonary blood flow from the right ventricle. This may be accomplished by performing a patch augmentation of the right ventricular outflow tract onto the main pulmonary artery across the atretic segment without cardiopulmonary bypass, which is a somewhat dangerous technique. Alternatively, a pulmonary artery homograft can be inserted between the right ventricle and pulmonary artery confluence using cardiopulmonary bypass, leaving the ventriculoseptal defect open.

STEAL PHENOMENON

If large aortopulmonary collateral arteries are not temporarily or permanently occluded before commencing cardiopulmonary bypass, a large amount of arterial blood return will run off through these vessels, creating low perfusion pressure to vital organ systems including the brain. This may lead to serious central nervous system deficits.

VENTRICULAR DISTENTION

If flow from the aortopulmonary collateral arteries has not been completely controlled, the excessive blood return to the left ventricle causes left ventricular distention. Therefore, a vent placed through the right superior pulmonary vein into the left atrium and left ventricle is usually required.

Complete repair in patients with absent true pulmonary arteries and large aortopulmonary collateral arteries can only be performed if adequate unifocalization of vessels supplying the majority of bronchopulmonary segments has been achieved. The repair then consists of connecting the unifocalized segments, closing the ventriculoseptal defect, and placing a valved conduit from the right ventricle to this connection.

Technique for Complete Repair

Standard aortic and bicaval cannulation is performed. Before commencing cardiopulmonary bypass, any previously placed systemic to pulmonary artery shunts are dissected. As cardiopulmonary bypass is being initiated, the shunt is occluded, usually with one or two large Ligaclips. The intraventricular repair is carried out as for tetralogy of Fallot (see previously). If the distance from the right ventricular outflow tract to the main pulmonary artery is less than 1.0 cm, the right ventriculotomy is extended across the atretic segment onto the main pulmonary artery (Fig. 21-10A). Any stenoses of the left and right pulmonary arteries are managed as described previously for tetralogy of Fallot. A rectangular graft of autologous pericardium or GORE-TEX or a monocusp patch is used to close the opening in the pulmonary artery and right ventricle, using running 5-0 or 6-0 Prolene suture and placing the stitches through the epicardial edges of

the incised atretic connection between the right ventricle and pulmonary artery. If the distance between the top of the right ventricle and pulmonary artery is too great or the pulmonary arteries are small, a homograft valve conduit is used. A valve conduit is also necessary if an anomalous left anterior descending artery from the coronary artery crosses the right ventricular outflow tract, precluding a transannular patch. In this case, before aortic cross-clamping, the pulmonary artery confluence must be dissected free of the aorta. An appropriately sized aortic or pulmonary homograft is then prepared. The distal main pulmonary artery or pulmonary artery confluence is then opened, and the distal anastomosis performed in an end-to-end fashion between the homograft and pulmonary artery, using a running 6-0 Prolene technique. The proximal end of the homograft is then sewn directly to the upper margin of the right ventriculotomy incision. Suturing is begun at the heel of the anastomosis and continued on both sides of the homograft until one-third to one-half of the circumference of the homograft has been anastomosed to the right ventricular opening. A hood-shaped patch of autologous pericardium or GORE-TEX is then sewn to the anterior portion of the homograft circumference and to the remaining opening in the right ventricle, using running 5-0 or 6-0 Prolene suture (see Figs. 25-5 through 25-8 in Chapter 25). The remainder of the procedure is completed as for tetralogy of Fallot.

GRADIENT ACROSS TRANSANNULAR PATCH

The patch must be sufficiently generous in the area of the atretic segment to ensure that an adequately sized Hegar's dilator can pass through the completed pericardial tube graft that results from this anastomosis.

HYPOPLASTIC PULMONARY ARTERY CONFLUENCE

Small confluent pulmonary arteries should be opened widely, extending the incision on the anterior surface of the left and right pulmonary arteries out to the hila of both lungs. A separate rectangular patch of autologous pericardium is then anastomosed to the edges of this opening, using running 6-0 or 5-0 Prolene suture. The distal end of the homograft is then inserted into an opening in the patch itself. Alternatively, a pulmonary artery homograft can be used, and the bifurcation portion of the homograft can be used to augment the hypoplastic pulmonary-arterial confluence.

ANEURYSM OF A PULMONARY HOMOGRAFT

If distal pulmonary artery stenoses are present, the thin-walled pulmonary homograft may dilate and even become aneurysmal. In these cases, an aortic homograft may be preferable.

REOPERATION FOR A FAILED HOMOGRAFT

Both aortic and pulmonary homografts may calcify and become stenotic. Recent information suggests that pulmonary homografts remain unobstructed for a longer period of time.

Absent Pulmonary Valve Syndrome

Absent pulmonary valve syndrome occurs in approximately 3% of cases with tetralogy of Fallot. Characteristically, there is failure of development of the pulmonary valve leaflets. The pulmonary valve annulus is normal or somewhat small, but the central pulmonary arteries are massively dilated. Patients who present as neonates or infants have severe respiratory symptoms related to compression of the main stem bronchi by the aneurysmal central pulmonary arteries. These infants require urgent surgical attention. Older children may have few if any symptoms and can be operated on electively. Complete surgical correction consists of closure of the ventriculoseptal defect, plication of the enlarged portions of the pulmonary artery, and placement of a homograft between the right ventricle and pulmonary artery.

Technique

A median sternotomy is performed, and most of the thymus gland is removed to aid in exposure of the central pulmonary arteries. A patch of pericardium is harvested and fixed with 0.6% glutaraldehyde solution. The aorta is then dissected free from the main and right pulmonary arteries, and the pulmonary arteries are mobilized out to the hilum of the lung on each side. Aortic cannulation is performed near the takeoff of the innominate artery on the right-hand side of the aorta to keep the cannula away from the operative site. Bicaval cannulation is performed, and cardiopulmonary bypass is established. Systemic cooling to 28°C is carried out. The aorta is cross-clamped, and cardioplegic arrest of the heart is achieved by infusion of cold blood cardioplegic solution into the aortic root. A high vertical right ventriculotomy is made that can be extended if the need arises. The hypertrophied infundibular muscles are divided and resected. This brings the ventricular septal defect into view, and its closure is thus facilitated and subsequently completed as described earlier. The abnormally enlarged main pulmonary artery is then dissected free posteriorly and transected just above the pulmonary valve annulus and divided distally at the level of its bifurcation, resecting redundant portions of the inferior wall of both the right and left pulmonary arteries (Fig. 21-11). The defect on the right and left pulmonary arteries is then partially closed with running 6-0 or 5-0 Prolene sutures. These suture lines are continued until the area of confluence of the pulmonary arteries is reached, leaving an opening

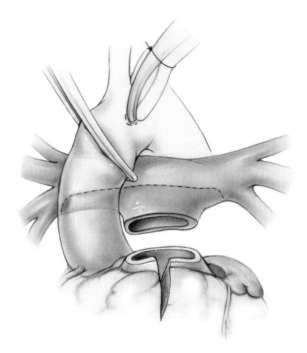

FIG. 21-11. Absent pulmonary valve syndrome: ventriculotomy and resection of dilated portions of main and branch pulmonary arteries.

large enough to accommodate the appropriately sized homograft. The suture lines are then secured with an additional interrupted suture (Fig. 21-12).

The homograft is then prepared, and the distal anastomosis to the opening in the pulmonary artery is com-

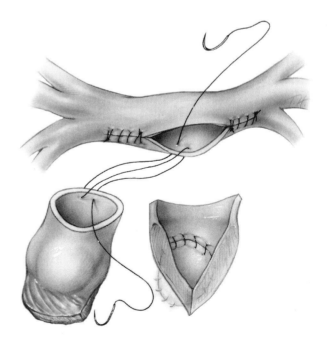

FIG. 21-12. Absent pulmonary valve syndrome: reconstruction of the right and left pulmonary arteries and insertion of a homograft.

pleted with continuous 5-0 Prolene suture. The proximal end of the homograft is then tailored and sewn to the transected pulmonary valve annulus, using running 6-0 or 5-0 Prolene sutures. The suture line is continued around to the anterior edges of the right ventriculotomy where it is secured with an additional interrupted suture. The resulting defect between the homograft and the right ventriculotomy is covered with a hood-shaped patch of autologous pericardium or GORE-TEX, which is then anastomosed to the anterior portion of the homograft and edges of the right ventriculotomy. The remainder of the procedure is completed as described for tetralogy of Fallot (see previously).

KINKING OF THE HOMOGRAFT
The homograft should not be left too long because this causes it to kink and create a gradient from the right ventricle to the pulmonary artery.

RESIDUAL AIRWAY OBSTRUCTION
The pressurized posterior wall of the pulmonary artery confluence may continue to compress the main stem bronchi after surgery. The bifurcation should be dissected completely away from the underlying posterior structures, and any fibrous bands between the pulmonary artery and bronchi should be divided.

COMPRESSION OF THE HOMOGRAFT BY THE STERNUM
If reapproximating the two sternal edges appears to compress the homograft, the sternotomy should be

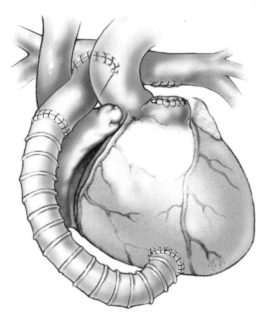

FIG. 21-13. Placement of a homograft with a tube graft extension from the diaphragmatic surface of the right ventricle along the right atrium to the right pulmonary artery. Oversewing of the native right ventricular outflow tract.

reopened and the left pleural cavity opened widely. This allows the homograft to shift toward the left where it will not be compressed by sternal closure. If it appears at the time of surgery that the homograft will lie immediately under the sternum, the operation can be planned to avoid compression. One approach is to sew the distal end of the homograft onto an opening in the left pulmonary artery rather than the confluence. A second option is to use an aortic rather than a pulmonary homograft and orient the homograft so that the curve lies toward the left-hand side. Finally, the homograft extended by a tube graft can be anastomosed to a separate opening on the diaphragmatic surface of the right ventricle, positioned along the right atrium and sewn into an opening on the right pulmonary artery (Fig. 21-13).

PULMONARY ATRESIA, INTACT VENTRICULAR SEPTUM

Patients usually present with cyanosis on the first day of life. Prostaglandin E_1 is begun to maintain patency of the ductus arteriosus. The diagnosis is made by echocardiography, which demonstrates the size of the right ventricular cavity, the size and competence of the tricuspid valve, the size of the pulmonary arteries, and the size of the interatrial communication. The size of the right ventricle in this anomaly ranges from diminutive to larger than normal. Ten percent of patients have major obstructions of one or more coronary arteries with fistulous communications from the right ventricular cavity to the distal coronary arteries. Cardiac catheterization is required to identify these abnormalities of coronary circulation.

The initial management of these patients depends on the anatomy that is present. Patients with a small right ventricle whose tricuspid valve diameter is less than 6 to 8 mm should undergo a modified Blalock-Taussig shunt. Similarly, patients with enlarged right ventricles and severe tricuspid regurgitation and those with significant stenoses involving more than one of the three major epicardial coronary systems should also undergo a shunt procedure (see Chapter 16).

Patients with larger right ventricles and competent tricuspid valves should undergo a pulmonary valvotomy with or without patch enlargement of the outflow tract. If the right ventricle is only mildly hypoplastic, a concomitant systemic to pulmonary artery shunt may not be required. However, the majority of these patients are best served by combined pulmonary valvotomy or outflow tract patch and a GORE-TEX interposition shunt from the innominate artery to the proximal right pulmonary artery.

Surgical Technique

A median sternotomy incision is used. A piece of pericardium is harvested and prepared with 0.6% glutaraldehyde. If use of a monocusp patch is planned, an appropriate pulmonary homograft piece is now thawed. The aorta is cannulated, and a single straight or right-angled cannula is placed through the right atrial appendage for venous drainage. The ductus arteriosus is dissected and looped with a heavy silk tie. Cardiopulmonary bypass is commenced, and the ductus arteriosus is ligated. Because a patent foramen ovale is always present, the aorta should be cross-clamped and cardioplegia given to prevent systemic air embolism. Traction sutures are placed on the main pulmonary artery, and a vertical arteriotomy is performed. The pulmonary valve dimple is visualized; if the infundibulum is patent and the annulus is of good size, a valvotomy or valvectomy may be performed. Otherwise, the incision is carried down across the atretic annulus and onto the right ventricle. The previously prepared patch of pericardium or monocusp patch is sewn into place, using running 7-0 Prolene suture. The systemic to pulmonary artery shunt is constructed after removing the aortic cross-clamp. The right pulmonary artery between the aorta and superior vena cava is dissected, as is the takeoff of the innominate artery from the ascending aorta. A curved C clamp is then placed on the underside of the innominate artery, and a 3.5- or 4-mm GORE-TEX tube graft is cut in an oblique fashion. An incision is made on the anterior, inferior aspect of the innominate artery, and an end-to-side anastomosis, using running 7-0 Prolene suture, is performed between the GORE-TEX tube graft and the artery. The GORE-TEX tube graft is then trimmed to an appropriate length to just meet the superior aspect of the proximal right pulmonary artery. A second curved C clamp is placed on the most medial aspect of the right pulmonary artery, and an incision is made on the superior aspect of the pulmonary artery. The distal end of the GORE-TEX tube is anastomosed to this opening, using running 7-0 Prolene suture (see Chapter 16).

At this point, the heart is filled, ventilations are begun, and cardiopulmonary bypass is discontinued as the C clamps are removed. The patent foramen ovale is left open.

POSTOPERATIVE CYANOSIS

Right ventricular diastolic dysfunction increases right-to-left shunting at the atrial level across the patent foramen ovale. If transannular patching is performed without a shunt procedure, this may result in unacceptably low systemic oxygenation. If a shunt procedure is not performed, the ductus arteriosus should be left open and only temporarily occluded during cardiopulmonary bypass. Prostaglandin E_1 can be slowly withdrawn in the postoperative period and continued for as long as 3 to 4 weeks postoperatively, if required. If at the end of this period, inadequate oxygenation persists, the patient should be returned to the operating room for a systemic to pulmonary artery shunt.

Definitive Repair

At 1 to 2 years of age, these patients should be reevaluated in the cardiac catheterization laboratory. Patients with proven significant obstructive lesions in more than one of the major coronary arteries should be referred for cardiac transplantation or undergo a staged Fontan procedure (see Chapter 29). In other patients, the adequacy of the right ventricle and tricuspid valve needs to be evaluated. This can be accomplished by balloon occlusion of the intraatrial communication and the systemic to pulmonary artery shunt. If the right atrial pressure remains less than 20 mm Hg while maintaining an adequate systemic cardiac output, a two-ventricle system should be tolerated. If temporary occlusion of the septal opening and shunt is not tolerated, a Fontan procedure or a so-called one and one-half ventricular repair is indicated. The latter consists of combining a right ventricular to pulmonary artery connection with a bidirectional caval–pulmonary artery anastomosis (see Chapter 29).

For patients who can tolerate a two-ventricle approach, surgery consists of revising the right ventricular outflow patch if any residual obstruction is noted at the time of cardiac catheterization and closing the intraatrial communication and the systemic to pulmonary artery shunt (see Chapters 16 and 17). If the outflow patch is satisfactory, the atrial septal defect and shunt may be closed in the catheterization laboratory.

TRICUSPID REGURGITATION

If significant tricuspid regurgitation is present, a homograft valve should be placed in the right ventricular outflow tract and a tricuspid valve repair should be performed.

PULMONARY STENOSIS AND AN INTACT VENTRICULAR SEPTUM

Typically, the valve is dome shaped with its three leaflets fused, leaving a tiny central opening. Occasionally, the leaflets are thickened and dysplastic and produce obstruction by their bulkiness. The pulmonary valve annulus may be hypoplastic; however, it usually is of adequate size. At present, most of these patients can be managed in the cardiac catheterization laboratory by balloon valvuloplasty. However, occasionally surgical intervention is required.

Technique for Repair

In neonates, pulmonary valvotomy may be carried out without cardiopulmonary bypass. Most often it is preferable to perform a pulmonary valvotomy in all patients through a median sternotomy on cardiopulmonary bypass.

Aortic and bicaval cannulation is performed. After initiation of cardiopulmonary bypass, a longitudinal inci-

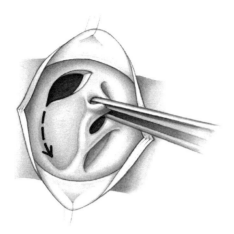

FIG. 21-14. Pulmonary valvulectomy.

sion is made on the anterior surface of the pulmonary artery. The commissures of the pulmonary valve are incised up to and including the annulus. The commissurotomy should be generous enough to produce some insufficiency. If the valve leaflets are thickened or dysplastic, then a valvulectomy is performed (Fig. 21-14).

Occasionally, the annulus of the pulmonary valve is hypoplastic. Under these circumstances, the arteriotomy is extended across the annulus onto the right ventricular outflow tract and the resulting opening is closed with a patch of autologous pericardium or monocusp, using 5-0 or 6-0 Prolene suture (Fig. 21-10).

APPENDIX

Hegar Dilation Sizing

The internal diameter of the narrowest part of the pulmonary outflow tract is determined by passing calibrated Hegar's dilators of increasing size through the pulmonary valve and into the dilated pulmonary artery. The largest size Hegar's dilator to fit snugly is used to predict the need for a transannular patch by referring to the data from Rowlatt et al. (Rowlatt UF, Rimoldi HJA, Lev M. The quantitative anatomy of the normal child's heart. *Pediatr Clin North Am* 1963;10:499).

With the diameters shown, only 15% probability exists that the right ventricular—left ventricular pressure ratio will be more than 0.65. If transannular patching is required, it can be sized by the correct Hegar's dilator to prevent the patch from being too patulous and interfering with effective forward flow.

Body Surface Area (m²)	Diameter (mm = Hegar size/3)
0.15	5.9
0.20	7.3
0.25	8.4
0.30	9.3
0.35	10.1
0.40	10.7
0.45	11.3
0.50	11.9
0.55	12.3
0.60	12.8
0.65	13.2
0.70	13.5
0.75	13.9
0.80	14.2
0.90	14.8
1.0	15.3
1.2	16.2
1.4	17.0
1.6	17.6
1.8	18.2
2.0	18.7

NB: The Hegar size is calculated by multiplying the diameter by 3.

CHAPTER 22

Left Ventricular Outflow Tract Obstruction

CONGENITAL AORTIC STENOSIS

Pathologic findings in congenital aortic stenosis can vary. The valve may be bicuspid, tricuspid, or unicuspid, and the commissures may be fused together in any combination. The functional orifice of the aortic valve, however, is usually between the left and noncoronary cusps, whereas the other cusp and commissures are fused and deformed to various degrees.

Infants or neonates with critical aortic stenosis may require urgent intervention. Neonates may present in extremis with marked metabolic acidosis. Infusion of prostaglandin E_1 may improve the circulation in these neonates by reopening the ductus arteriosus. It is critical in these cases to differentiate isolated, critical aortic stenosis from a form of hypoplastic left heart syndrome that requires a modified Norwood procedure (see Chapter 28). Although percutaneous balloon valvuloplasty for critical aortic stenosis in the neonate and infant is being performed with satisfactory results, surgery is still indicated for some patients.

Valvotomy Technique

A median sternotomy approach is used. Surgical valvotomy is performed on cardiopulmonary bypass. Cannulation is carried out with a standard aortic cannula and a single venous cannula in the right atrial appendage. Cardiopulmonary bypass is begun, and the ductus arteriosus is closed with a heavy tie or metal clip. The aorta is cross-clamped, and cardioplegic solution is administered (see Chapter 3). The aorta is incised transversely, the aortic valve is exposed, and its anatomy is studied closely. A no. 15 blade is used to incise the fused commissures to within 2 mm of the aortic annulus (Fig. 22-1).

🚫 *AORTIC INSUFFICIENCY*
The purpose of the operation is to relieve obstruction to the left ventricular outflow tract in these very sick infants as effectively as possible, without producing aortic insufficiency. Therefore, overzealous incision of the commissures or division of a nonexistent or rudimentary raphe only results in gross aortic insufficiency and may necessitate aortic valve replacement (Fig. 22-2).

🚫 *INADEQUATE RELIEF OF OBSTRUCTION*
Conversely, inadequate relief of the obstruction may not help the child very much. Experience provides the good judgment required to incise to just the right extent at the precise area of a grossly deformed aortic valve.

NB *EXPOSING THE AORTIC VALVE*
When the aorta is small, an oblique rather than transverse aortotomy provides better exposure of the aortic valve.

🚫 *AWARENESS OF SUBVALVULAR OBSTRUCTION*
It is of paramount importance to inspect the aortic subvalvular area and rule out the presence of a fibrous diaphragm or other forms of left ventricular outflow tract obstruction. A Hegar's dilator of appropriate size can be used for precise evaluation of the valvular orifice and the left ventricular outflow tract.

🚫 *SEVERELY DEFORMED OR MALDEVELOPED AORTIC LEAFLETS*
A satisfactory commissurotomy with long-lasting good results depends on how well-formed the valve was initially. When there is severe deformity and maldevelopment of the aortic valve, surgical relief of left ventricular outflow tract obstruction is only temporary and palliative. These subgroups of patients should be followed so that a more definitive form of treatment can be planned for them when they are older, before permanent left ventricular dysfunction ensues.

263

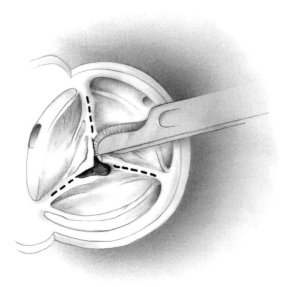

FIG. 22-1. Technique for an aortic commissurotomy.

FIG. 22-2. Overzealous incision of the commissures, causing gross aortic insufficiency.

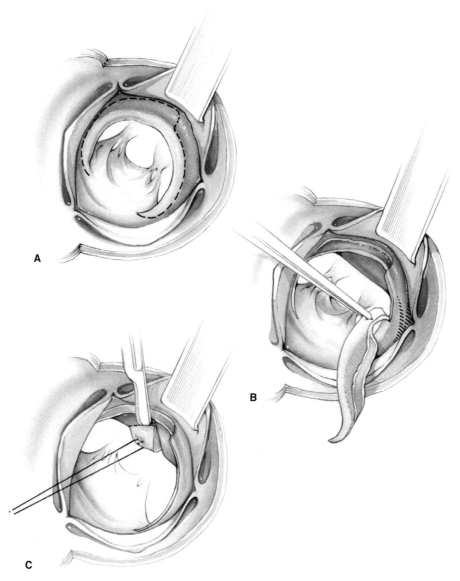

FIG. 22-3. Resection of the subvalvular diaphragm. **A:** Dashed line depicts the extent of resection. **B:** Only the white fibrous tissue is resected near the penetrating bundle. **C:** As an extra precaution against inadequate relief of an obstruction, a limited myectomy is also carried out.

RESECTION OF THE SUBVALVULAR DIAPHRAGM

A fibrous muscular or membranous rim of tissue arising from the anterior two-thirds of the left ventricular outflow tract may be present within 1 cm below the aortic annulus. The aortic valve leaflets are retracted gently with narrow ribbon retractors. The fibromuscular diaphragm is then excised with a no. 15 blade (Fig. 22-3A, B). This shelf of abnormal tissue can also be mobilized and enucleated in its whole circumference with an endarterectomy spatula.

NB *MYOTOMY OR MYECTOMY*
A myotomy or a limited myectomy involving the bulging septum is recommended to prevent the possible persistence of a significant residual obstruction (Fig. 22-3C). This may also help to prevent recurrence of the membrane, the incidence of which is higher the younger the patient is when the initial operation is performed.

⊘ *INTERVENTRICULAR SEPTAL DEFECT*
A substantial segment of the abnormal fibromuscular tissue can be excised and removed from the septal area without producing a defect in the interventricular septum. If such a complication does occur, the defect must be identified and closed. Pledgeted sutures are essential to protect the friable muscular tissue.

⊘ *INJURY TO CONDUCTION TISSUE*
Only the white fibrous tissue should be mobilized and removed from the area immediately below the right and noncoronary cusps adjacent to the bundle branches to avoid injury to the conduction tissue and consequent heart block (Fig. 22-3B).

⊘ *VALVULAR INSUFFICIENCY*
Occasionally, the membranous tissue is adherent to the underside of the right coronary leaflet of the aortic valve. It must then be meticulously dissected free without damaging the aortic valve to avoid producing valvular insufficiency.

⊘ *INJURY TO THE MITRAL VALVE*
Occasionally, the lesion may extend and become adherent to the anterior leaflet of the mitral valve; in this case, it should be dissected free with the utmost care. Injury to the mitral valve near its annulus may result in an opening into the left atrium.

HYPERTROPHIC OBSTRUCTIVE CARDIOMYOPATHY

Hypertrophic obstructive cardiomyopathy is usually not a surgical lesion. When indicated, however, the excess septal muscle can be excised to relieve obstruction of the left ventricular outflow tract. A relatively thick segment (1 cm deep by 1.5 cm wide) of septal wall is excised and removed (Fig. 22-4).

⊘ *SEPTAL DEFECT FROM TOO AGGRESSIVE AN EXCISION*
Too aggressive an excision may result in the creation of a ventriculoseptal defect, which must be closed with pledgeted sutures.

NB *EXCISION OF THE MITRAL VALVE*
When systolic anterior motion of the anterior leaflet of the mitral valve is a significant component of the left ventricular outflow obstruction, mitral valve replacement with a low-profile valve resecting the entire anterior subvalvular apparatus may be indicated. In younger patients, abnormal chordal attachments from the anterior leaflet to the septum may create outflow tract obstruction. Oftentimes, these attachments can be taken down without causing significant mitral insufficiency. When combined with a myectomy, this can result in relief of the obstruction.

⊘ *EMBOLISM FROM MUSCLE FRAGMENTS FALLING INTO THE VENTRICULAR CAVITY*
During the process of excising the hypertrophied muscle, fragments may fall into the left ventricular cavity, resulting in a subsequent embolism. This can be prevented to some degree by pulling on the desired segment to be excised with a 4-0 or 5-0 Prolene stitch (see Fig. 22-4). Care should be taken to remove all debris from within the left ventricular cavity.

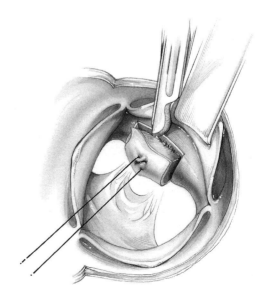

FIG. 22-4. Myectomy for idiopathic hypertrophic subaortic stenosis.

NB *INADEQUATE EXPOSURE*
Exposure may be inadequate through the retracted aortic leaflets. The obstructing muscle may then be removed through a left atriotomy working through the mitral valve.

The long-term surgical results in this disease are not uniformly satisfactory. Some postoperative patients do respond to adjunctive medical therapy, including β-adrenergic blockers, calcium channel blockers, and, occasionally, dual-chamber pacemakers.

LEFT VENTRICULAR TUNNEL OBSTRUCTION

When the left ventricular outflow tract is diffusely obstructed by a congenital narrow tunnel, none of the aforementioned techniques is helpful to any significant degree. A left ventricular apical conduit to the ascending or descending aorta is an alternative, but not a favored one. The Rastan-Konno aortoventriculoseptoplasty, although a somewhat radical procedure, provides satisfactory results. In infants and children, a Ross-Konno procedure (replacing the aortic root with the pulmonary autograft, completing the ventriculoseptoplasty, and reconstructing the right ventricular outflow tract with a pulmonary homograft) is the operation of choice for this diagnosis.

Rastan-Konno Aortoventriculoseptoplasty

Bicaval and aortic cannulations are made in the usual manner. On cardiopulmonary bypass with moderate cooling, the aorta is cross-clamped and cardioplegic arrest of the heart is achieved by the usual techniques (see Chapter 3). The aorta is incised anteriorly in a longitudinal direction. The incision is then extended downward under direct vision into the root of the aorta.

 DIRECTION OF THE AORTOTOMY
The direction of the aortotomy should be as far as possible to the left of the right coronary artery ostium, but not reaching the commissure between the right and left sinuses. This prevents injury to the ostium of the right coronary artery.

The anterior surface of the right ventricular outflow tract is then incised obliquely downward from the aortic root for a distance sufficient to provide good exposure of the interventricular septum (Fig. 22-5). Alternatively, the right ventriculotomy is made first and then extended upward into the aortic root.

 ABNORMAL DISTRIBUTION OF RIGHT CORONARY ARTERY BRANCHES
The possibility of abnormal distribution of right coronary artery branches crossing the right ventric-

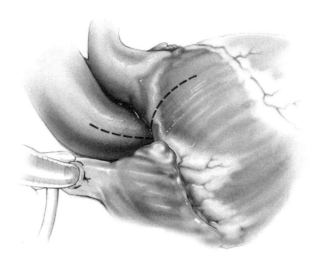

FIG. 22-5. Oblique incision downward from the aortic root to expose the interventricular septum in the Rastan-Konno aortoventricular septoplasty.

ular outflow tract to supply the left ventricular mass must be borne in mind when incising the infundibulum to prevent ischemic injury to the heart.

The aortotomy is then continued obliquely downward across the aortic annulus onto the massively thickened interventricular septum (Fig. 22-6). The distorted aortic leaflets are then removed.

 SEPTAL INFARCTION
Division of an aberrant septal artery may result in a septal infarction.
An appropriately sized, oval Hemashield patch of generous width is sewn on the right ventricular side of the interventricular septum, up to the level of the annulus of the resected aortic valve (Fig. 22-7).

 REINFORCING THE SUTURES ON THE INTERVENTRICULAR SEPTUM
The interventricular septum is thick and friable; a continuous Prolene suture may tear through it, causing suture leaks and a resulting shunt across the septum. The suture line can be reinforced by buttressing the sutures over a strip of Teflon felt or pledgets on the left or right ventricular side (or both) of the septum (Fig. 22-7). Using interrupted sutures buttressed with pledgets results in surface-to-surface coaptation of the patch to the septum, thus reducing the possibility of leaks (Fig. 22-7B).

NB *MAXIMIZING THE ROOT ENLARGEMENT*
To maximize the root enlargement, the Hemashield patch graft is sewn onto the right ventricular side of the septum.

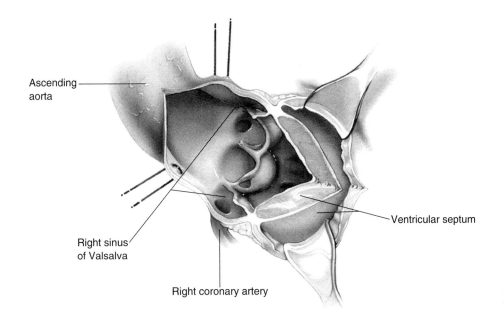

Ascending aorta

Right sinus of Valsalva

Right coronary artery

Ventricular septum

FIG. 22-6. Continuation of the oblique aortotomy on the interventricular septum.

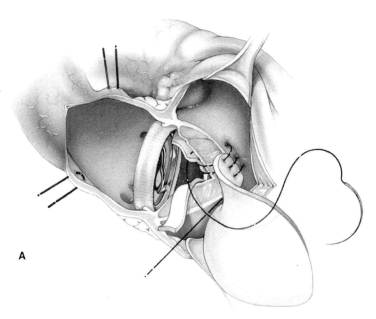

A

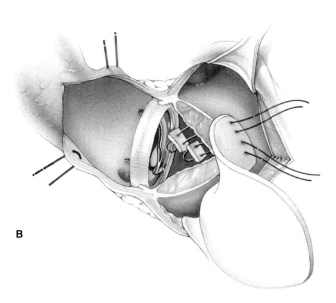

B

FIG. 22-7. Oval patch sewn on the right ventricular side of the interventricular septum, across the prosthetic ring and upward along the aortotomy. **A:** A continuous suture line is reinforced with a strip of Teflon felt. **B:** An alternate technique uses interrupted sutures buttressed with pledgets.

Interrupted valve sutures are inserted into the aortic annulus and through the patch at the level of the annulus (see Chapter 5). After the sutures are inserted through the prosthetic sewing ring, the prosthesis is seated satisfactorily into position (Fig. 22-7). The prosthesis can be sewn to the Hemashield with either continuous or interrupted sutures.

APPROPRIATENESS OF VALVE TYPES
Because of their early calcification in children, stented tissue valves are not used. Low-profile disc or bileaflet mechanical valves are the preferred prostheses if a pulmonary autograft is not available or contraindicated.

SUTURE LINE
A new continuous suture should be started at the valve sewing ring and should proceed so that the patch is laid onto the aortotomy incision. Thus, the septal suture line is tied snugly at the prosthetic level. This entails separating the suture that closes the interventricular septum from the suture that closes the aortotomy (Fig. 22-8).

A triangular, appropriately generous patch of Hemashield, bovine pericardium, or autologous pericardium is sewn to the edges of the incision on the right ventricular outflow tract and across the first patch at the level of the prosthetic valve (Fig. 22-9). Alternatively, a large pericardial patch is sewn onto the right ventricle and is extended over the aortic patch to secure hemostasis.

REINFORCING THE SUTURE LINE
The suture line can be reinforced with Teflon felt if the right ventricular wall appears to be thin and friable.

Once the aortotomy closure is completed, the heart is filled and standard deairing maneuvers are carried out (see Chapter 4).

NB EXTENDED AORTIC ROOT REPLACEMENT WITH AN AORTIC HOMOGRAFT OR PULMONARY AUTOGRAFT
There are many problems associated with mechanical valves in infants and children. An alternative technique is to combine the concept of aortic root replacement with reimplantation of the coronary arteries and the concept of aortoventriculoplasty. The aortic, right ventricular, and septal incisions are similar to those described earlier for the Rastan-Konno procedure. The coronary arteries are excised with a generous cuff of aortic wall and mobilized. The aortic valve and proximal ascending aorta are excised. If an aortic homograft is used, it is oriented so that the attached anterior leaflet of the mitral valve can be used to patch the incision on the ventricular septum. If a pulmonary autograft is used, a triangular piece of the right ventricular wall can be left attached to the pulmonary valve annulus when harvesting the autograft. This muscle can then be used to patch the defect in the interventricular septum. Aortic root replacement and reimplantation of the coronary ostia are completed as described in

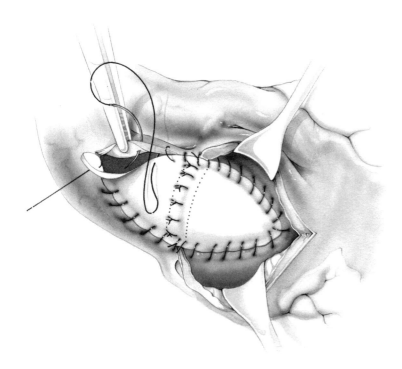

FIG. 22-8. A continuous suture is used to approximate the patch onto the aortotomy incision.

pulmonic valve (Fig. 22-5). This is extended to the level of the aortic annulus just to the left of the right coronary ostium. A longitudinal incision is made in the ventricular septum extending from just below the aortic annulus at the commissure between the left and right coronary sinuses proximally on the septum past the area of obstruction. The thickened septal muscle is resected from the left ventricular outflow tract. An oval patch of Hemashield is then used to close the defect, placing horizontal, pledgeted, interrupted mattress sutures from the left ventricle through the septum and then the patch on the right ventricular side (Fig. 22-10). The opening on the right ventricle is then closed with a pericardial patch.

 AORTIC VALVE INJURY
Before making the septal incision, a small aortotomy to allow visualization of the aortic valve and annulus may be useful. A right-angled clamp passed through the aortic valve can identify the appropriate location for the septal incision.

 INJURY TO THE CONDUCTION SYSTEM
The incision on the septum should be well to the left of the right coronary ostium to avoid the conduction system.

INADEQUATE SEPTAL OPENING
The incision on the ventricular septum must be extended far enough proximally to completely relieve the narrowing of the left ventricular outflow tract.

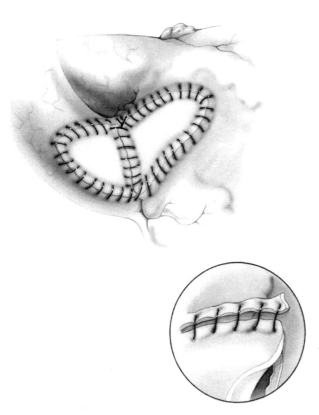

FIG. 22.-9. Sewing a triangular patch to the edges of the right ventricular outflow tract opening and the aortic root. **Inset:** Reinforcement of the suture line with Teflon felt.

Chapter 5. The defect in the right ventricle is then closed with a piece of autologous or bovine pericardium. The patch is sutured to the edges of the right ventriculotomy incision and along the annulus of the valve of the homograft or autograft.

ORIENTATION OF THE AORTIC HOMOGRAFT
When the anterior mitral leaflet is left attached to the aortic homograft and used to patch the ventricular septal defect, the homograft must be oriented in only one way. This may create complications for the reimplantation of the coronary ostia. Alternatively, the mitral leaflet can be excised and the ventricular septum enlarged with a triangular patch of Hemashield, which is then sewn to the annulus of the aortic homograft.

Modified Rastan-Konno Procedure

When there is diffuse long-segment tunnel stenosis with a competent aortic valve and adequately sized aortic annulus, a modified Rastan-Konno procedure is indicated.

Cardiopulmonary bypass with bicaval cannulation and aortic cross-clamping is used. An oblique incision is made in the infundibulum of the right ventricle below the

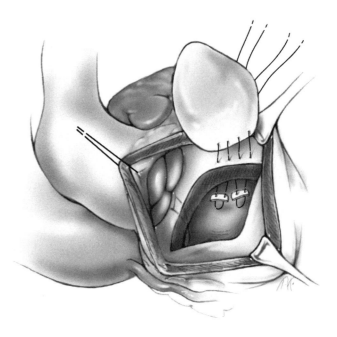

FIG. 22-10. Modified Rastan-Konno procedure: septal incision and placement of horizontal mattress sutures from the left ventricle to the right ventricle.

SUPRAVALVULAR AORTIC STENOSIS

An oblique aortotomy provides good exposure. If the stenosis involves only the ascending aorta, it can be conveniently managed by excising the fibrous ridge and sewing an appropriately sized, diamond-shaped Hemashield or GORE-TEX patch across the stricture to relieve the stenosis (Fig. 22-11). The type of supravalvular narrowing that is caused by a fibrous ridge usually extends onto the annulus and the commissures, however. This fibrous ridge must be meticulously excised to free the aortic leaflets.

 PATCH ENLARGEMENT OF THE ASCENDING AORTA

The supravalvular lesion may be extensive and affect major parts of the ascending aorta. This lesion may require extensive patch enlargement from the noncoronary sinus to the innominate artery. The width of the patch must be oversized, with allowance made for the eventual growth of the rest of the vascular system, to prevent the late recurrence of stenosis (Fig. 22-12). Patients with Williams syndrome may have long-segment narrowing of the entire ascending aorta, necessitating at times the replacement of the ascending aorta up to the innominate artery and possibly the aortic root as well.

 INJURY TO THE AORTIC LEAFLETS
While the fibrous ridge is being excised, the aortic valve leaflets must be protected. Any injury to the aortic leaflets can produce aortic insufficiency.

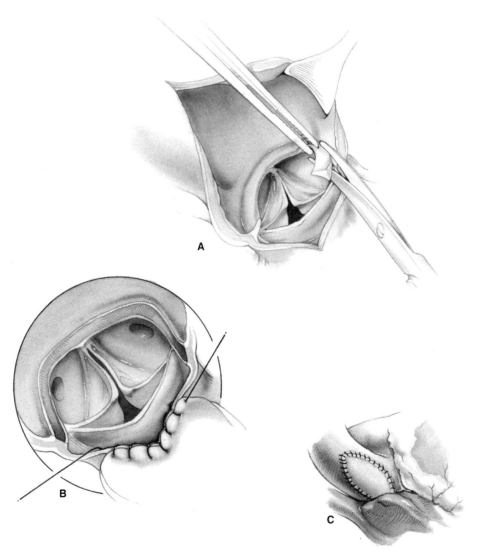

FIG. 22-11. Relief of supravalvular aortic stenosis. **A:** The shelf of fibrous tissue is excised. **B:** The aortic root is enlarged by extension of the aortotomy into the noncoronary sinus of Valsalva. **C:** The defect is covered with a large patch.

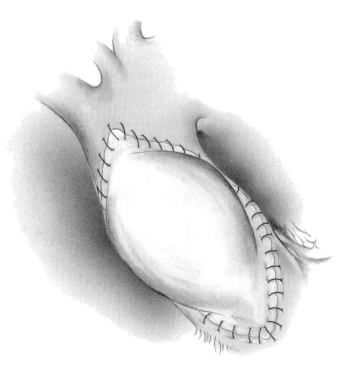

FIG. 22-12. Patch enlargement of the ascending aorta.

 OBSTRUCTION EXTENDING INTO THE AORTIC SINUSES

At times, the fibrous ridge continues into, narrows, and distorts one of the aortic sinuses. This must be dissected free, and sinus of Valsalva may need to be enlarged with a patch of autologous pericardium treated with glutaraldehyde or Hemashield to relieve the obstruction. Occasionally, more than one sinus of Valsalva may require patch enlargement (Fig. 22-13).

 INJURY TO THE LEFT CORONARY ARTERY OSTIUM

Removal of a fibrous ridge from the left coronary sinus region must be carried out carefully, always bearing in mind the possibility of injuring the left coronary ostium.

The degree of supravalvular obstruction may be so severe that a more extensive form of therapy is indicated. An effective technique was devised by Brom with excellent results. In this technique, the aorta is completely transected just above the stenotic segment (Fig. 22-14).

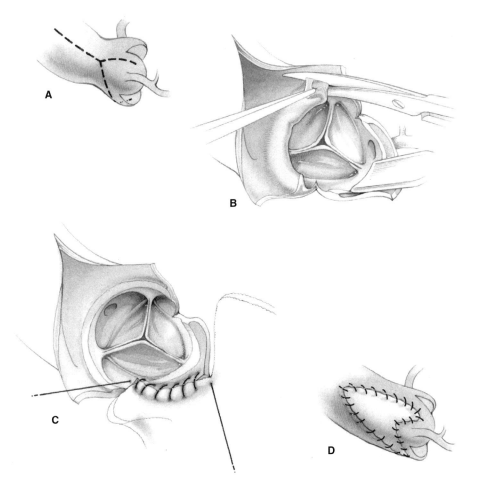

FIG. 22-13. Relief of an obstruction to the aortic sinuses. **A:** The aortotomy is extended down into the noncoronary and right sinus of Valsalva. **B:** The fibrous shelf is removed. **C and D:** Pericardium is incorporated as a patch to enlarge both aortic sinuses and the ascending aorta.

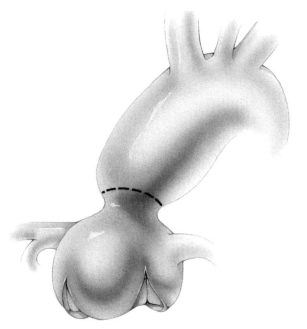

FIG. 22-14. Transection of the aorta above the stenotic segment.

The lumen of the stenosis is rarely larger than 6 to 8 mm in diameter, as measured with a Hegar's dilator; by a simple calculation, the circumference of the stenosis is therefore approximately 18 mm, and the width of each segment between the commissures is 6 to 8 mm.

The aortic root, sinus of Valsalva, and the coronary artery ostia are usually widely dilated. A short, vertical incision is made down into the noncoronary sinus to the level of maximal width of the proximal aorta (Fig. 22-15). This improves exposure and allows close inspection

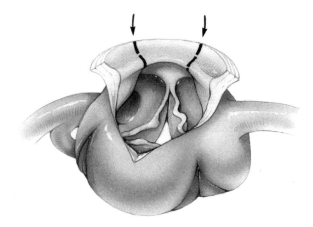

FIG. 22-16. Line of incision into the other two coronary sinuses.

of the lesion (Fig. 22-16). Similar incisions are made into the other two coronary sinuses; the stenotic lumen is now fully opened (Fig. 22-17).

 INCISIONS INTO THE CORONARY SINUSES
Incisions into the coronary sinuses should never extend beyond the point of maximal width of the proximal aortic segment (Fig. 22-15). If these incisions are made deeper than this level, the patches will distort the base of the valve and give rise to aortic incompetence.

Often, the ostia of the coronary arteries are greatly enlarged and occupy the entire area between the commis-

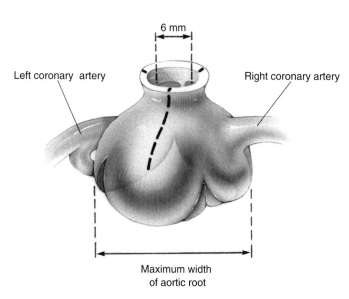

FIG. 22-15. Line of incision into the noncoronary sinus.

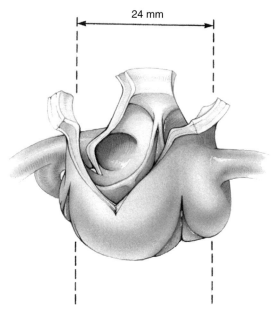

FIG. 22-17. Fully opened stenosis.

sures. Because of this enlargement, the incisions into the sinuses can be extended into the coronary orifices without producing ostial stenosis.

 DISTORTION OF THE CORONARY OSTIA
To prevent distortion of the coronary ostia with subsequent patch plasty, the incisions into the coronary sinuses and, whenever appropriate, into the coronary artery ostia should be to the right of the left coronary artery ostium and to the left of the right coronary ostium (Fig. 22-18).

The normal aortic valve annulus is measured with a Hegar's dilator of appropriate size. The circumference of the annulus is approximately three times its diameter or Hegar size. For example, if the aortic annular diameter (Hegar size) is 24 mm, its circumference will be 24 mm × 3 or 72 mm. If the lumen of the stenotic segment is 6 mm (Hegar size), its circumference is 6 mm × 3 or 18 mm.

It is clear from these observations and calculations that the stenotic aortic segment must be enlarged by 54 mm (72 mm − 18 mm) for it to match the size of the aortic valve annulus. Because this enlargement must be made among the three commissures, each pericardial patch must be 54 mm ÷ 3 or 18 mm wide along its superior rim (Fig. 22-19).

Autologous, glutaraldehyde-treated pericardium is used to prepare triangular patches with specific measurements; in this example, an isosceles triangle with a base of 18 mm and a height commensurate with the distance between the stenotic segment and the maximal width of the proximal aorta (Fig. 22-19) is the necessary size. The pericardial patches are then sewn in place with 6-0 or 7-0 Prolene sutures. The ostia of the coronary arteries, if they are enlarged, can be incorporated into the suturing process without the risk of producing subsequent ostial stenosis (Fig. 22-19).

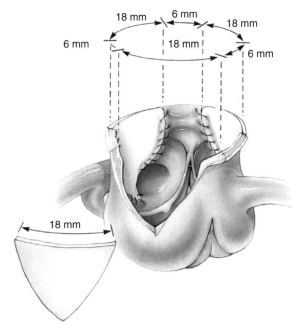

FIG. 22-19. An example of measurements needed for an accurate stenotic enlargement.

The two aortic ends are now anastomosed in an end-to-end fashion with Prolene suture in a continuous suturing technique (Fig. 22-20).

NB *NARROW DISTAL AORTIC SEGMENT NBH:*
Occasionally, the lumen of the distal ascending aorta, just above the stenotic segment, may be small

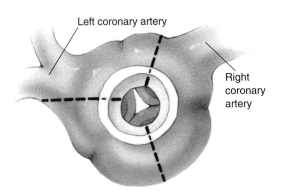

FIG. 22-18. Placement of an incision to prevent distortion of the ostia of the coronary arteries.

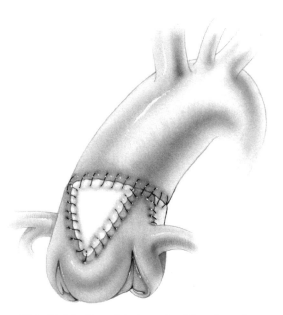

FIG. 22-20. Completed repair of the stenosis.

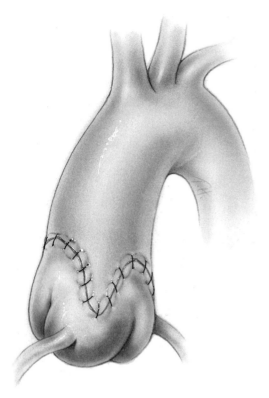

FIG. 22-21. Completed repair of the end-to-end reconstruction of the aorta.

compared with the newly constructed proximal aorta. This discrepancy can be rectified by further resection of the distal aorta or a vertical incision into its lumen.

In select group of patients, it may be possible to perform end-to-end reconstruction of the aorta without the use of pericardial patches. The distal aorta is anastomosed to the aortic root by making appropriate counter-incisions to provide three tongues of aortic tissue (Fig. 22-21).

NB *TENSION ON THE ANASTOMOSIS*
The aorta must be well mobilized to provide adequate length, thus minimizing any tension on the anastomosis.

CHAPTER 23

Transposition of the Great Vessels

Transposition of the great arteries generally connotes a congenital malformation in which the heart has atrioventricular concordance and ventriculoarterial discordance. Therefore, the clinical findings are an anterior aorta that originates from the right (morphologic) ventricle and a pulmonary artery that originates from the left (morphologic) ventricle. Other congenital defects can also be associated with transposition of the great arteries.

At present, anatomic correction of transposition of the great arteries with or without ventricular septal defect is the procedure of choice. When the interventricular septum is intact, the arterial switch operation must be performed while the left ventricle is still prepared to handle systemic pressures. After 2 to 3 weeks of age, changes in the left ventricular wall thickness and geometry may preclude a successful arterial switch procedure. If the left ventricular pressure is less than 60% systemic, a two-staged approach involving initial pulmonary artery banding with or without a systemic to pulmonary artery shunt followed by an arterial switch procedure when the left ventricle becomes prepared is required. Alternatively, a so-called atrial switch procedure (Mustard or Senning operation) may be undertaken.

The Senning and Mustard procedures were designed to achieve a rerouting of the venous returns in the two atria; this entails channeling the systemic venous return from the caval veins into the left atrium and across the mitral valve into the left ventricle and through the pulmonary artery to the lungs. Similarly, pulmonary venous return from the pulmonary veins is directed into the right atrium across the tricuspid valve into the right ventricle, which functions as the systemic ventricle, pumping blood into the aorta. Except for the torn fossa ovalis, which is found if a palliative balloon septostomy has been performed, the surgical anatomy of both the right and left atria is essentially normal. The long-term follow-up of patients who underwent Senning and Mustard procedures has shown a high incidence of atrial arrhythmias and a significant rate of late right ventricular dysfunction. However, physio-logic repair with one of these two procedures may be indicated in patients with transposition of the great vessels and associated pulmonary valve stenosis, nonresectable left ventricular outflow tract obstruction, or some abnormalities of the coronary arteries that may prohibitively increase the risk of anatomic repair. An atrial switch procedure may be part of the surgical approach in patients with some complex congenital heart lesions, and therefore every surgeon dealing with patients with congenital heart disease should have the Senning and Mustard procedures as part of his or her surgical armamentarium.

SURGICAL ANATOMY

In hearts with transposition of the great arteries, the right ventricular wall thickness is greater than normal at birth and increases progressively thereafter. If the ventricular septum is intact and no pulmonary stenosis exists, the left ventricular wall thickness does not increase after birth, and within 2 to 3 months, the left ventricle is relatively thin walled.

The aorta is most commonly directly anterior to the pulmonary artery, although occasionally the great vessels are side by side with the aorta to the right. The coronary arteries usually arise from the aortic sinuses facing the pulmonary artery. Thus, the nonfacing sinus is most often anterior. According to the Leiden convention, sinus 1 is on the right hand side and sinus 2 is the next sinus counterclockwise to sinus 1, as viewed from the nonfacing noncoronary sinus. Approximately 70% of patients have the left anterior descending and circumflex coronary arteries arising as a single trunk from sinus 1 and a right coronary artery from sinus 2 (Fig. 23-1A). The left anterior descending arises from sinus 1, and the right coronary artery and circumflex originate together from sinus 2 in approximately 15% of cases (Fig. 23-1B). Rarely, all three main coronary arteries arise from a single sinus, most commonly sinus 2. In some of these cases, the left

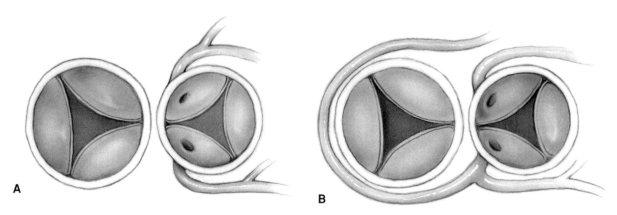

FIG. 23-1. A,B: Coronary artery configuration (see text).

anterior descending or left main coronary artery may be intramural.

Surgical Anatomy of the Right Atrium

Although the right atrium is morphologically molded into a single chamber, it is formed by two components: the sinus venarum and the right atrial appendage (sometimes referred to as the body of the atrium). Systemic venous return flows in from opposite directions through the superior and inferior venae cavae into the sinus venarum. This smooth-walled area is the most posterior portion of the right atrium and stretches between the orifices of the caval veins. From the viewpoint of the surgeon looking down into the right atrium, the sinus venarum is more or less horizontal, with the superior

vena cava entering from the left and the inferior vena cava entering (bounded by the eustachian valve) from the right (Fig. 23-2).

Just below and medial to the orifice of the superior vena cava arises the crista terminalis, a muscle bundle that springs into prominence as it circles the orifice of the superior vena cava to the right lateral wall of the atrium and continues inferiorly toward the inferior vena cava, thus forming the boundary between the sinus venarum and the atrial appendage. This muscle bundle is evidenced on the outside of the atrium by a groove, the sulcus terminalis. Lying subepicardially in the sulcus terminalis, just below the entrance of the superior vena cava, is the sinoatrial node, which may be vulnerable to injury from the various surgical incisions and cannulations that are commonly performed on the right atrium. The

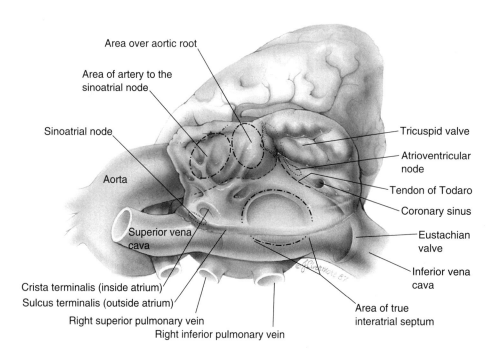

Area over aortic root
Area of artery to the sinoatrial node
Sinoatrial node
Aorta
Superior vena cava
Crista terminalis (inside atrium)
Sulcus terminalis (outside atrium)
Right superior pulmonary vein
Right inferior pulmonary vein
Tricuspid valve
Atrioventricular node
Tendon of Todaro
Coronary sinus
Eustachian valve
Inferior vena cava
Area of true interatrial septum

FIG. 23-2. Surgical anatomy of the right atrium.

remainder of the right atrium is made up of the atrial appendage, which begins at the crista terminalis and extends anteriorly (upward from the surgeon's perspective) to surround the tricuspid valve and form an expanded chamber.

In contrast to the smooth-walled sinus venarum, the lateral wall of the atrial appendage is ridged by multiple narrow bands of muscle, the musculi pectinati. These bands arise from the crista terminalis and pass upward to the most anterior part of the atrium. Functionally, they supply the right atrium with enough pumping capacity to propel the venous inflow through the tricuspid valve into the right ventricle.

Just above the sinus venarum in the center of the medial wall is the fossa ovalis, an elliptical or horseshoe-shaped depression. The true interatrial septum consists of the fossa ovalis with variable contributions from the superior, anterior, and inferior limbic muscle bundles that surround it. The aortic root is hidden behind the antero-medial atrial wall between the fossa ovalis and the termination of the heavily trabeculated right atrial appendage. Segments of the noncoronary and right sinus of Valsalva are in close apposition to the atrial wall in this area. Their locations may be manifested by the aortic mound, a bulge above and slightly to the left of the fossa ovalis. The presence of the aortic valve here can be more clearly visualized if one takes into consideration its continuity, through the central fibrous body, with the adjacent tricuspid valve annulus.

Also invisible to the surgeon is the artery to the sinoatrial node, which runs through this same area. Although its origin and exact location are unpredictable, the sinoatrial node takes a variable course toward the superior cavoatrial angle and the sinus node.

The tricuspid valve is located anteroinferiorly in the right atrium, where it opens widely into the right ventricle. The annulus of the tricuspid valve crosses over the membranous septum, dividing it into atrioventricular and interventricular segments. The membranous, or fibrous, septum is a continuation of the central fibrous body, through which the tricuspid, mitral, and aortic valves are connected.

Immediately below the upper or atrioventricular section of the membranous septum lies the hidden atrioventricular node. It is situated at the apex of Koch's triangle, the boundaries of which are the annulus of the septal leaflet of the tricuspid valve, Todaro's tendon (running intramyocardially from the central fibrous body to the eustachian valve of the inferior vena cava), and its base, the coronary sinus. Anderson describes Todaro's tendon as a fibrous extension of the commissure between the eustachian valve (of the inferior vena cava) and the thebesian valve (of the coronary sinus). Conduction tissue passes from the atrioventricular node as His's bundle below the membranous septum and down into the muscular interventricular septum. The coronary sinus, draining the cardiac veins, is situated alongside Todaro's tendon, between it and the tricuspid valve.

THE ARTERIAL SWITCH OPERATION

Incision

A median sternotomy is performed, and most or all of the thymus is removed.

Preparation

A rectangular piece of pericardium is harvested and attached to a piece of cardboard from a suture pack using metal clips. It is placed in 0.6% glutaraldehyde solution for 5 to 6 minutes and then rinsed in saline. The relationship of the great vessels and coronary anatomy can be confirmed at this point.

Cannulation

The ascending aorta is cannulated as far distally as possible. Direct caval cannulation is carried out except in very small neonates weighing less than 2 kg in whom a single venous cannula through the right atrial appendage is used. With commencement of cardiopulmonary bypass, the ductus arterious is occluded at its aortic end with a heavy tie or Ligaclip. The ductus arteriosus is later divided, oversewing the pulmonary artery side with 6-0 or 7-0 Prolene suture. During cooling, the ascending aorta is dissected free from the main pulmonary artery and the right and left pulmonary arteries are mobilized out to the first branches in the hilum of each lung. Most or all of the dissection is accomplished with an electrocautery on low current.

 FLOODING OF THE PULMONARY BED
As soon as cardiopulmonary bypass is instituted, the ductus arterious must be occluded to prevent runoff of aortic cannula return into the lungs.

Continuous cardiopulmonary bypass is used with tapes tightened around the venous cannulae during closure of the atrial defect and ventricular septal defect, if present. A small vent may be placed through the right superior pulmonary vein. Alternatively, in very small infants, low-flow cardiopulmonary bypass can be conducted by directing the single venous cannula in the right atrial appendage toward the superior vena cava to minimize air in the venous return. A brief period of hypothermic arrest is used to close the septal defect(s).

Transection of the Great Arteries

If low-flow or circulatory arrest is required, the patient is cooled for at least 10 minutes. The aortic cross-clamp is applied just proximal to the aortic cannula. A dose of cold blood cardioplegic solution is administered through a butterfly needle into the ascending aorta approximately 1 cm above the valve. The aorta is then transected at this level, and traction sutures are placed just above the three commissures of the aortic root and tagged (Fig. 23-3). The pulmonary artery is transected at the level of the takeoff of the right pulmonary artery, and traction sutures are placed at the commissures and tagged. The pulmonary valve is inspected to rule out significant abnormalities because this will be the new aortic valve.

NB *PULMONARY VALVE ABNORMALITIES*
The status of the pulmonary valve is usually defined by the preoperative transthoracic echocardiogram and intraoperative transesophageal echocardiogram. A sufficiently competent and non-stenotic valve must be confirmed before excising the coronary arteries.

The pulmonary artery confluence is brought anterior to the distal ascending aorta (Fig. 23-4). The most proximal portion of the transected distal aorta is then grasped with

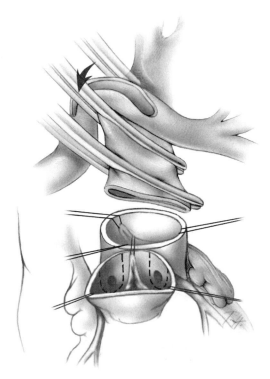

FIG. 23-4. The LeCompte maneuver: pulmonary artery confluence is brought in front of the aorta and a second aortic clamp is applied. Arrow shows distal aortic clamp reapplied below the pulmonary artery confluence. Dotted lines indicate excision for the coronary tongues.

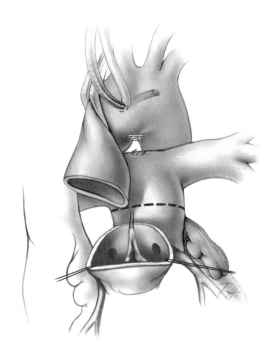

FIG. 23-3. The ascending aorta has been transected. Note the divided ductus arteriosus and line of transection on the main pulmonary artery.

a forceps or straight vascular clamp. The initial cross-clamp is then reapplied proximal to the pulmonary artery confluence as high as possible on the ascending aorta (Fig. 23-4B). This technique, often referred to as the LeCompte maneuver (after the surgeon who originally described it), avoids the need for an interposition conduit to connect the new pulmonary artery base to the pulmonary artery confluence.

 DISTORTING THE DISTAL ASCENDING AORTA
When repositioning the aortic cross-clamp, care must be taken not to twist the aorta and create torsion at the aortic suture line.

 EXCISION OF THE CORONARY OSTIA
The coronary ostia and at least 2 to 3 mm of surrounding aortic wall are excised as tongues of tissue (Fig. 23-4). The proximal coronary arteries are mobilized from the epicardium for several millimeters using an electrocautery on low current.

 KINKING OF CORONARY ARTERIES
Adequate dissection of the coronary arteries must be carried out to allow successful translocation of

the coronary ostium to the corresponding sinus of the pulmonary artery. Insufficient mobilization may lead to tension on the coronary anastomosis or kinking of the coronary artery.

 MOBILIZATION OF THE RIGHT CORONARY ARTERY
Conal branches may rarely need to be ligated and divided to allow adequate mobilization of the right coronary artery.

 JUXTACOMMISSURAL OSTIA
When one or both coronary ostia arise immediately adjacent to the commissure, the adjacent commissure must be excised along with the coronary ostia. This may lead to mild neopulmonary valve insufficiency.

INTRAMURAL CORONARY ARTERY
A generous cuff of aortic wall must be included in the tongue of tissue containing the coronary ostium to avoid injury to the intramural portion of the coronary artery.

Coronary Artery Reimplantation

The reimplantation sites for the coronary ostia are determined by holding the mobilized coronary arteries up against the anterior facing sinuses of the pulmonary root, ensuring that no distortion of the proximal course of the coronary arteries is created. The coronary arteries can be reimplanted into the pulmonary root as tongues of tissue by making a U-shaped incision in the appropriate location (Fig. 23-5). Alternatively, the coronary flaps are reattached as buttons of tissue, trimming the distal end of the flap before completing the suture line. In this case, a small slit is made at the appropriate location for coronary reimplantation in the pulmonary root. A small aortic punch is introduced into this hole and used to create an appropriately sized opening. The coronary artery is sutured to the opening in the pulmonary root using 7-0 or 8-0 Prolene suture (Fig. 23-6). After each coronary anastomosis, cold blood cardioplegic solution is infused directly into each coronary ostium with a 2-mm olive-tipped cannula, allowing assessment of any kinking or distortion of the coronary artery. If any problems are detected, they should be rectified now by either freeing up any restrictive adventitial or epicardial bands or redoing the anastomosis.

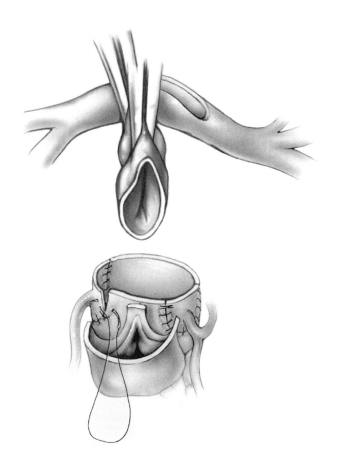

FIG. 23-5. Reattachment of the coronary tongues to the pulmonary root.

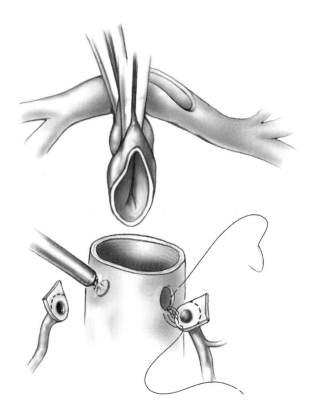

FIG. 23-6. Reattachment of the coronary ostia as buttons to the pulmonary root.

TORSION OF THE CORONARY ARTERY
Some surgeons prefer to excise the coronary ostia as buttons, instead of tongues, of tissue from the aortic root. When this technique is used, extreme care must be taken to prevent rotation and distortion of the coronary artery button during reimplantation.

 CIRCUMFLEX CORONARY ARTERY ARISING FROM THE RIGHT CORONARY ARTERY
If the circumflex coronary artery arises from the right coronary artery, a trapdoor may be created in the neoaorta to prevent kinking of the takeoff of the circumflex branch (Fig. 23-7). Alternatively, the right coronary artery ostium may be implanted higher on the neoaorta. When the circumflex arises from the right coronary artery, the pulmonary artery should be transected as far distally as possible to allow a high reimplantation of the right coronary button. Occasionally, the anastomosis must be performed on the ascending aorta distal to the suture line joining the neoaortic root to the distal aorta (Fig. 23-8).

INTRAMURAL CORONARY ARTERY
A shallow, U-shaped incision is made in the proximal neoaortic segment corresponding to the location of the previously prepared aortic button con-

taining the involved coronary ostium or ostia. The upper edge of the aortic button is then sutured to the lower portion of the U-shaped opening in the neoaortic root with 7-0 Prolene suture (Fig. 23-9A). After completing all but this portion of the suture line joining the neoaortic root to the ascending aorta, a piece of autologous pericardium is cut and sewn into place to create a convex roof over the remaining opening (Fig. 23-9B). This technique allows the coronary artery to remain *in situ* and minimizes the risk of twisting or tension on the proximal course of the coronary artery.

 INJURY TO THE NEOAORTIC LEAFLETS
Care must be taken when making the opening in the neoaortic root first with the knife blade and then with the punch to protect the valve leaflets from injury. The assistant may gently retract the leaflet with the back of a fine forceps.

Reconstructing the Aorta

The distal ascending aorta is anastomosed to the neoaortic root with running 6-0 or 7-0 Prolene suture (Fig. 23-10).

 SIZE DIFFERENCE BETWEEN THE NEOAORTIC ROOT AND ASCENDING AORTA
If a discrepancy between the diameter of the distal ascending aorta and neoaortic root exists, the excess tissue can usually be gathered in the posterior suture line. Gathering tissue anteriorly can distort the coronary artery anastomoses. This is espe-

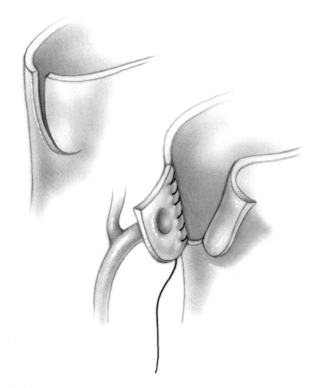

FIG. 23-7. Trapdoor technique: attachment of the circumflex coronary artery arising from the right coronary artery to the neoaorta.

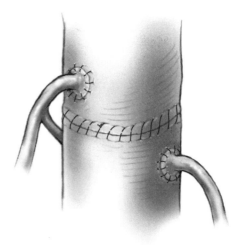

FIG. 23-8. Placing an anastomosis of the right coronary artery above an anastomosis of the neoaortic root to the ascending aorta.

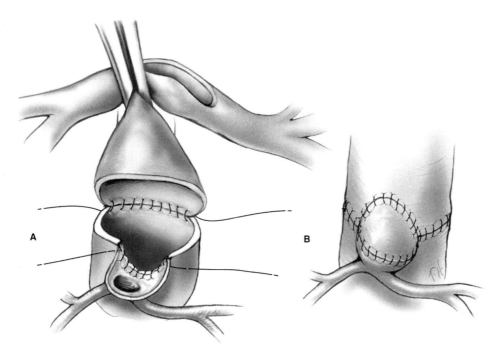

FIG. 23-9. A: Anastomosing a single intramural coronary artery to the neoaorta leaving the coronary tongue *in situ*. **B:** Using a pericardial hood to complete the anastomosis.

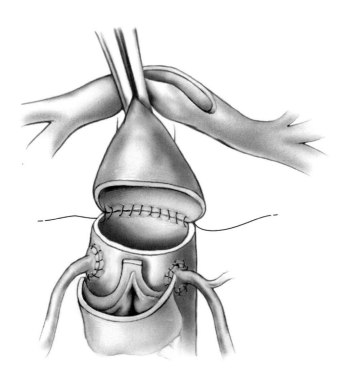

FIG. 23-10. Anastomosis of the neoaortic root to the distal aorta.

cially true if the coronary arteries have been reimplanted as flaps.

NB *HEMOSTASIS OF THE POSTERIOR SUTURE LINE*
Care must be taken to ensure hemostasis of the aortic suture line, especially posteriorly, because this is relatively inaccessible after the repair is completed.

NB *SIDE-BY-SIDE GREAT VESSELS*
When the aorta and pulmonary artery are side by side, the LeCompte maneuver may not have to be performed. The distal ascending aorta is simply mobilized laterally and anastomosed to the neoaortic base.

Intracardiac Repair

At this point, the atrial septal defect or balloon atrial septostomy and a ventricular septal defect, if present, are closed through a right atriotomy incision (see Chapters 18 and 19). Alternatively, a ventricular septal defect can be closed through one of the semilunar valves. If this is done through the posterior (pulmonary) valve, great care must be taken to avoid the conduction system. After closing the right atrium, the aortic cross-clamp may be removed or left in place until the pulmonary artery reconstruction is finished. If it is left in place, another dose of cardioplegia is given through a butterfly needle in the aortic root, allowing the surgeon to check the lie and filling of the coronary arteries as well as the suture lines for bleeding.

Reconstructing the Pulmonary Artery

If the aorta is to remain clamped, the clamp must now be moved back above the pulmonary artery confluence. The defect created in the neopulmonary base is filled with a rectangular patch of glutaraldehyde-treated pericardium. The patch should be approximately twice as long as the remaining neopulmonary sinus. A slit-like or V-shaped excision is made halfway along the long edge of this rectangular patch. This fits into the posterior commissure of the neopulmonary base. The patch is sewn into place with running 6-0 or 7-0 Prolene sutures. The resultant neopulmonary root is then anastomosed to the pulmonary artery confluence with 6-0 Prolene suture (Fig. 23-11).

 SUPRAVALVULAR PULMONARY STENOSIS
A well-recognized late complication of arterial switch procedures is supravalvular pulmonary stenosis. This can be avoided by leaving a generous

cuff of pericardium when reconstructing the neopulmonary root.

NB *SIDE-BY-SIDE GREAT VESSELS*
When the LeCompte maneuver is not performed, the pulmonary artery confluence is oversewn with 6-0 Prolene suture. A longitudinal opening is made on the underside of the right pulmonary artery. The reconstructed neopulmonary artery base is anastomosed to this opening in the right pulmonary artery with 6-0 Prolene suture.

Completing the Operation

The aortic cross-clamp is removed, and deairing carried out through the cardioplegic needle hole, which is subsequently closed with a 7-0 horizontal mattress suture. When rewarming is completed, the patient is weaned off cardiopulmonary bypass, taking care not to overfill the heart.

NB *EXAMINING CORONARY PERFUSION*
After the aortic cross-clamp is removed, the heart is examined for perfusion in all coronary distribu-

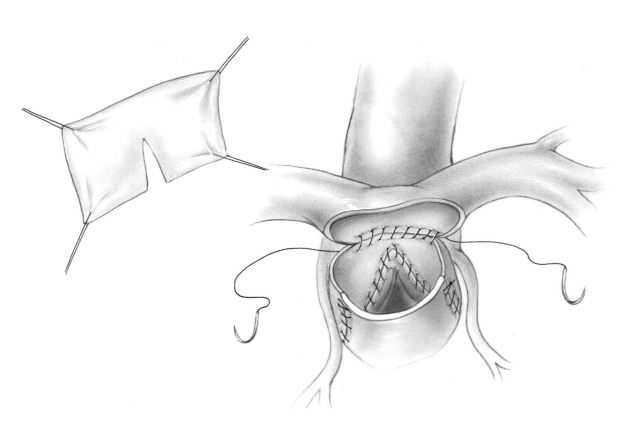

FIG. 23-11. Reconstruction of the neopulmonary root with pericardium and its attachment to the pulmonary artery confluence.

tions. Abnormalities of perfusion must be corrected. Further mobilization of the coronary artery in question may be required, or a coronary anastomosis may need to be repositioned.

DYSRHYTHMIAS

Rhythm disturbances during rewarming or soon after cardiopulmonary bypass is discontinued are most often secondary to coronary perfusion problems. The cause must be determined and corrected promptly.

STRETCHING OF THE CORONARY ARTERIES

Overdistention of the heart in the immediate post-bypass period may stretch the transposed coronary arteries. This can lead to decreased coronary flow. Therefore, volume administration must be done cautiously in these patients for the first 24 to 48 hours postoperatively to avoid this potentially fatal complication.

SUTURE LINE BLEEDING

Bleeding can be a problem because of extensive suture lines. Hemostasis should be checked after removing the aortic cross-clamp. Bleeding sites should be carefully sutured with adventitial horizontal mattress 7-0 Prolene sutures. If bleeding from the aorta is noted after discontinuation of cardiopulmonary bypass, reinstitution of bypass may be required. Takedown of the pulmonary artery anastomosis to allow access to the aortic suture line may be necessary.

CORONARY ARTERY SPASM

The transposed coronary arteries are susceptible to spasm in the postbypass and early postoperative periods. Intravenous nitroglycerin infusion is indicated in these patients. Intravenous calcium solution should be given very cautiously to prevent coronary artery spasm.

SENNING PROCEDURE

Incision

Both a right anterior thoracotomy and median sternotomy provide satisfactory exposure for the performance of the Senning operation, although most surgeons prefer a median sternotomy (see Chapter 1).

Cannulation

The anterosuperior aspect of the ascending aorta is cannulated as described previously (see Chapter 2). Generally, candidates for this procedure are infants younger than 6

months of age and of relatively low weight. The operation is generally performed with cardiopulmonary bypass, deep hypothermia, and total circulatory arrest. Some surgeons, however, prefer not to use circulatory arrest and perform the operation with deep hypothermia and low flow.

A single cannula through the right atrial appendage suffices to initiate cardiopulmonary bypass in preparation for total circulatory arrest. If total circulatory arrest is not contemplated, the superior and inferior venae cavae can be directly cannulated with right-angled cannulae. The site of the superior vena cava cannula should be as high as possible above the cavoatrial junction (Fig. 23-12). Individual caval cannulation must be done carefully to minimize interference with venous return and avoid hypotension and serious dysrhythmias. Partial cardiopulmonary bypass may be initiated after one cannula, usually in the inferior vena cava, is inserted.

A 5-0 Prolene purse-string suture is applied to the superior and inferior venae cavae, and right-angled cannulae of appropriate size are introduced by the bayonet technique (Fig. 23-12, inset) (see the discussion in Chapter 2 of caval cannulation). Aortic cross-clamping in the usual manner followed by infusion of cold blood cardioplegic solution results in cardioplegic arrest of the heart.

Atrial Incision

Access to the inside of the right atrium is gained through a longitudinal incision made 3 to 4 mm anterior and parallel to the sulcus terminalis (Fig. 23-13).

INCISION LENGTH

The incision should be well away from the sinoatrial node, and its cranial extension should be limited to 0.5 cm from the superior margin of the right atrium. If additional length is required, the incision can be extended ventrally into the right atrial appendage (Fig. 23-13).

NB *DIRECTION OF THE INCISION*

Only after the surgeon has inspected the inside of the right atrium should the incision be extended caudally so that it can be directed toward the lateral insertion of the valve of the inferior vena cava (eustachian valve) (Fig. 23-13).

The Atrial Septum

The fossa ovalis is usually torn if a balloon septostomy has been performed earlier. The trapezoid septal flap is developed starting in the most anterior part of the foramen ovale and is incised cranially for a distance of

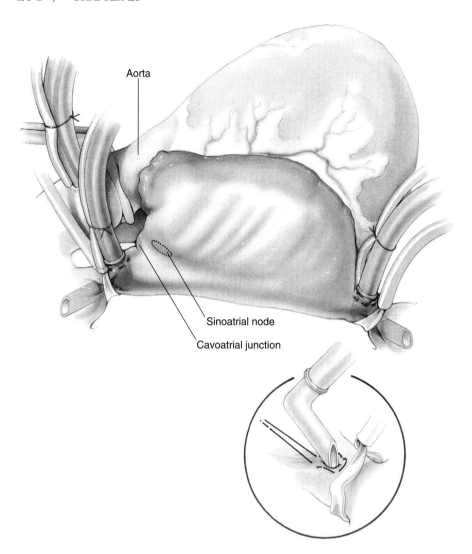

Aorta

Sinoatrial node

Cavoatrial junction

FIG. 23-12. Technique for caval cannulations. **Inset:** Direct cannulation using a right-angled cannula.

approximately 7 mm. The direction of the incision is then changed dorsally toward the superior margin of the right superior pulmonary vein and extends to the base of the interatrial septum. Similarly, an incision from the lower part of the fossa ovalis is continued downward toward the inferior margin of the right inferior pulmonary vein (Fig. 23-14). The raw margins of the septum are then endothelialized with interrupted sutures of 5-0 or 6-0 Prolene taking superficial bites and approximating endothelium (Fig. 23-14, inset). This atrial septal flap is now connected only at its base, which corresponds outside the atria with the interatrial groove.

⊘ *INJURY TO THE SINOATRIAL NODE ARTERY*

The artery to the sinoatrial node traverses the anterosuperior quadrant of the medial wall of the right atrium. Development of the atrial septal flap should spare the vascular supply of the sinoatrial node by not deviating the cranial extension of the incision anteriorly.

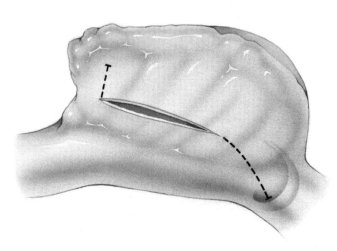

FIG. 23-13. Atriotomy.

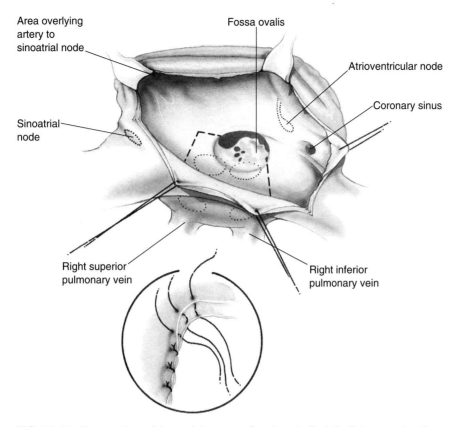

Area overlying
artery to
sinoatrial node

Fossa ovalis

Atrioventricular node

Coronary sinus

Sinoatrial
node

Right superior
pulmonary vein

Right inferior
pulmonary vein

FIG. 23-14. Preparation of the atrial septum flap. **Inset:** Endothelial approximation.

⊘ *PERFORATION OF THE MEDIAL WALL OF THE RIGHT ATRIUM*

Similarly, the direction of the cranial extension in the septum is significant. If this incision is deviated anteriorly toward the muscular aortic mound, it may lead into the pericardium outside the heart. If this happens, it must be immediately detected and the defect reapproximated with multiple fine Prolene sutures.

⊘ *PREFERENTIAL CONDUCTION TRACTS*

There are three main preferential conduction tracts or muscle bands joining the sinoatrial node to the atrioventricular node (Fig. 23-15). These probably correspond to the crista terminalis and limbic muscle bundles. The anterior conduction tract passes anterior to both the fossa ovalis and coronary sinus. The middle tract also lies anterior to the fossa ovalis but may pass through or just posterior to the

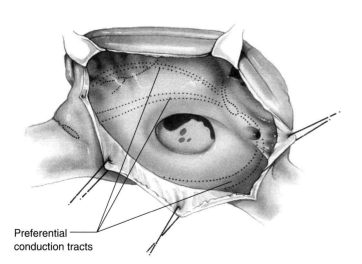

Preferential
conduction tracts

FIG. 23-15. The three main preferential conduction tissue pathways joining the sinoatrial node to the atrioventricular node.

coronary sinus. The posterior preferential tract crosses the posterior wall of the right atrium between the venae cavae and then curves forward toward the coronary sinus. During the development of the flap, the middle tract will be sacrificed in most cases. Great care should be taken to prevent injury to the other conduction pathways.

The defect in the flap from the fossa ovalis is filled by attaching an appropriately sized patch of GORE-TEX or glutaraldehyde-treated autologous pericardium. The size of the atrial septal flap thus developed is remarkably constant and has a base of approximately 3 cm, a height of 2 cm, and an anterior side of 1.5 to 2 cm in infants 6 to 12 months of age.

NB *INADEQUATE FLAP SIZE*

The flap, if not of adequate size (and it rarely is), can be enlarged by attaching a patch of appropriately sized GORE-TEX or autologous pericardium previously treated with glutaraldehyde with continuous suture of 5-0 Prolene (Fig. 23-16).

 TEARING THE FOSSA OVALIS

A segment of the fossa ovalis is usually torn open by an earlier balloon septostomy. It is also thin and sometimes full of perforating holes. This segment should be excised because it may tear at the suture line and produce a defect in the newly constructed atrial septum.

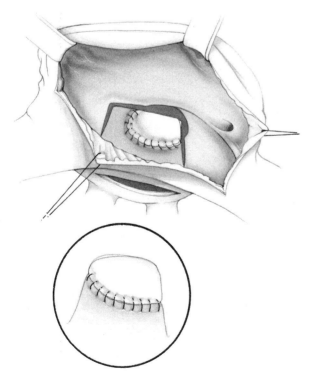

FIG. 23-16. Enlarging the septal flap with a patch of autologous pericardium or GORE-TEX.

The interatrial groove is dissected to free as much of the posterior atrial walls as possible. Traction on the septal flap brings the left atrium and pulmonary veins into view. A longitudinal incision is made parallel with and posterior to the groove into the left atrium (Fig. 23-16).

 SMALL LEFT ATRIAL OPENING

A transverse incision may be made down into the right superior pulmonary vein or between the right superior and inferior pulmonary veins to ensure a larger left atrial opening.

The Septal Flap

The septal flap must be mobile enough so that it can be slightly rotated without causing any tension. The midpoint of the anterior margin of the flap is sutured to the left atrial wall behind the left auricle just in front of and between the left superior and inferior pulmonary veins with double-armed, continuous sutures of 5-0 Prolene. The suture line is continued both superiorly and inferiorly along the posterior wall of the left atrium to the base of the flap.

 OBSTRUCTION OF THE LEFT PULMONARY VEINS

The flap must be of adequate size or it will be under tension and cause obstruction of the left pulmonary veins at their orifices.

 SUTURE LINE BREAKS

The suture line should be checked for leaks with a nerve hook to prevent any postoperative shunting.

Sewing the Anterior Edge of the Posterior Segment

The anterior edge of the posterior segment of the right atrium is sutured to the anterior part of the septal defect between the mitral and tricuspid valves. Suturing is continued superiorly and inferiorly around the lateral margins of the orifices of the superior and inferior venae cavae (Fig. 23-17).

 INJURY TO THE ATRIOVENTRICULAR NODE

The suture line, when continued down toward the inferior vena cava, should pass either below or posterior to the coronary sinus to avoid any injury to the atrioventricular node.

OBSTRUCTION OF THE INFERIOR VENA CAVA

The medial aspect of the eustachian valve of the inferior vena cava, when well developed, is an important landmark because it signifies the medial limit of the orifice of the inferior vena cava. The approximation of the atrial wall flap to the medial margin of the eustachian valve ensures an adequate inflow channel for the inferior vena cava.

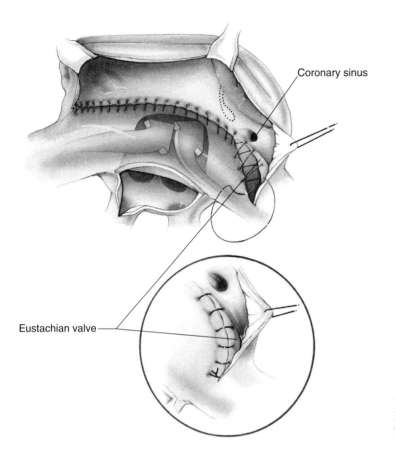

Coronary sinus

Eustachian valve

FIG. 23-17. Direction of the suture line to prevent injury to the atrioventricular node. **Inset:** Close-up of the suture line below the coronary sinus.

⊘ *UNDERDEVELOPED OR ABSENT EUSTACHIAN VALVE*

If the eustachian valve is absent or underdeveloped, a venous cannula of appropriate size may be introduced through the left auricle and the newly constructed atrial septal defect into the inferior vena cava. The atrial wall flap is then sutured in place using the cannula as a stent. This cannula can also be used as a means of venous drainage during the warming phase of the procedure (Fig. 23-18).

⊘ *CAVAL OBSTRUCTION*

If suturing impinges on the orifices of the superior or inferior vena cava, the resultant constriction may cause obstruction to the venous return. This can be particularly troublesome with the superior vena cava (Fig. 23-19).

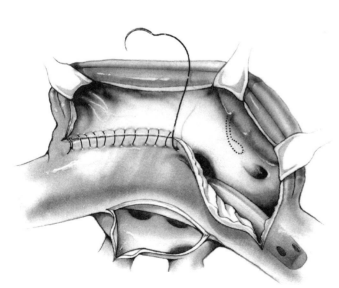

FIG. 23-18. Introduction of a venous cannula into the inferior vena cava when the eustachian valve is absent or underdeveloped to ensure adequate flow.

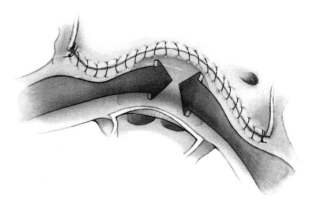

FIG. 23-19. Obstruction to venous return owing to constriction at the orifices of the vena cava.

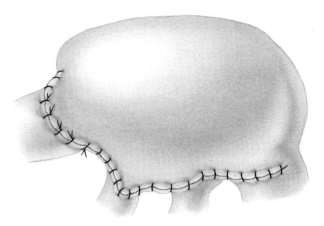

FIG. 23-20. Closure of the right atrium.

Sewing the Posterior Edge of the Anterior Segment

The posterior edge of the anterior segment of the right atrial wall is now sewn to the left atrial opening and the right atrial wall around the caval channel (Fig. 23-20).

 INJURY TO THE SINOATRIAL NODE
To prevent injury to the sinoatrial node, suturing is done with interrupted sutures 0.5 to 1 cm above the superior cavoatrial junction. If time is a limiting factor, continuous suturing with 6-0 or 7-0 Prolene taking small bites is an alternative technique.

 CAVAL CONSTRICTION
The caval snares are loosened so that both cavae become filled, fully distended, and stretched before suturing is continued. This prevents any caval constriction.

🚫 *INADEQUATE RIGHT ATRIAL WALL*
Occasionally, the anterior part of the right atrial wall may not be adequate to provide a satisfactory

roof over the new caval drainage chamber and allow comfortable approximation to the left atrial opening. This problem can be overcome by adding a patch of pericardium or GORE-TEX to enlarge the atrial wall (Fig. 23-21). This is particularly useful when the auricles (atria) are juxtaposed. In these cases, there is always too little atrial wall, and enlargement with a patch becomes mandatory.

MUSTARD PROCEDURE

Incision

A right anterior thoracotomy or median sternotomy provides exposure for performance of the Mustard operation, although most surgeons prefer a median sternotomy (see Chapter 1).

The Baffle

The pericardium is dissected free from the thymus gland and pleural reflections, and a large segment of it is removed with care to avoid injury to the phrenic nerves (Fig. 23-22). The pericardium is then cut into an appropriate size and shape. The rectangular shape used in the past has gradually been replaced by a wedge or a dumbbell shape. Brom's trouser-shaped baffle has the advantage of taking all the detailed intraatrial dimensions into consideration (Fig. 23-23).

The major complication of the Mustard procedure, apart from dysrhythmia, has been obstruction to both systemic and pulmonary venous systems, which can be attributed to baffle malfunction. Therefore, a clear and accurate understanding of the functional anatomy of Mustard's procedure is essential to prevent subsequent complications. The atrial septum must be excised as completely as possible (taking care not to injure the sinoatrial

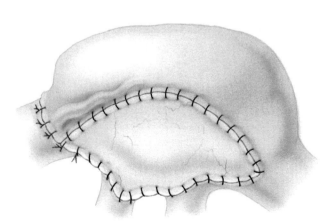

FIG. 23-21. Use of a patch of pericardium or GORE-TEX to enlarge the atrial wall.

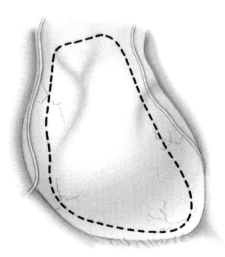

FIG. 23-22. Segment of pericardium for use as a baffle in the Mustard procedure.

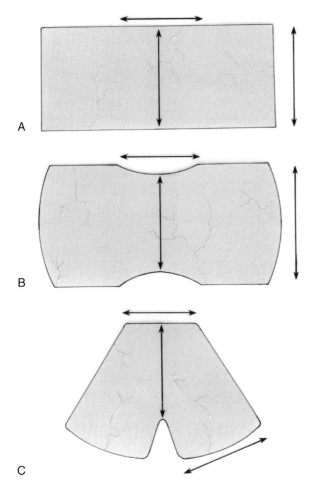

FIG. 23-23. Appropriate sizes and shapes of pericardium for a baffle. **A:** Traditional rectangle shape. **B:** Dumbbell shape. **C:** Trouser shape. See legend to Fig. 23-24 for explanation of dimensions.

node artery and the preferential conduction pathways; see hazards in Senning Procedure section). The baffle then becomes the new interatrial septum and functions as part of the inflow tract for drainage from the caval system into the mitral valve.

NB *THE DORSAL MARGIN OF THE BAFFLE*
The dorsal margin of the baffle should be 0.5 cm longer than the combined diameters of both left pulmonary veins (they can each be measured with calibrated Hegar's dilators). In small infants younger than 6 months of age or weighing less than 5 kg, the pulmonary veins measure approximately 7 mm in diameter. Thus, the dorsal margin of the baffle in the small infant is 2 to 2.5 cm (Fig. 23-24).

NB *WIDTH OF THE BAFFLE*
The distance from the left pulmonary veins to the atrial septal remnant at its midpoint is the width of the lateral wall of the new systemic venous atrium. The width of the baffle should be the same because

the baffle will now function as the interatrial septum and form part of the inflow tract for drainage of the superior and inferior venae cavae into the new pulmonary ventricle through the mitral valve. This distance is 3 cm in infants and 3.5 to 5 cm in older children (Fig. 23-24).

Technique for Preparing the Baffle

The size of the caval openings should be noted, and the two limbs of the baffle should be wide enough to be sewn well away from the caval orifices. This is usually 2.5 to 4 cm, depending on the size of the patient (Fig. 23-24). Regardless of the baffle material used, proper shape and size are significant factors in the prevention of baffle complications. For this reason, Brom designed metallic patterns for different age groups. This pattern is placed on the sheet of pericardium, and the baffle is prepared by cutting around the pattern with a knife. Dacron velour and GORE-TEX are easier to handle than pericardium and probably will not undergo shrinkage or deformation; for these reasons, they are the materials of choice for many surgeons. Untreated pericardium may shrink to approximately two-thirds of its original size. However, when autologous pericardium is pretreated with glutaraldehyde, it becomes fixed and changes minimally over time. Nevertheless, the normal atrial wall should dilate and enlarge to maintain adequate atrial volumes. In any case, baffle shrinkage is generally limited to a great extent by the degree of tension created by a secure suture line. Therefore, only attention to detail in preparing a baffle of adequate shape and size and meticulously suturing it in place will prevent many of the complications usually associated with this procedure.

Cannulation

The anterosuperior aspect of the ascending aorta is cannulated as described earlier (see Chapter 2). Most patients who are candidates for the Mustard operation are younger than 1 year old and have already undergone a balloon septostomy. In small infants, deep hypothermia and total circulatory arrest may be used and a single atrial cannula is sufficient. Direct bicaval cannulation with continuous cardiopulmonary bypass is used in most patients.

Right Atrial Incision

The right atrium is opened with an oblique incision, anterior to and parallel with the sulcus terminalis, and its edges are suspended to the pericardium or skin towels.

 INJURY TO THE SINOATRIAL NODE
The sinoatrial node is always prone to injury from cannulation, passage of tape around the superior vena cava, and atriotomy. The incision should be

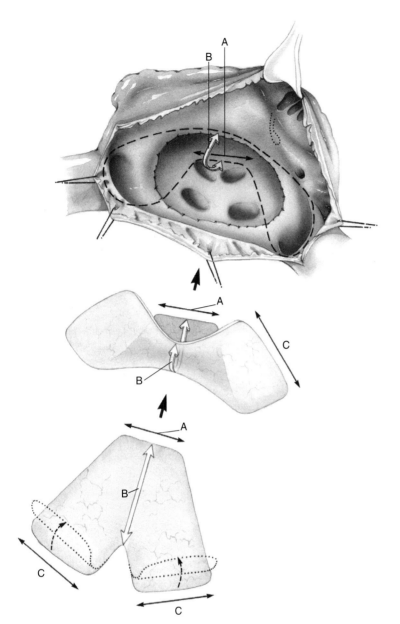

FIG. 23-24. Size of the baffle corresponding to the age of the patient. The dorsal margin *(A)* in small infants is 2 to 2.5 cm. The width of the baffle *(B)* is approximately 3 cm in infants and 3 to 5 cm in older children. Caval openings *(C)* are 2.5 to 4 cm.

well away from the sinoatrial node, and its cranial extension should be limited to 0.5 cm from the superior margin of the right atrium. If additional length is required, the incision can be extended anteriorly into the right atrial appendage (Fig. 23-13).

Excision of the Atrial Septum

The atrial septum, including the fossa ovalis (which may have already been torn by a previous balloon septostomy), is now partially excised. The line of incision begins in the foramen ovale and is extended cranially toward the center of the superior vena cava orifice for a short distance (approximately 7 mm). It is then continued dorsally toward the base of the interatrial septum and is finally curved caudally (parallel with the septum) (Fig. 23-25). The ventral or

anterior margin of the fossa ovalis is also cut caudally, avoiding the coronary sinus and extending toward the ostium of the inferior vena cava. The septal remnant is now removed, and the raw edges of the septum are endothelialized using interrupted sutures of 6-0 Prolene (Fig. 23-25, inset). This technique ensures safe removal of as large a segment of atrial septum as possible.

 EXCISION OF THE SEPTUM
The artery to the sinoatrial node traverses the anterosuperior quadrant of the atrial wall. Excision of the septum should spare the vascular supply of the sinoatrial node. This can be achieved by starting the excision through the foramen ovale cranially and then continuing it dorsally toward the interatrial groove (Fig. 23-25).

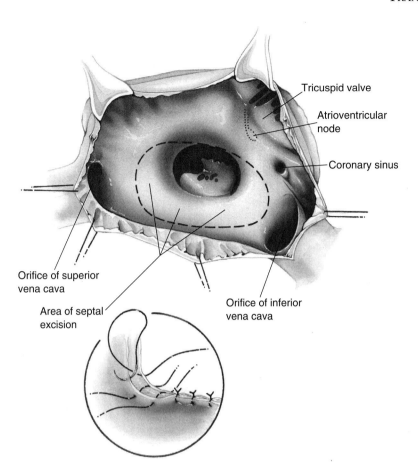

Tricuspid valve

Atrioventricular node

Coronary sinus

Orifice of superior vena cava

Orifice of inferior vena cava

Area of septal excision

FIG. 23-25. Excision of the atrial septum. **Inset:** Endothelialization of the edges of the septum.

⊘ *PREFERENTIAL CONDUCTION TRACTS*
There are three main preferential conduction tracts joining the sinoatrial node to the atrioventricular node (Fig. 23-15). These probably correspond with the crista terminalis and limbic muscle bundles. The anterior tract passes anterior to both the fossa ovalis and coronary sinus. The middle tract also lies anterior to the fossa ovalis but may pass through or just posterior to the coronary sinus. The posterior preferential tract crosses in the posterior wall of the right atrium between the cavae and then curves forward toward the coronary sinus. Although the middle tract and the posterior tract are more likely to be sacrificed during excision of the atrial septum, every precaution should be made not to injure or traumatize the anterior conduction tract.

Baffle Insertion

The baffle is sutured in place with 5-0 continuous Prolene suture starting between the left superior pulmonary vein and the left atrial appendage. The suture line continues along the posterior wall of the left atrium toward the base of the most lateral aspect of the superior vena cava and then curves gradually onto the right atrial wall around the orifice of the superior vena cava before continuing back along the edge of the already cut atrial septum (Fig. 23-26).

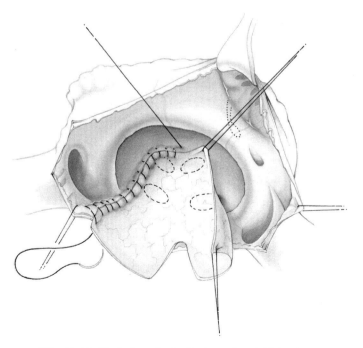

FIG. 23-26. Technique for baffle insertion: initial sutures.

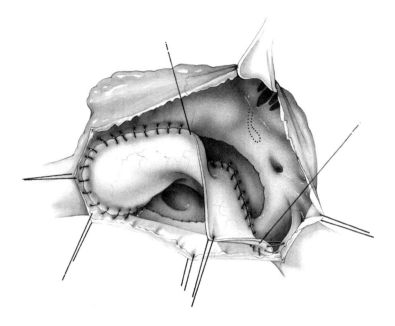

FIG. 23-27. Technique for baffle insertion: completing the sutures.

Similarly, the other end of the suture is continued along the margin of the left inferior pulmonary vein and the posterior atrial wall and toward the lateral margin of the eustachian valve of the inferior vena cava. It then curves around the orifice of the inferior vena cava onto the right atrial wall before returning along the cut edge of the atrial septum behind the coronary sinus to be tied to the other end of the suture (Fig. 23-27).

 DIRECTION OF THE CAVAL LEGS OF THE BAFFLE
The caval legs of the baffle should extend obliquely toward the base of lateral margins of the superior and inferior venae cavae to lessen the possibility of pulmonary vein obstruction as a result of future baffle constriction (Fig. 23-28).

 POSITIONING OF THE SUTURE LINE
The suture line should be a good distance away from the margin of the pulmonary veins so as not to encroach on their lumina and give rise to possible pulmonary venous obstruction.

 PREVENTING OBSTRUCTION TO THE SUPERIOR VENA CAVA
Special care should be taken to ensure a wide superior vena cava opening while suturing some distance away from the margin of the orifice. Small bites of the right atrial wall followed by relatively larger bites on the baffle result in balloon-

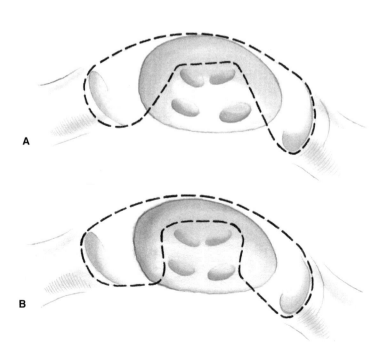

FIG. 23-28. Direction of the caval legs of the baffle. **A:** Correct. **B:** Incorrect.

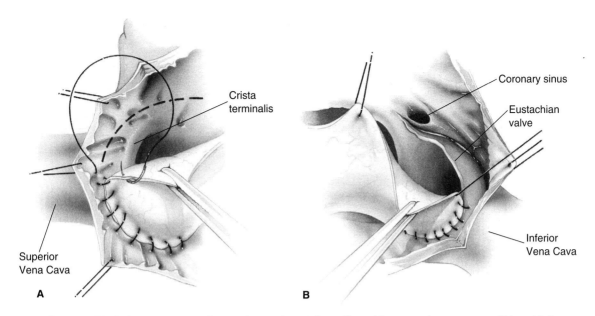

FIG. 23-29. Technique to prevent future obstruction at the orifice of the superior vena cava **(A)** and inferior vena cava **(B)**.

ing of the baffle, lessening the possibility of future obstruction to the superior vena cava (Fig. 23-29A).

 PREVENTING OBSTRUCTION TO THE INFERIOR VENA CAVA
The same precautions should be taken to prevent obstruction to the inferior vena cava. The suture line of the baffle is continued along the border of the eustachian valve so as not to impinge on the inferior vena cava orifice (Fig. 23-29B).

 RELATIONSHIP OF THE CORONARY SINUS TO THE BAFFLE
Because of the close proximity of the conduction tracts and atrioventricular node to the coronary sinus, the baffle suture line is continued behind the coronary sinus. This allows its drainage to mix with the pulmonary venous return (Fig. 23-30).

SUTURE LINE LEAKS
With the aid of a fine nerve hook, the surgeon must check the suture line for possible leaks that could

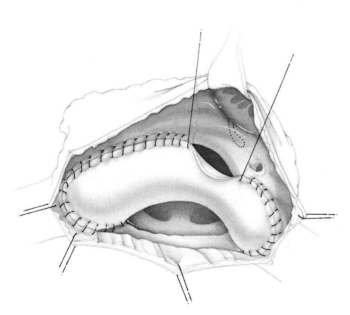

FIG. 23-30. Relationship of the coronary sinus to the baffle.

be corrected with additional sutures at this time to prevent postoperative shunting. This can also be accomplished by releasing the caval tapes if the patient is on cardiopulmonary bypass and occluding the venous cannula. The baffle will balloon out and reveal any possible leaks, providing an opportunity to judge the caval drainage visually.

⊘ OBSTRUCTION OF THE MITRAL VALVE BY REDUNDANT BAFFLE

If there is some gross redundancy of the baffle, it can obstruct the mitral valve orifice during diastole. Excess baffle material should be noted and excised (Fig. 23-31).

Management of Late Complications of the Mustard Procedure

Hemodynamic Deterioration

Episodic hemodynamic deterioration in the immediate postoperative period may be owing to baffle redundancy that may intermittently protrude into the mitral valve and obstruct the venous return (Fig. 23-31A). This problem can easily be diagnosed by two-dimensional echocardiography. The patient must undergo another operation as soon as possible, and redundancy must be excised and the defect sutured together (Fig. 23-31B).

Baffle Leaks

Minor leaks are relatively common in most patients. Occasionally, the leak is large enough to warrant reoperation. At the time of surgery, primary closure may be possible, but more commonly a patch of GORE-TEX or pericardium is used to make up for the shrunken pericardium and to reduce tension on the suture line (Fig. 23-32).

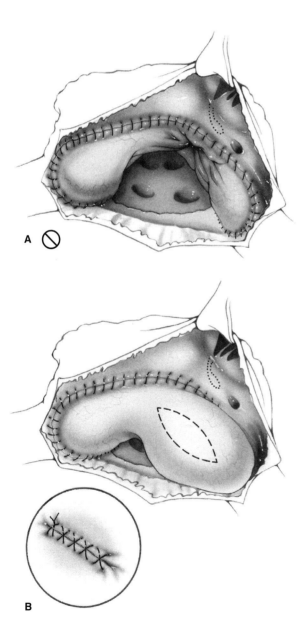

FIG. 23-31. A: Mitral valve obstruction from the baffle redundancy. **B:** Excision of gross redundancy of the baffle to prevent obstruction of the mitral valve orifice during diastole.

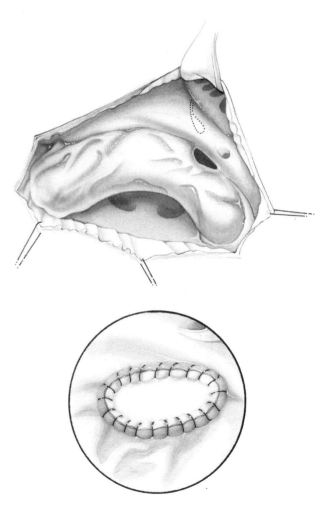

FIG. 23-32. Patching a baffle leak.

Obstruction to the Superior Vena Cava

Obstruction to the superior vena cava may have important implications owing to elevated central venous pressure in the upper body. Obstruction is usually owing to inadequate width and length of the superior limb of the baffle or to suturing too close to the ostium of the superior vena cava. Unless the gradient across the caval ostium is minimal, these patients should undergo surgical correction of the obstruction. At the time of reoperation, the baffle looks thickened, shrunken, and wrinkled. It is incised longitudinally, and the superior vena cava inflow is enlarged by suturing an appropriately sized GORE-TEX patch in place. The right atrium is also enlarged with the same patch material (Fig. 23-33).

Obstruction to the Inferior Vena Cava

Obstruction to the inferior vena cava is rarely seen, but when it occurs, it can be approached in the same fashion as obstruction to the superior vena cava.

Obstruction to the Pulmonary Veins

Fibrosis and cicatrization around the lumen of the right pulmonary veins may cause obstruction to the pulmonary venous return. These patients should undergo surgical correction. The technique entails extension of a transverse right atriotomy that crosses the interatrial groove between the superior and inferior pulmonary veins for a short distance. The defect can be repaired by an appro-

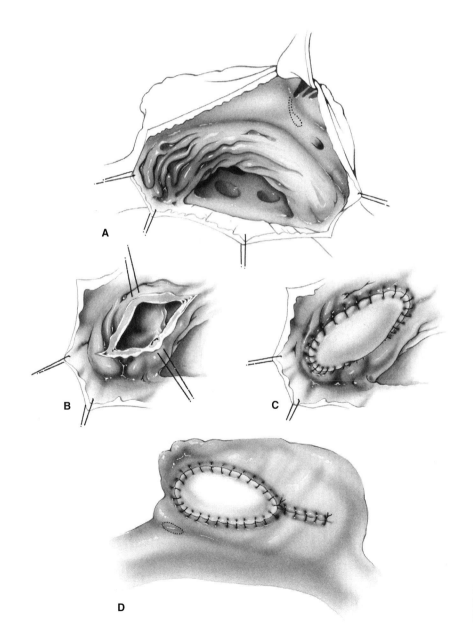

FIG. 23-33. A–D: Stepwise technique for a patch enlargement of an obstructive baffle.

priately sized patch; alternatively, the parietal pericardium can be sewn to the edges of the atriotomy to a point well above the right pulmonary veins. This substantially enlarges the pulmonary inflow tract. The remaining right atriotomy can be closed either directly or with a separate patch of pericardium or GORE-TEX. Alternatively, if the pulmonary venous obstruction has led to pulmonary hypertension, the left ventricle may be prepared for an arterial switch procedure. If the pulmonary artery pressure is at least two-thirds systemic, a combined arterial switch procedure and removal of the interatrial baffle and atrial reseptation can be performed in one stage.

CHAPTER 24

Aortopulmonary Window

An aortopulmonary window is a relatively rare anomaly that can occur either as an isolated defect or in association with other congenital lesions, such as ventriculoseptal defect, atrioseptal defect, patent ductus arteriosus, and tetralogy of Fallot. The defect classically occurs between the main pulmonary artery and aorta just above the level of sinus of Valsalva (Fig. 24-1A). Occasionally, the defect may be at the origin of the right pulmonary artery (Fig. 24-1B). Rarely, the right pulmonary artery may actually have a separate anomalous origin from the aorta (Fig. 24-1C).

Although simple ligation or division between clamps has been successfully performed in the past, closure of the defect under direct vision with the aid of cardiopulmonary bypass or total hypothermic arrest is now the method of choice. This prevents serious hemorrhagic complications that can occur as a result of the fragility of the great vessel walls and allows precise closure of the various forms of the defect.

INCISION

A median sternotomy provides excellent exposure. The aorta and both venae cavae are cannulated in preparation for cardiopulmonary bypass. A single atrial cannula is used when hypothermic arrest is used.

TECHNIQUE

On cardiopulmonary bypass with moderate hypothermia, the ascending aorta is clamped just below the aortic cannula. Cardioplegic solution is administered into the aortic root, and the ascending aorta is then incised longitudinally between two traction sutures of fine Prolene. The defect is identified, and a patch of autologous pericardium prepared with glutaraldehyde or GORE-TEX is used to close the defect with 5-0 or 6-0 continuous Prolene sutures (Fig. 24-2). The aortotomy is then closed with continuous sutures of fine Prolene.

Alternatively, an incision is made through the anterior part of the window itself. The opening of the right pulmonary artery and the ostia of the left and right coronary arteries are identified. A patch of pericardium or GORE-TEX is then sewn to the posterior, superior, and inferior edges of the window. At the edges of the incision, the suture is continued, passing through the pulmonary artery edge, the patch, and then the aortic wall until the entire opening is closed. In this fashion, the patch is sandwiched between the aorta and pulmonary artery to close the window (Fig. 24-3).

The patient is rewarmed. All air is evacuated, and the aortic clamp is removed.

 AORTIC CANNULATION
Aortic cannulation must be done high on the ascending aorta so that cross-clamping will still allow good visualization of the defect.

 OCCLUDING THE PULMONARY ARTERIES
Both right and left pulmonary arteries must be occluded with snares immediately before initiation of cardiopulmonary bypass to prevent flooding of the pulmonary circulation. The snares must be kept in place while cardioplegia is delivered into the aortic root.

 DAMAGE TO THE LEFT CORONARY OSTIUM
The lower margin of the defect may be in close proximity to the left coronary artery ostium; therefore, closure of the defect must be performed in such a manner as to avoid damaging the coronary ostium.

⊘ ***ANOMALOUS ORIGIN OF THE CORONARY ARTERIES***
Occasionally, the right coronary artery, and rarely the left coronary artery, may arise from the pulmonary trunk close to the edge of the defect. In these cases, the patch must be modified to baffle the coronary opening into the aorta.

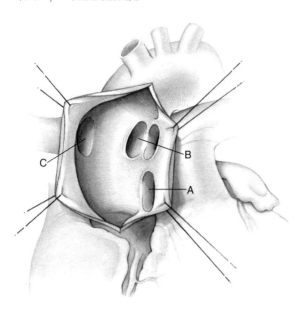

FIG. 24-1. Types of aortopulmonary window. Defect just above the level of the sinuses of Valsalva; *(A)*. Defect at the origin of right pulmonary artery; *(B)*. Anomalous origin of the right pulmonary artery from the aorta *(C)*.

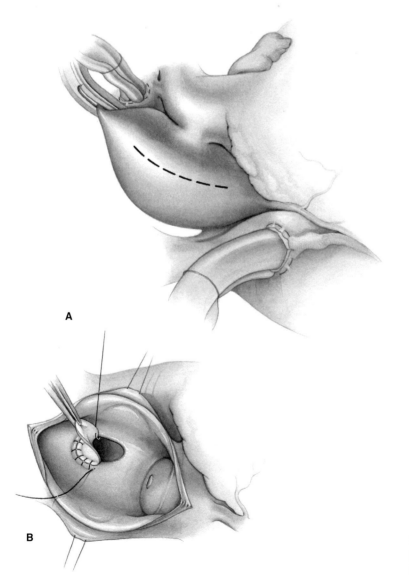

FIG. 24-2. Technique for closure of an aortopulmonary window. **A:** Incision of the aorta. **B:** Patch closure of the defect.

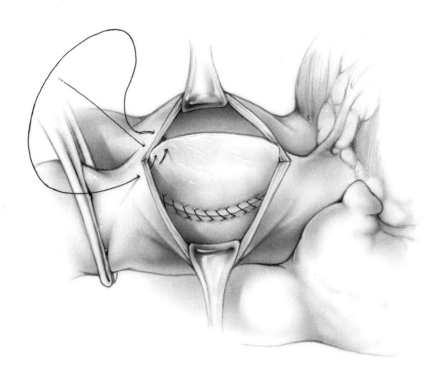

FIG. 24-3. Sandwich patch closure of an aortopulmonary window.

PULMONARY ARTERY STENOSIS
When the defect involves the origins of both pulmonary arteries, the patch inside the aorta must be sewn well away from the margins of the defect to prevent stenosis of the right or left pulmonary artery.

NB ### ANOMALOUS ORIGIN OF THE RIGHT PULMONARY ARTERY FROM THE AORTA
If the right pulmonary artery has an anomalous origin from the aorta, it is detached from the aorta and anastomosed to the main pulmonary artery with continuous 6-0 Prolene sutures. The resulting defect in the aorta is then closed with an appropriately sized patch of GORE-TEX or piece of pulmonary homograft.

POOR EXPOSURE OF THE DEFECT
It may be difficult to adequately expose and repair the defect with the aortic cross-clamp in place. In these cases, a brief period of hypothermic arrest allows the cross-clamp to be removed to identify and patch the defect precisely.

CHAPTER 25

Truncus Arteriosus

Persistent truncus arteriosus is characterized by the emergence of a single common arterial trunk from the left ventricle. The main pulmonary artery or the right and left pulmonary arteries originate from the side or posterior aspect of the truncal artery at various distances above the truncal valve. Most commonly, the truncal valve is trileaflet and semilunar and overrides a high ventricular septal defect. Nearly one-half of the valves have two or four leaflets; all truncal valves exhibit varying degrees of dysplasia and may be regurgitant, stenotic, or both. Often, the main pulmonary artery originates from the left side of the truncus arteriosus and divides into left and right branches that traverse in the usual fashion to their respective lungs. This form has been classified as type I by Collett and Edwards. In type II, the right and left pulmonary arteries originate adjacent to each other from the side or back of the truncal artery. In type III, each pulmonary artery originates from different parts of the truncal artery (Fig. 25-1). Type IV, when the lungs are supplied by two pulmonary arteries originating in the descending thoracic aorta, is now considered not a true truncus arteriosus but a form of pulmonary atresia with a ventricular septal defect.

In most infants, the truncus arteriosus should undergo correction within the first 2 to 3 months of life to avoid the development of irreversible pulmonary vascular disease. Pulmonary artery banding is no longer recommended in infancy because it carries a high mortality and experience has shown that it is not beneficial. In symptomatic infants with congestive heart failure, surgery may be performed any time after 2 to 3 weeks of age when the pulmonary vascular resistance has fallen.

INCISION

A median sternotomy is the approach of choice.

TECHNIQUE

A high aortic cannulation is made. A single atrial cannulation is adequate if total circulatory arrest is contemplated. Some surgeons prefer direct cannulation of the superior vena cava and low atrial cannulation just above the inferior vena cava. The anatomy is well evaluated, and the aorta and pulmonary arteries are dissected free and mobilized. Tapes are passed around the pulmonary arteries so that they can be occluded just before the initiation of cardiopulmonary bypass.

 AORTIC CANNULA POSITION
The aortic cannula should be placed at the level of the innominate artery to ensure adequate exposure of the pulmonary arteries after the cross-clamp is applied. Alternatively, the aortic cannula can be removed and the innominate and left carotid arteries snared after circulatory arrest is achieved.

 FLOODING OF THE LUNGS
It is essential to dissect the pulmonary artery and both its branches so that they can be encircled and occluded as soon as cardiopulmonary bypass is initiated. This prevents runoff of arterial flow from the pump into the lungs, which may lead to inadequate systemic perfusion and flooding of the pulmonary circulation.

Cardiopulmonary bypass is initiated, the pulmonary artery snares are tightened, and systemic cooling is begun.

 TRUNCAL VALVE INSUFFICIENCY
If significant truncal valve insufficiency is present, the heart may distend as soon as cardiopulmonary bypass is begun. A vent should be immediately placed through the right superior pulmonary vein into the left ventricle (see Chapter 4). If regurgitation is severe, a large amount of the aortic line return may be retrieved by the left ventricular vent, leading to inadequate systemic perfusion. In this case, the truneal artery must be clamped immedi-

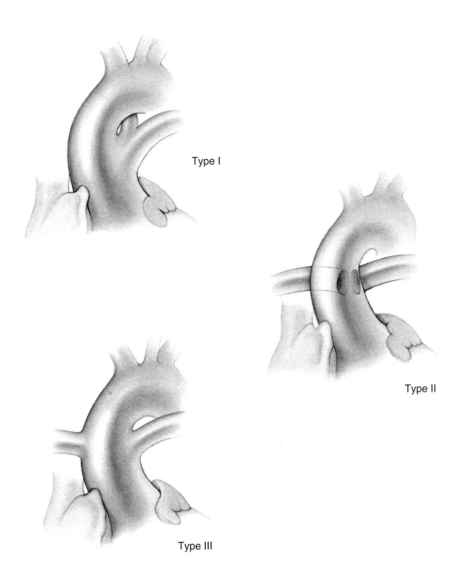

Type I

Type II

Type III

FIG. 25-1. Forms of truncus arteriosus.

ately and cardioplegic solution may have to be administered directly into the coronary arteries.

The truncus is cross-clamped, and cardioplegic solution is administered in the usual manner. The main pulmonary artery is detached from the truncal artery (Fig. 25-2A), and the defect is closed with two layers of continuous 6-0 or 5-0 Prolene sutures (Fig. 25-2B). In type II or III defects, the pulmonary arteries are similarly detached, leaving a rim of aortic tissue attached to their origins, and the resulting defect in the truncal artery is closed.

 TOO LARGE A DEFECT ON THE AORTA
If the defect is too large and direct closure of the truncal artery (now the aorta) will result in supravalvular stenosis, an autologous pericardial or GORE-TEX patch of appropriate size is used to close the defect (Fig. 25-2C).

 ADEQUATE TISSUE SURROUNDING THE PULMONARY ARTERIES
The main or right and left pulmonary arteries must be excised in continuity with adequate surrounding tissue. Often, this can be best accomplished by transecting the truncal artery just above the pulmonary arteries, excising the orifices of the pulmonary arteries, and then performing an end-to-end anastomosis of the ascending aorta to the truncal root. This technique necessitates adequate mobilization of the distal ascending aorta, aortic arch, and arch vessels to prevent undue tension on the aortic suture line.

 INJURY TO THE CORONARY OSTIUM
The left coronary artery may be located high on the posterior wall of the truncal root. Care must be taken when closing the aortic defect to not injure the left coronary artery.

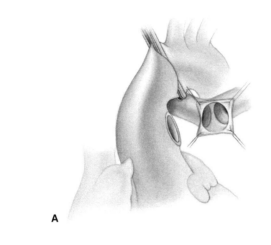

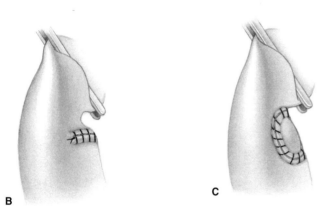

FIG. 25-2. A: Detachment of the pulmonary artery from the truncal artery. **B:** Direct closure of the resulting defect. **C:** Patch closure of the defect.

INADEQUATE CARDIOPLEGIC PROTECTION
The snares on the pulmonary arteries must be kept in place until after the cardioplegic solution has been delivered. Otherwise, the cardioplegia will run off into the pulmonary circulation and inadequate amounts will reach the coronary bed. When significant truncal valve insufficiency is present, cardioplegic solution should be delivered directly into the coronary ostia or retrograde into the coronary sinus (see Chapter 3).

A high, longitudinal right ventriculotomy is made, and the ventriculoseptal defect is identified. Usually, the septal defect is a subarterial infundibular type with a thick lower rim (Fig. 25-3). Occasionally, it may be a large perimembranous type extending to the rim of the tricuspid valve.

ABNORMAL CORONARY ARTERY BRANCHES
Ventriculotomy should attempt to spare any major coronary arteries on the anterior surface of the right ventricle. The left anterior descending coronary artery is particularly at risk when it takes origin from the right coronary artery.

TOO HIGH RIGHT VENTRICULOTOMY
Care must be taken when extending the ventriculotomy superiorly to avoid cutting or injuring the truncal valve and annulus.

The ventriculoseptal defect is then closed with a Dacron velour patch, using continuous 5-0 Prolene sutures (Fig. 25-4). The superior edge of the patch meets the upper edge of the ventriculotomy and will be incorporated into the suture line of the right ventricular–pulmonary artery conduit. The air may be removed from the aortic root and the aorta unclamped at this time to shorten the ischemic time. If hypothermic arrest has been used, the heart is now filled with saline and cardiopulmonary bypass is recommenced.

LEFT VENTRICULAR DISTENTION
If significant aortic regurgitation is present, left ventricular distention may occur when the cross-clamp is removed. This may respond to manual decompression until the heart is warm enough to eject.

NB *TRUNCAL VALVE REPAIR*
If truncal regurgitation is mild to moderate, most surgeons recommend a conservative approach. The sinotubular junction can be narrowed if it appears that this will improve the coaptation of dysplastic valve leaflets. The aorta is transected just above the sinotubular ridge. After excising the pulmonary arteries, a wedge of tissue is removed anteriorly from the distal aorta so that, when closed, the new diameter of the distal aorta will be the new sinotubular diameter. The aortic root is symmetrically gathered during the suturing process, bringing the proximal and distal aortic segments together. Occasionally, if there are more than three valve leaflets, one entire leaflet and the attached aortic wall may be excised and the resulting defect reapproximated with 5-0 or 6-0 Prolene suture. This reduces the size of the annulus and sinotubular junction (Fig. 25-5). The distal aorta is reduced in size by resecting a wedge of tissue of similar width and the two ends reanastomosed. Only if severe regurgitation persists should valve replacement with a homograft be carried out (see Chapter 5).

NB *PATENT FORAMEN OVALE*
In a patient younger than 2 to 3 months of age, a patent foramen ovale is normally left open to provide decompression of the right-sided circulation during the early postoperative period.

Ideally, a pulmonary or aortic homograft is used as the conduit. More recently, bovine jugular vein conduits have

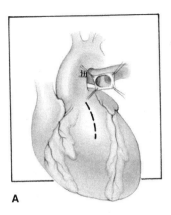

A

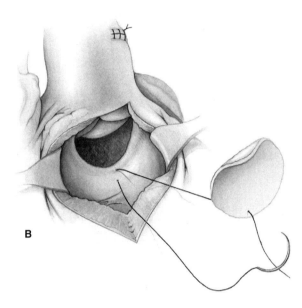

B

FIG. 25-3. Technique for closure of the associated ventricular septal defect. **A:** Right ventriculotomy. **B:** Patch closure of the ventricular septal defect.

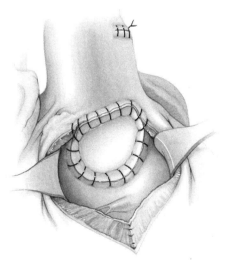

FIG. 25-4. Superior edge of the ventricular septal defect patch meets the upper edge of the ventriculotomy (see text).

been used , and porcine aortic roots such as the Freestyle valve are available in smaller sizes (see Chapter 5). The distal pulmonary artery is appropriately tailored. Four traction sutures are used on its adventitia to maintain the correct orientation.

⊘ *NONVALVED RIGHT VENTRICULAR TO PULMONARY ARTERY CONNECTIONS*
Nonvalved tube grafting and reconstruction of right ventricular to pulmonary artery continuity using autologous tissue and a pericardial patch have been done. Both approaches leave the infant with wide open pulmonary insufficiency that is poorly tolerated.

⊘ *TOO SMALL A PULMONARY ARTERY LUMEN*
The lumen of the pulmonary artery can be enlarged by extending the opening onto both its branches.

The homograft or conduit is cut to the appropriate length and anastomosed to the pulmonary artery with 5-

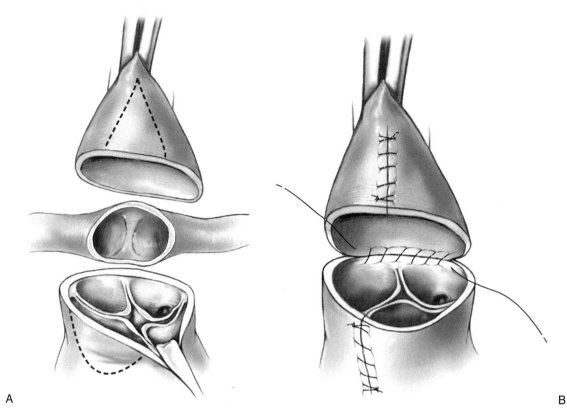

A   B

FIG. 25-5. Truncal valvuloplasty. **A:** Excision of one leaflet and the attached aortic wall. **B:** Reconstruction of a new truncal root, tailoring the distal ascending aorta. Anastomosis of the reconstructed root and ascending aorta.

0 or 6-0 Prolene suture. The posterior layer of the anastomosis is completed first (Fig. 25-6).

 HOMOGRAFT LENGTH
The homograft should be trimmed at a level just above the commissures of the valve. If the homograft is left too long, it will produce kinking of the pulmonary artery bifurcation.

 ANASTOMOTIC LEAKS FROM THE POSTERIOR WALL
An anastomotic leak from the posterior wall is practically impossible to control once the operation has been completed. For this reason, small bites close to each other should be taken.

The anterior distal anastomosis is then completed. The proximal end of the homograft is anastomosed to the right ventriculotomy beginning posteriorly, using 5-0 Prolene running sutures (Fig. 25-7). After approximately 40% of the circumference of the homograft has been attached in this fashion, the remainder of the opening is closed with a triangular patch of autologous pericardium prepared with glutaraldehyde solution, using running 5-0 or 6-0 Prolene sutures, attaching the patch along the anterior circumference of the homograft and the remainder of the right ventriculotomy opening (Fig. 25-8, inset). If an aortic homo-

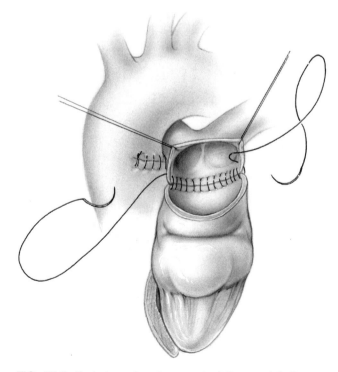

FIG. 25-6. Technique for placement of the conduit (homograft) from the right ventricle to the pulmonary artery. Posterior aspect of a distal anastomosis.

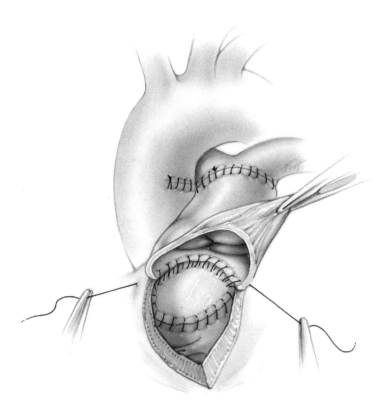

FIG. 25-7. Technique for placement of a homograft from the right ventricle to the pulmonary artery.

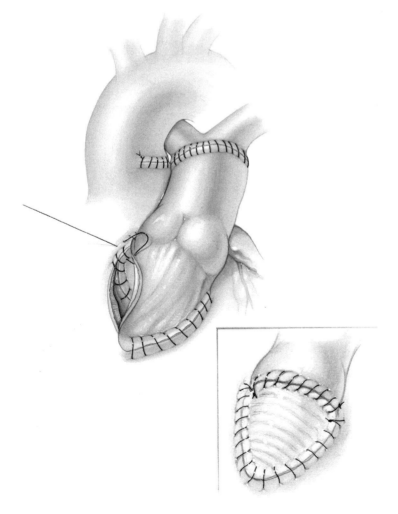

FIG. 25-8. Completion of placement of the aortic homograft conduit from the right ventricle to the pulmonary artery. **Inset:** Augmentation of a proximal anastomosis with pericardium when using a pulmonary homograft.

graft is used, it may be oriented so that the attached anterior leaflet of the mitral valve is lying anteriorly. This tissue may be used instead of a triangular patch of pericardium to close the remaining right ventriculotomy (Fig. 25-8).

NB *AORTIC HOMOGRAFT ORIENTATION*
Alternatively, it may be advantageous to orient the aortic homograft so that its greater curvature is leftward. This may prevent compression of the homograft when the chest is closed, thus avoiding valvular insufficiency and stenosis of the conduit.

 TWISTING OF THE CONDUIT
Care must be taken when performing the proximal anastomosis to maintain the correct orientation of the homograft to avoid distortion of the pulmonary artery confluence.

When the procedure is completed and the patient is warmed, the process of air removal is meticulously carried out and the patient is gradually weaned off bypass. Chest tubes are inserted, and the sternotomy is closed in the usual fashion.

CHAPTER 26

Ebstein's Anomaly

Ebstein's anomaly is a rare disease. The pathologic anatomy consists of displacement of part or all of the tricuspid valve orifice into the right ventricle. Attachments of all valve leaflets are abnormal, especially the septal and posterior leaflets, which are dysplastic and displaced downward. This gives rise to the extension of the right atrium into the right ventricle, resulting in an "atrialized" portion of the right ventricle above the valve. The anterior leaflet is large and usually has an abnormal insertion, sometimes producing obstruction in the right ventricular cavity. The atrioventricular node and conduction bundle lie within Koch's triangle as in the normal heart, but because of the downward displacement of the valve below the true atrioventricular junction, the atrialized ventricle separates the penetrating bundle from the valve proper. An atrioseptal defect or a patent foramen ovale is usually present (Fig. 26-1).

PRESENTATION

There is a wide range of anatomic variations of Ebstein's anomaly. The least severe form has a true right ventricle with adequate volume. These patients have very mild cyanosis and may be asymptomatic even as adults.

The most severe form consists of nearly complete atrialization of the right ventricle. These patients present as neonates with massive cardiomegaly and hypoplasia of both lungs. Because there is no forward flow from the right ventricle, there is functional pulmonary atresia. Ductal patency is therefore required for survival in these neonates.

SURGERY FOR THE NEONATE

Neonates who demonstrate a need for mechanical ventilation and dependence on prostaglandin E_1 to maintain ductal patency have a universally poor outcome with medical management. The surgical approach is designed to create a reliable source of pulmonary flow, reduce the massive cardiomegaly, and prevent severe tricuspid insufficiency. This operation creates a single ventricle physiology and allows a future Fontan procedure (see Chapter 29).

Incision

A median sternotomy is used, resecting most or all of the thymus.

Cannulation

The ascending aorta is cannulated. Bicaval cannulation or a single cannula in the right atrium with a period of circulatory arrest for the intracardiac portion of the procedure is usually used.

Technique

The ductus arteriosus is ligated with the institution of cardiopulmonary bypass. Cooling is carried out. The aorta is cross-clamped, and cold blood cardioplegic solution is administered into the aortic root. The operation can be carried out with a short period of deep hypothermic circulatory arrest. Alternatively, tapes around the cavae are snared snugly and cardiopulmonary bypass is continued with low perfusion flow. The right atrium is then opened through an oblique incision. The atrioseptal defect is enlarged. A piece of autologous pericardium treated with glutaraldehyde and rinsed in saline is then used to patch the tricuspid valve opening with running 6-0 Prolene suture, placing the coronary sinus beneath the patch (Fig. 26-2).

 INJURY TO THE CONDUCTION SYSTEM
By placing the coronary sinus on the right ventricular side of the pericardial patch, the risk of heart block is minimized.

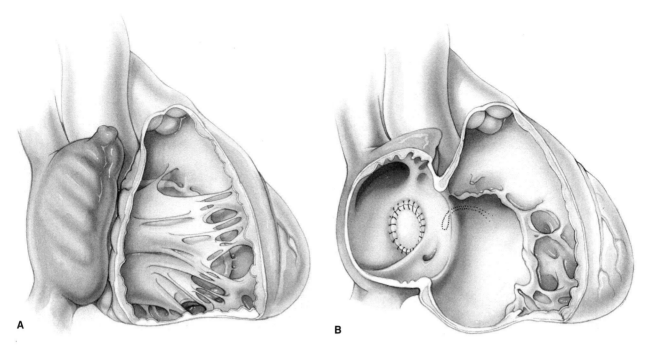

FIG. 26-1. Surgical view of Ebstein's anomaly. **A:** Right anterior oblique view of the heart with the anterior wall of the right ventricle cut away. The abnormally large anterior leaflet with its multiple anomalous attachments, as shown in this heart, sometimes impedes blood flow into the distal ventricle and pulmonary outflow tract. **B:** Same view as in **A** but with the anterolateral wall of the right atrium and the anterior tricuspid leaflet removed to show the dilated area of the atrialized ventricle and the displaced remnants of the septal and posterior tricuspid leaflets. The atrial septal defect has been closed with a patch.

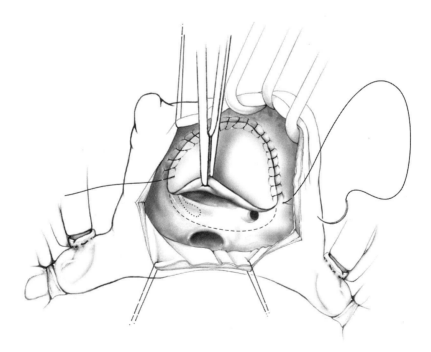

FIG. 26-2. The pericardial patch is sewn around the right ventricular orifice deviating into the true right atrium in the area of the conduction system (*dotted line*).

The excessively enlarged right atrium is reduced in size by excision of a segment of its free wall. The atriotomy is then closed with running 6-0 Prolene sutures. At this point, if circulatory arrest has been used, the heart is filled with saline and cardiopulmonary bypass is recommenced; the aortic cross-clamp is removed, and the usual deairing procedures are carried out. If continuous low-flow cardiopulmonary bypass has been used, the aortic cross-clamp can now be removed. During the rewarming phase, a 3.5- to 4.0-mm GORE-TEX interposition graft is constructed between the ascending aorta and main pulmonary artery or the innominate and right pulmonary artery. This shunt remains clamped until just before cardiopulmonary bypass is discontinued.

 RIGHT VENTRICULAR DISTENTION
These patients require significant inotropic support, usually including epinephrine to increase right ventricular contractility and thereby prevent distention of the right ventricle from coronary sinus return and blood from the thebesian veins.

 ANATOMIC PULMONARY ATRESIA
If anatomic pulmonary atresia is present, this operation should not be performed because fatal right ventricular distention results.

These patients subsequently become candidates for a staged Fontan procedure. A bidirectional cavopulmonary anastomosis is performed at 6 to 9 months followed by completion Fontan at 2 to 3 years of age (see Chapter 29).

NB *FORWARD FLOW THROUGH THE PULMONARY VALVE*
It is most important to bear in mind that when a Fontan procedure is to be performed in these patients, the right ventricular pulmonary arterial communication must be maintained to allow egress of the coronary sinus and thebesian vein blood flow.

SURGERY BEYOND INFANCY

Most patients do not become symptomatic until adolescence or adulthood. Symptoms include progressive heart failure and cyanosis secondary to severe, chronic tricuspid insufficiency.

Incision

A median sternotomy is the usual approach.

Cannulation

Bicaval cannulation is required and is most often accomplished with right-angled cannulae in the superior vena cava and the inferior vena cava–right atrium junction. The ascending aorta is cannulated for arterial return, and cardiopulmonary bypass is initiated. Myocardial preservation is accomplished with cold blood potassium cardioplegic solution administered into the aortic root after aortic cross-clamping. This may be complemented by the retrograde technique (see Chapter 3).

Exposure of Tricuspid Valve

A longitudinal atriotomy is made 1 cm posterior to and parallel with the atrioventricular groove. The atriotomy edges are retracted with sutures, and exposure of the tricuspid valve is further facilitated by means of appropriately sized Cooley or Richardson retractors.

Repair of the Tricuspid Valve

When the anterior leaflet is large and has a relatively normal attachment, tricuspid insufficiency is the essential hemodynamic abnormality. During the operation, the displaced posterior and septal annuli (up to a point adjacent to the coronary sinus) are pulled upward into the right atrium proper to the level of the atrioventricular junction by means of interrupted 3-0 Ticron sutures buttressed with Dacron or pericardial pledgets on both the atrial and ventricular sides of the sutures (Fig. 26-3).

 RIGHT CORONARY ARTERY INJURY
The ventricular plication sutures must be placed carefully after identifying the posterior descending and other large branches of the right coronary artery to avoid direct injury to or distortion of the coronary arteries, which can result in myocardial infarction.

 INJURY TO CONDUCTION TISSUE
Because of the proximity of the atrioventricular node to His's bundle, placement of sutures that extend between the septal leaflet and the true right atrium is hazardous, particularly to the left of the coronary sinus.

 CREATION OF AN ANEURYSMAL CAVITY
The mattress sutures are woven in and out of the atrialized portion of the right ventricle so that when they are tied, the atrialized ventricle is completely obliterated and no aneurysmal chamber is formed (Fig. 26-3).

NB *BICUSPIDIZATION*
Depending on the local anatomy, it is sometimes possible to exclude the posterior leaflet by a modified annuloplasty converting the tricuspid valve into a bicuspid valve (or if the septal leaflet is very dysplastic, a monocuspid valve) and thus eliminate

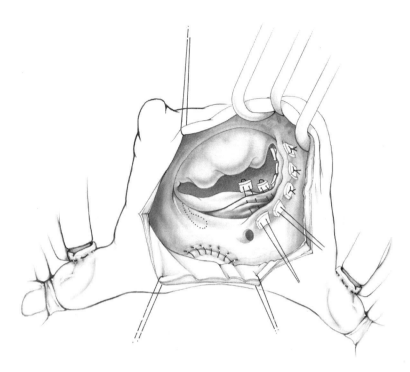

FIG. 26-3. Repair of the tricuspid valve with pledgeted sutures.

any tricuspid insufficiency (Fig. 26-4). This is achieved by constricting the posterior segment of the annulus with interrupted sutures of 3-0 Ticron buttressed with pledgets.

An alternate technique championed by Carpentier entails temporary detachment of the anterior leaflet and adjacent part of the posterior leaflet, allowing them to slide for ease of reconstructing a competent tricuspid valve (Fig. 26-5A). One-third of the anterior leaflet attachment proximal to the anterior septal commissure is left intact. Extensive mobilization is achieved by dividing the fibrous band connections of the leaflets to the muscular wall of the right ventricle. The interchordal spaces on the leaflets may require conservative fenestration.

The atrialized segment of the right ventricle can now be clearly visualized. It is plicated with multiple interrupted sutures of 3-0 Ticron, and the posterior annulus is similarly reduced in size to achieve a relatively normal right ventricular geometry. The redundant atrial wall behind the coronary sinus may also need to be plicated with continuous suture of 4-0 Prolene.

The anterior leaflet and posterior leaflet are then reattached to the fibrous annulus using continuous 5-0 Prolene suture. This repair is always reinforced with an annuloplasty ring (Fig. 26-5B).

 EXCESS TRACTION ON THE LEAFLETS
If the anterior papillary muscle is malpositioned, it must be cut at its base and reimplanted at a higher level in the septum or the ventricular wall with pledgeted 3-0 Prolene sutures.

 INJURY TO THE CONDUCTION SYSTEM
The right atrial plication must be accomplished to the right side of the coronary sinus to avoid the conduction system.

Tricuspid Valve Replacement

When the abnormality produces obstruction within the right ventricle, the tricuspid valve is excised and replaced

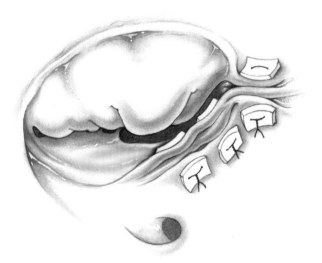

FIG. 26-4. Converting the tricuspid valve to a bicuspid valve.

with an appropriate prosthesis. The septal and posterior leaflet tissues are resected, but the anterior leaflet tissue is often incorporated in the suture technique of anchoring the prosthesis. Because of the ambiguous location of the conduction system owing to displacement of the tricuspid valve, the true atrial wall above the coronary sinus is used to construct a new annulus to which the prosthesis is sutured with multiple, interrupted, everting mattress sutures of 2-0 Tevdek buttressed with pledgets (see Chapter 8).

 INJURY TO CONDUCTION TISSUE
Incorporating the true atrial wall, rather than the septal annulus, in the suturing process prevents damage to the conduction system.

⊘ **FAILURE TO CLOSE THE ATRIAL SEPTAL DEFECT**
After correction of the tricuspid valve abnormality, the patent foramen ovale or atrioseptal defect must be securely closed with a patch of pericardium or GORE-TEX (see Chapter 18).

If the right ventricle is markedly hypoplastic because of excessive atrialization from an extensive tricuspid valve abnormality or when outflow obstruction has resulted from a grossly redundant anterior tricuspid leaflet, a modified Fontan procedure should be considered (see Chapter 29).

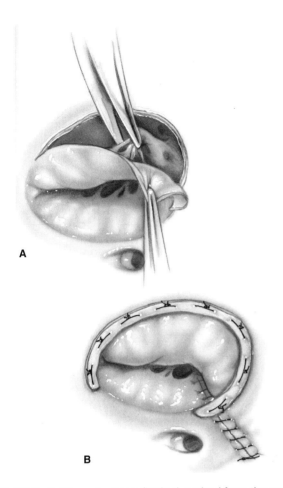

FIG. 26-5. A: The anterior leaflet is detached from the annulus to expose and divide the fibrous band. **B:** The atrialized ventricle and redundant atrial tissue are plicated. The anterior leaflet is reconstructed, and the annulus is reinforced.

CHAPTER 27

Interrupted and Hypoplastic Aortic Arch

INTERRUPTED AND HYPOPLASTIC AORTIC ARCH

Interruption of the aortic arch is a rare condition that is nearly always associated with a ventricular septal defect and patent ductus arteriosus. The ventricular septal defect may be associated with left ventricular outflow obstruction owing to malalignment of the infundibular septum. Other associated anomalies include a bicuspid aortic valve, truncus arteriosus, and aortopulmonary window. The aortic arch may be interrupted at one of three sites. The interruption may be just distal to the left subclavian artery (type A), between the left carotid and left subclavian arteries (type B), or between the innominate and left carotid artery (type C) (Fig. 27-1). Type B is the most common form of interrupted aortic arch, and type C is very rare.

Hypoplastic Aortic Arch

Hypoplasia of the aortic arch may occur with or without a discrete coarctation. Hypoplasia of the proximal arch between the innominate and left carotid arteries is defined as a diameter less than 60% of that of the ascending aorta. The distal arch between the left carotid and left subclavian arteries is considered hypoplastic if the diameter is less than 50% that of the ascending aorta. A hypoplastic aortic arch may be associated with a ventricular septal defect and other congenital heart lesions.

Patients with an interrupted or hypoplastic aortic arch usually present as neonates when the ductus arteriosus closes and flow to the descending aorta ceases or is severely restricted. Low cardiac output with metabolic acidosis is soon evident. Infusion of prostaglandin E_1 is immediately started to reopen the ductus arteriosus to perfuse the distal aorta. When the patient's general condition has improved and the low output state has been corrected, semiurgent surgical intervention is contemplated.

TOTAL CORRECTION

Incision

A median sternotomy is performed. Most of the thymus gland is removed to allow adequate mobilization of the branches of the aortic arch.

Cannulation

A purse-string suture is placed on the ascending aorta at a site just opposite where the intended anastomosis will be made. This is near the origin of the innominate artery on the right lateral aspect of the ascending aorta. In patients with an interrupted aortic arch, a second purse-string suture is placed on the proximal main pulmonary artery. The right and left pulmonary arteries are dissected and encircled with Silastic tourniquets. Dual arterial cannulation is carried out using a Y connector on the arterial line for interrupted aortic arch. Single aortic cannulation is used with a hypoplastic aortic arch. The right atrial cannula is then placed through a purse-string suture on the right atrial appendage, and cardiopulmonary bypass is established. The snares on the right and left pulmonary arteries are tightened to prevent flooding of the pulmonary bed. If intracardiac defects need to be addressed, bicaval cannulation is performed, and after repair of the arch, cardiopulmonary bypass can be recommenced, the aorta cross-clamped, and the remainder of the operation completed on full-flow bypass.

Technique

While cooling is being carried out, the innominate artery, left common carotid artery, and left subclavian arteries are mobilized and snares are placed around them. The ductus arteriosus is also dissected. After 10 to 15 minutes of cooling, with a core temperature below 18°C, circulatory arrest is established and the patient's blood volume is emptied into the pump oxygenator. The aorta is cross-clamped, and cold

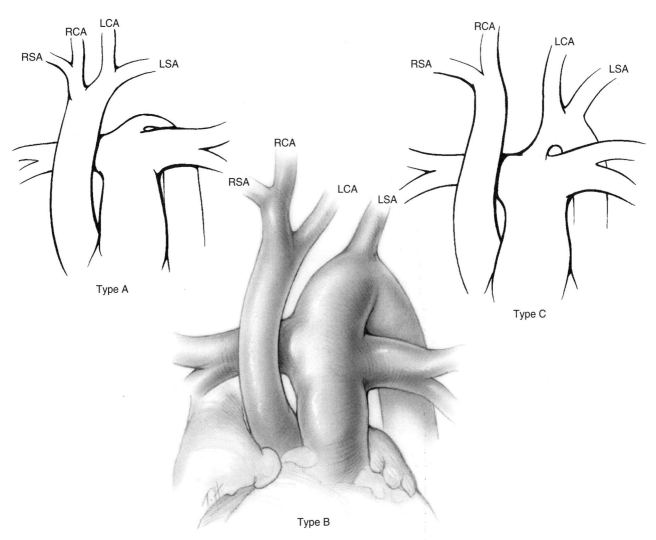

FIG. 27-1. Interrupted arch, types A, B, and C. RSA, right subclavian artery; RCA, right carotid artery; LSA, left subclavian artery; LCA, left carotid artery.

blood potassium cardioplegic solution is infused into the aortic root. At this point, the innominate and left carotid artery tourniquets are tightened. Cannulae are removed from the aorta, pulmonary artery, and right atrium; the aortic cross-clamp is also removed.

Interrupted Aortic Arch

The ductus arteriosus is divided and its pulmonary artery end is oversewn with 6-0 or 7-0 Prolene suture. The remaining ductal tissue on the aortic end is removed, and the distal aorta is dissected free and fully mobilized. An incision is made along the left posterolateral aspect of the ascending aorta; it is enlarged to approximate the lumen of the distal aorta. A small, vascular, curved C clamp is placed on the descending aorta and used to hold the descending aorta next to the proximal aortic segment without tension. The two aortic segments are then anastomosed together with continuous 6-0 Prolene sutures in an end-to-side fashion (Fig. 27-2).

⊘ *ANOMALOUS RIGHT SUBCLAVIAN ARTERY*
Frequently, the right subclavian artery arises from the upper descending aorta with a type B interrupted aortic arch; it must be dissected and divided between ligatures. This aids in mobilization of the descending aortic segment and prevents undue tension on the anastomosis.

⊘ *RESIDUAL TENSION ON THE ANASTOMOSIS*
If continued tension on the anastomosis is noted, the left subclavian artery may be ligated and divided, freeing up the distal aortic segment (Fig. 27-2).

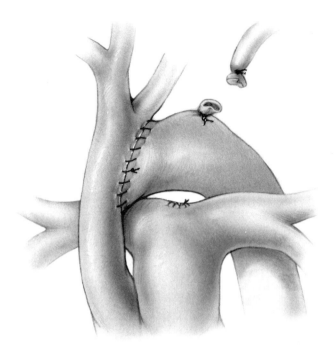

FIG. 27-2. Complete primary repair of type B interrupted arch. Note the division of the ductus arteriosus and left subclavian artery for full mobilization of the aorta.

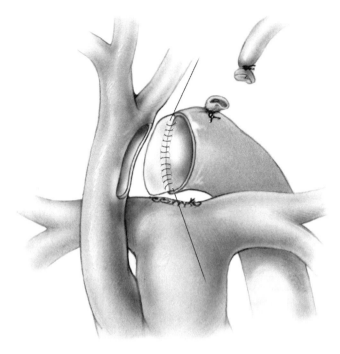

FIG. 27-3. Augmentation of the posterior aspect of the descending-to-ascending aortic anastomosis with a pulmonary homograft patch.

GROWTH OF THE SUTURE LINE
Some surgeons use polydioxanone suture for this anastomosis. There is no evidence that use of this suture results in a lower incidence of anastomotic stenosis. Prolene suture has less tissue drag and therefore can be followed more easily to allow even distribution of tension throughout the suture line with decreased risk of bleeding. It is believed that 6-0 and 7-0 Prolene sutures break or unravel as the child grows.

NB *LEFT BRONCHIAL OBSTRUCTION*
The left main bronchus passes under the arch of the aorta. A bowstring effect over the left main bronchus may be caused by inadequate mobilization of the ascending and descending aorta before direct anastomosis.

NARROWING OF THE AORTOPULMONARY WINDOW
If it appears that bringing the distal aorta up to the side of the ascending aorta will result in narrowing of the aortopulmonary window, a patch of pulmonary homograft can be used to lengthen the posterior aspect of the distal aorta before completing the ascending-to-descending aortic anastomosis (Fig. 27-3). This may well prevent compression of the left bronchus.

Hypoplastic Aortic Arch

After achieving hypothermic arrest as described previously, the ductus arteriosus is divided and the pulmonary end oversewn with fine Prolene suture. The opening on the underside of the aortic arch is now extended distally onto the descending aorta after mobilizing the distal aorta and placing a C clamp on it. Reverse Potts's scissors or a Beaver blade is used to incise the underside of the arch from the ductal opening back to the ascending aorta (Fig. 27-4). All the ductal tissue must be excised. Then a rectangular patch of pulmonary homograft is sewn into the opening beginning at the descending aortic end with 7-0 Prolene sutures (Fig. 27-5). The posterior suture line is completed first.

After the patch is sewn into place, the aortic and venous cannulae are reinserted and cardiopulmonary bypass is reinstituted. The snares are removed from the innominate, left carotid, and left subclavian arteries, and rewarming is begun.

RESIDUAL DUCTAL TISSUE
Leaving ductal tissue behind in the aortic arch may lead to bleeding from the suture line or even dehiscence of the patch from this area owing to friability. Residual ductal tissue also may lead to late constriction and stenosis of the aortic arch.

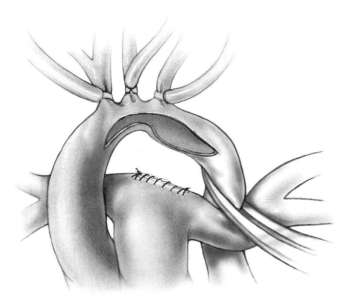

FIG. 27-4. Hypoplastic aortic arch: division and resection of ductal tissue and opening on the inferior aspect of the arch.

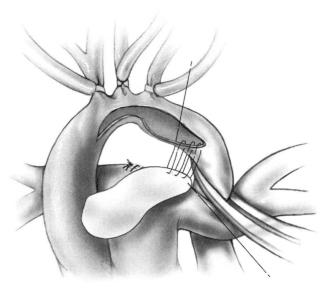

FIG. 27-5. Pulmonary homograft patch enlargement of the aortic arch.

NB *DISCRETE COARCTATION*

If a discrete coarcted segment of aorta is present, it may be resected and the superior aspect of the distal aorta anastomosed to the aortic arch before placing the patch. This may decrease the incidence of recoarctation.

Completion of the Operation

If intracardiac defects are present, they are most often addressed on full-flow bypass with aortic cross-clamping and cardioplegic arrest of the heart. If only a patent foramen ovale is present, this is closed during the period of hypothermic arrest before replacing the cannulae. After rewarming has been completed, cardiopulmonary bypass is discontinued in the usual fashion.

BLEEDING

If there is excessive tension on the arch anastomosis, bleeding is fairly common. Tissue friability also contributes to the risk of bleeding, and often retention of ductal tissue in the suture line is the cause. Systemic administration of clotting factors, including platelets and cryoprecipitate, may be helpful in controlling these bleeding sites. In addition, topical application of a fibrin glue made of equal parts of thrombin and cryoprecipitate may be useful.

INJURY TO RECURRENT LARYNGEAL AND PHRENIC NERVES

Both these nerves are at risk during repair of an interrupted and hypoplastic aortic arch. Identification and meticulous care of these nerves should be accomplished.

CHAPTER 28

The Norwood Principle

Hypoplastic left heart syndrome, in which there is only one fully developed ventricle, is the most common form of congenital heart disease and is the fourth most common congenital heart defect presenting in the first year of life. The anatomic features include aortic valve atresia or severe stenosis, with marked hypoplasia or absence of the left ventricle. The ascending aorta is small, usually only 2 to 3 mm in diameter, and the mitral valve is hypoplastic or atretic. A patent ductus arteriosus is the only route for adequate systemic perfusion.

Other single ventricle complexes may present with evident or potential left ventricular outflow tract obstruction. These include tricuspid atresia with transposition of the great arteries and single ventricles with left ventricular outflow chambers. Narrowing of the bulboventricular foramen may cause subaortic obstruction. Pulmonary artery banding in this subgroup of patients may predispose to the development of subaortic obstruction.

The Norwood principle connotes the creation or preservation of optimal hemodynamics and anatomy in patients with single-ventricle morphology and real or potential obstruction to systemic flow in preparation for a successful Fontan procedure.

There are three important basic concepts in the initial palliation phase:

1. The aorta must be associated directly with the single ventricle in such a way as to provide unobstructed flow from the single ventricle to the systemic circulation and to allow potential for growth.
2. Pulmonary blood flow must be regulated to avoid the development of pulmonary vascular disease and minimize the volume load on the single ventricle to preserve long-term ventricular function. This must be achieved without distorting the pulmonary arteries.

3. When there is stenosis or atresia of the left-sided atrioventricular valve, a large interatrial communication must be created to avoid the development of pulmonary venous obstruction and hypertension.

STAGE I: PALLIATIVE RECONSTRUCTION FOR HYPOPLASTIC LEFT HEART SYNDROME

Preoperative management includes continuous infusion of prostaglandin E_1 to maintain patency of the ductus arteriosus. Cardiac catheterization is almost never indicated because two-dimensional echocardiography is diagnostic. A balanced pulmonary and systemic circulation is critical to the survival of these patients. A restrictive interatrial communication limits pulmonary overcirculation, and a balloon atrial septostomy or blade septectomy may result in hemodynamic deterioration and should be avoided. In addition, hyperventilation and increased inspired oxygen concentrations may decrease pulmonary vascular resistance, leading to decreased systemic perfusion. Hypoventilation with room air is most often indicated in these patients.

Incision

A median sternotomy is performed, and most of the thymus is excised.

Cannulation

Purse-string sutures of 6-0 Prolene are placed in the anterior wall of the main pulmonary artery, approximately 1 cm above the level of the valve and in the right atrial appendage. Heparin is administered directly into the right atrium through the purse-string suture. A no. 11 blade is used to make a short incision within the purse-string suture on the pulmonary artery. A no. 8F or 10F straight arterial cannula is introduced several millimeters within the lumen and the purse-string suture is tightened. A no. 16F straight venous cannula is placed in the right atrial appendage, cardiopulmonary bypass is begun, and cooling is undertaken. The right and left pulmonary artery branches are mobilized quickly and encircled with Silastic tapes that are placed on traction to prevent pulmonary blood flow and ensure satisfactory systemic perfusion. During the 10- to 15-minute cooling period, the ascending aorta is dissected away from the main pulmonary artery and the branch vessels of the aortic arch are mobilized. The innominate, left carotid, and left subclavian arteries are looped with Silastic tapes on tourniquets. The distal aortic arch is mobilized down to the proximal descending thoracic aorta.

Procedure

After cooling for 10 to 15 minutes to at least 18°C by rectal probe, the previously placed tourniquets are used to occlude the branch vessels of the aortic arch. The circulation is discontinued, and blood is emptied into the venous reservoir. The arterial and venous cannulae are removed (Fig. 28-1).

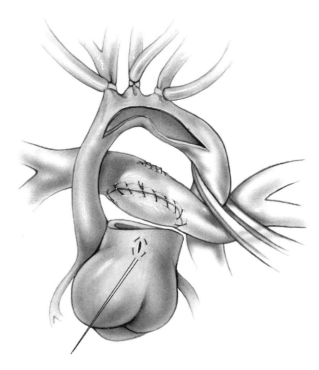

FIG. 28-2. Transection of the main pulmonary artery and a patch closure of the confluence. Oversewing of the pulmonary arterial end of the ductus arteriosus and opening of the proximal descending aorta and arch.

Myocardial Preservation

The first assistant occludes the descending thoracic aorta with a forceps, and cold blood cardioplegic solution is infused into the cannulation site of the main pulmonary artery, thus perfusing the myocardium by retrograde flow through the ductus and ascending aorta.

The septum primum is excised, either through the right atrial cannulation site or preferably through a small right atriotomy.

The ductus arteriosus is transected, and the pulmonary end is oversewn with a running 6-0 Prolene suture. The main pulmonary artery is transected at the level of the takeoff of the right pulmonary artery (Fig. 28-1). The defect in the distal pulmonary artery is then closed with a small patch of pulmonary homograft or autologous pericardium to prevent stenosis of the confluence of the right and left branch pulmonary arteries (Fig. 28-2).

The aortic opening of the ductus arteriosus is extended distally for 10 to 15 mm into the descending thoracic aorta. The opening is carried proximally along the inferior aspect of the aortic arch to the level of the innominate artery (Fig. 28-2).

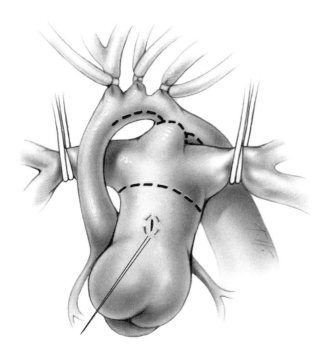

FIG. 28-1. Occlusion of the pulmonary arteries during cooling. The innominate, left carotid, and left subclavian arteries are snared down when circulation is discontinued. Dotted lines represent proposed incisions.

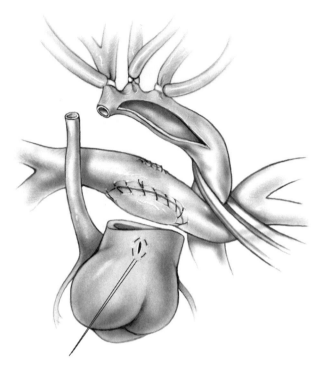

FIG. 28-3. Transecting the small ascending aorta. The distal opening may be connected to the incision on the inferior aspect of the aortic arch.

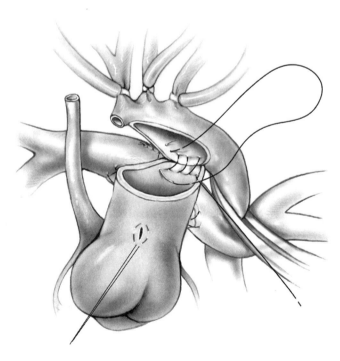

FIG. 28-4. All autologous tissue Norwood anastomosis joining the pulmonary artery base to the underside of the arch. Note the C clamp on the descending aorta.

NB *SMALL ASCENDING AORTA*
If the ascending aorta is less than 3 to 4 mm in diameter, it is transected distally near the takeoff of the innominate artery and the distal opening is connected to the aortic arch incision or is closed with a separate running suture (Fig. 28-3).

The pulmonary artery base is now brought up to the opening in the aortic arch. If the main pulmonary artery is of good length, it can be anastomosed directly into the opening on the aortic arch with no patch material (Fig. 28-4). This theoretically should allow optimal growth of the connection and prevent recoarctation or arch stenosis. The suture line is begun at the distal opening on the descending aorta using double-armed 7-0 Prolene suture. The needle is first passed from inside to outside on the pulmonary artery base and then outside to inside on the aorta. This suturing is continued along the posterior aspect until the proximal arch opening is reached. The second needle is used to complete the suture line anteriorly starting inside to outside on the descending aorta and continuing along the arch until the first suture line is met.

 INADEQUATE MOBILIZATION OF THE DESCENDING AORTA
The descending aorta must be aggressively mobilized at least 1 cm beyond the ductal insertion to allow a tension-free anastomosis. A C clamp placed on the descending aorta helps to hold it in place and provides improved exposure for the distal extent of the anastomosis (Fig. 28-4).

 INADEQUATE LENGTH OF THE MAIN PULMONARY ARTERY
The takeoff of the right pulmonary artery is variable in its proximity to the pulmonary valve. When it is located more proximally, the transected main pulmonary artery may not be long enough to reach the aortic arch. A rectangular or oval piece of pulmonary homograft is then used to augment the posterior aspect of the opening in the arch and descending aorta (Fig. 28-5). The pulmonary base can then be sewn to the pulmonary homograft patch posteriorly and directly to the aortic arch anteriorly.

 INADEQUATE AORTOPULMONARY WINDOW
A direct anastomosis of the pulmonary base to the arch or augmenting the anastomosis anteriorly instead of posteriorly can result in narrowing of the aortopulmonary window. This can result in compression of the left pulmonary artery or left bronchus with dire consequences.

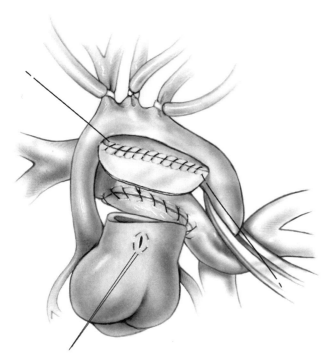

FIG. 28-5. Augmenting the posterior aspect of the aortic arch opening with a patch of pulmonary homograft.

NB *INCOMPLETE RESECTION OF DUCTAL TISSUE*
Residual ductal tissue in the aortic arch and descending aorta must be completely excised or excluded in the suturing process. Sewing to ductal tissue may result in bleeding from the suture line or even dehiscence of a portion of the anastomosis. In addition, residual ductal tissue can lead to late stenosis of the reconstructed arch.

NB *MYOCARDIAL PROTECTION*
At 20-minute intervals, cold blood cardioplegia is delivered into the ascending aorta by introducing an olive-tipped catheter either retrogradely through the aortic arch opening or into the ostium of the transected aorta.

If the ascending aorta has been transected, it is now trimmed to a length of 10 to 15 mm and the open end is beveled (Fig. 28-6). A 2.8-mm aortic punch is used to create a circular opening of the appropriate size on the posterolateral aspect of the main pulmonary artery. The anastomosis is performed in an end-to-side fashion using 7-0 or 8-0 Prolene.

⊘ *TOO LONG AN ASCENDING AORTA*
If the diminutive aorta is left too long, it may kink, thus causing coronary ischemia.

⊘ *PURSE-STRINGING THE ANASTOMOSIS*
When the ascending aorta is 2 mm or less in diameter, the suture line of the main pulmonary artery to aortic arch may be left untied. When the ascending aortic anastomosis is complete, a 1.5- or 2-mm coronary probe is passed through the arch anastomosis into the ascending aorta, and the suture is tied over the probe to avoid purse-stringing the anastomosis (Fig. 28-6).

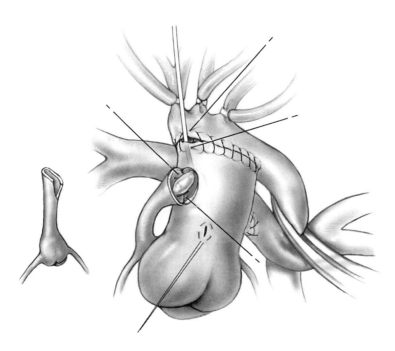

FIG. 28-6. Anastomosing the diminutive ascending aorta to the posterolateral aspect of the main pulmonary artery (neoaortic root). Note the probe introduced through the open arch anastomosis to prevent purse-stringing of the ascending aortic suture line.

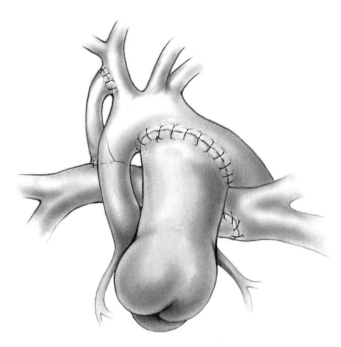

FIG. 28-7. Completed aortic reconstruction when the ascending aorta is not diminutive. GORE-TEX tube graft from the innominate to proximal right pulmonary arteries.

The aortic cannula is reinserted into the neoaortic root, and pump flow is resumed slowly after which the venous cannula is replaced. Cardiopulmonary bypass is recommended. The tourniquets are released from the branch vessels of the aortic arch, and rewarming is begun.

The shunt is now performed using a 3.5- or 4.0-mm GORE-TEX interposition graft from the innominate artery to the proximal right pulmonary artery, using partial occlusion clamps on the innominate artery. Both suture lines are performed in an end-to-side fashion with running 7-0 or 8-0 Prolene sutures (Fig. 28-7). The shunt is then clamped with a bulldog vascular clamp for the remainder of the rewarming period.

After rewarming is completed, the shunt is opened and the patient is weaned off cardiopulmonary bypass. Pulmonary vascular resistance is often high for the first 15 to 30 minutes after weaning off bypass. It may be necessary to hyperventilate the patient aggressively during this time with 100% FIO_2. Nitric oxide may be useful in these patients. The oxygen saturation may be as low as 50% to 60% during this period. If adequate ventricular function appears to be maintained, these low saturations should be tolerated.

 PERSISTENT LOW OXYGEN SATURATION
If very low oxygen saturations persist, the cause must be determined. One cause of low systemic oxygen saturation is low cardiac output with very low mixed venous saturations. Direct visualization of the heart or, preferably, transesophageal assessment of ventricular function is useful. If decreased function is noted, an increase in inotropic support may improve the situation. If the myocardial contractility remains poor, extracorporeal membrane oxygenator support may be indicated.

If shunt flow is thought to be inadequate, the patient should be placed back on cardiopulmonary bypass and the shunt revised. If a 3.5-mm shunt was used, a 4-mm shunt can be inserted.

 PERSISTENT HIGH OXYGEN SATURATIONS
High oxygen saturations greater than 85% usually indicate excessive pulmonary blood flow and may lead to progressive hypotension and metabolic acidosis. This may respond to modest hypoventilation with a PCO_2 of 45 to 50 mm Hg and maintaining an inspired O_2 concentration of 21%. If it becomes clear that the problem is excessive shunt size, the shunt should be replaced with a 0.5-mm smaller GORE-TEX interposition graft.

 RESIDUAL ARCH OBSTRUCTION
Stenosis of the reconstructed aortic arch may lead to high systemic oxygen saturations because more blood will be directed to the innominate artery and through the shunt. Lower and upper body blood pressures should be checked if this possibility is considered. If a pressure difference greater than 10 mm is present, the patient should be placed back on cardiopulmonary bypass and recooled so that the arch anastomosis can be revised.

In nearly every case, the sternum should be left open. An oval patch of Silastic is sutured to the skin edges over the mediastinal chest tube. Betadine ointment is applied to the suture line, and the entire chest is covered with a Betadine-impregnated Vi-drape.

 DISTAL SHUNT PLACEMENT
The distal end of the shunt should be placed as centrally as possible, close to the oversewn ductus on the proximal pulmonary. This theoretically should allow more uniform growth of both pulmonary arteries. In addition, it may allow the bidirectional Glenn procedure to be performed without cardiopulmonary bypass (see Chapter 29).

NB Recently, some surgeons have been placing a valved or nonvalved conduit from the right ventricle to the pulmonary artery confluence instead of placing a systemic to pulmonary artery shunt. This avoids the relatively low systemic diastolic pressures seen with a shunt, which can lead to coronary perfusion problems.

DYSRHYTHMIAS

After weaning off cardiopulmonary bypass, dysrhythmias often indicate inadequate coronary perfusion. If discoloration of the ventricle is observed or inadequate coronary arterial filling is noted, cardiopulmonary bypass should be recommenced. The proximal anastomosis between the ascending aorta and proximal main pulmonary artery may need to be revised. If the ascending aorta was left in continuity with the aortic arch, it should now be transected and sewn into the side of the neoaorta.

DAMUS-KAYE-STANSEL PROCEDURE

Patients with a single ventricle and mild or potential obstruction to systemic blood flow probably are best served by application of the Norwood principle. Banding the pulmonary artery in such patients may encourage the development of a subaortic obstruction and should be avoided. In these cases, two outlets for systemic perfusion are created by anastomosing the pulmonary artery to the ascending aorta, often referred to as the Damus-Kaye-Stansel procedure. Controlled pulmonary blood flow is then established by interposing a GORE-TEX graft from the innominate artery to the right pulmonary artery.

Incision

A median sternotomy is performed. The thymus is excised, and a patch of autologous pericardium is harvested and prepared in 0.6% of glutaraldehyde solution.

Cannulation

The ascending aorta and right atrium are cannulated, and the ductus arteriosus is dissected free from surrounding structures.

Procedure

Cardiopulmonary bypass is commenced with systemic cooling, and the ductus arteriosus is occluded with a medium-sized metal clip. The procedure can be carried out under hypothermic arrest or low-flow cardiopulmonary bypass. After a period of cooling, the aortic cross-clamp is applied and cardioplegic solution is infused into the aortic root.

The main pulmonary artery is divided just proximal to the bifurcation. The distal opening is closed with an oval pericardial or pulmonary homograft patch with continuous 6-0 Prolene sutures.

An incision is then made on the ascending aorta along its medial aspect adjacent to the pulmonary artery. This should begin just above the commissures of the aortic valve and extend nearly to the level of the origin of the innominate artery. The proximal pulmonary artery is then opened longitudinally adjacent to the incision in the aorta (Fig. 28-8).

The proximal portion of the anastomosis is started at the lowest aspect of the line of incision on the sides of aorta and pulmonary artery with a running 6-0 or 7-0 Prolene suture. To prevent distortion of the pulmonary root, the distal aspect of the anastomosis is completed by using a hemicone-shaped patch of pericardium or pulmonary homograft (Fig. 28-9, inset) to augment the pulmonary artery to aorta confluence, again using a continuous 6-0 or 7-0 Prolene suture (Fig. 28-9).

TENSION ON THE VALVULAR APPARATUS

Care must be taken not to distort either the pulmonary or aortic valves when performing this anastomosis. Any tension on the valve annulus may result in valvular insufficiency.

INJURY TO THE VALVE

When opening the ascending aorta, it is important to keep the incision above the commissures of the valve to avoid valvular insufficiency.

BLEEDING

While performing the posterior aspect of the aorta to pulmonary artery anastomosis and patch augmentation, it is important to ensure complete hemostasis. Bleeding in this area after cessation of cardiopulmonary bypass is difficult to control. Cardiopulmonary bypass must be recommenced if additional adventitial sutures are to be placed in this situation.

ALTERNATIVE TECHNIQUE

Both the pulmonary artery and ascending aorta can be transected just above the sinotubular ridge. The adjacent edges of the two vessels are sewn together for approximately one-third to one-half of their circumferences (Fig. 28-10A). Then the distal ascending aorta is anastomosed to the posterior aspect of the double-barrel root with 5-0 or 6-0 sutures. The anterior opening is then closed with an oval piece of pulmonary homograft (Fig. 28-10B).

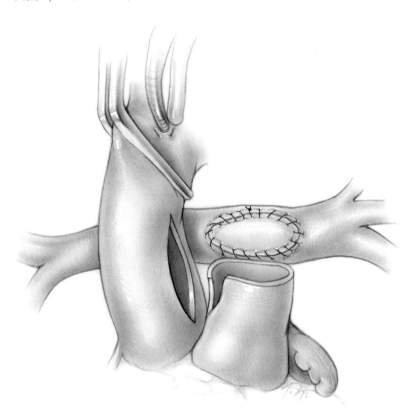

FIG. 28-8. Damus-Kay-Stansel procedure. The distal pulmonary artery opening is closed with a patch. The medial aspect of the aorta is opened, and a corresponding opening is made in the proximal pulmonary artery.

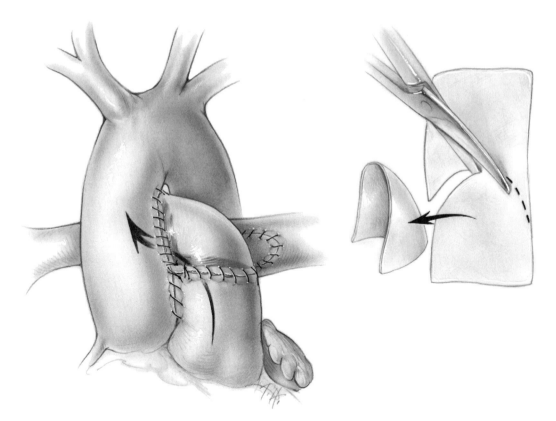

FIG. 28-9. The completed Damus-Kay-Stansel anastomosis. **Inset:** Fashioning the hemicone-shaped patch to complete the pulmonary artery–aorta anastomosis.

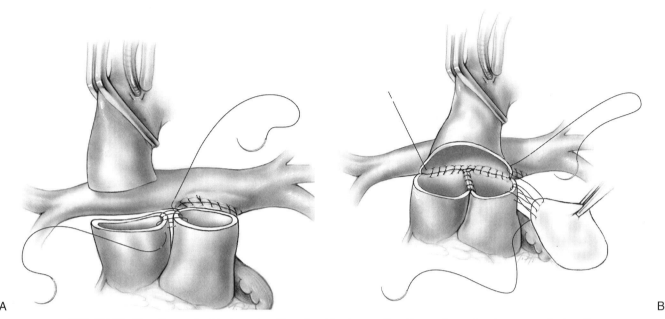

FIG. 28-10. Creating a double-barrel outflow tract by transecting the aorta and pulmonary arteries. **A:** The two roots are anastomosed together along adjacent sides and then attached to the ascending aorta. **B:** The anterior opening is closed with a patch of a pulmonary homograft.

Completion of the Operation

If the aortic arch is also hypoplastic, the pulmonary base can be anastomosed to an incision on the inferior aspect of the arch as described previously for the stage I palliation for hypoplastic left heart syndrome. After removal of the aortic cross-clamp, a modified Blalock-Taussig shunt using a 3.5- or 4.0-mm GORE-TEX tube graft is performed between the innominate and right pulmonary arteries during systemic rewarming. The shunt should be clamped until cardiopulmonary bypass is discontinued, at which point the shunt is opened. Vigorous hyperventilation may be required in the early postbypass period because pulmonary vascular resistance is often elevated during this time.

CHAPTER 29

The Fontan Principle

Fontan circulation connotes the diversion of the systemic venous return directly into the pulmonary arterial system, bypassing the right ventricle. The Fontan procedure was originally introduced for the surgical management of patients with tricuspid atresia. However, a wide range of other congenital heart defects functionally have a single ventricular chamber. Therefore, the Fontan procedure and its modifications are currently used for many of these anomalies.

PATHOPHYSIOLOGY OF A SINGLE VENTRICLE

The patient with a single ventricle may present in a variety of ways depending on the presence or absence of obstruction to pulmonary or systemic flow. Severe obstruction to pulmonary flow results in cyanosis. Obstruction to systemic flow may lead to inadequate systemic perfusion and a low cardiac output state. The flow of blood through a patent ductus arteriosus bypasses the obstruction in either the pulmonary or systemic circulation, ensuring a clinically stable state. However, when the ductus starts to close, clinical deterioration becomes evident. In a small group of patients, there is no or minimal obstruction to systemic or pulmonary blood flow. Initially, these patients may demonstrate well-balanced pulmonary and systemic circulations. However, as the pulmonary vascular resistance diminishes over the first several weeks of life, pulmonary blood flow increases and congestive heart failure develops. If pulmonary venous obstruction is present, the patient may be cyanotic owing to increased pulmonary vascular resistance.

Management of the neonate with a single ventricle is directed at achieving adequate systemic oxygenation while preventing the development of pulmonary vascular disease. Relatively unimpeded outflow into the systemic circulation from the single ventricle must be ensured. These hemodynamics allow the patient to become a candidate for a subsequent Fontan procedure.

Surgical Management

Infants younger than 3 to 4 months old with inadequate pulmonary blood flow require a systemic to pulmonary artery shunt. A 3.5-mm GORE-TEX modified Blalock-Taussig shunt or a 3.0-mm GORE-TEX central shunt is indicated to limit pulmonary blood flow (see Chapters 16 and 28).

Infants who manifest excessive pulmonary blood flow with no obstruction to systemic outflow require early intervention aimed at reducing the volume load on the systemic ventricle and reducing pulmonary blood flow to prevent pulmonary vascular disease. In the past, pulmonary artery banding has been used to accomplish these goals (see Chapter 14). However, pulmonary artery banding may not limit pulmonary blood flow sufficiently or may result in distortion of the right or both pulmonary arteries. Therefore, many surgeons believe that division and oversewing of the proximal main pulmonary artery followed by placement of a 3.5-mm GORE-TEX interposition tube graft between the innominate and right pulmonary arteries through a median sternotomy is the best palliation in these cases.

Patients who have both excessive pulmonary blood flow and obstruction to systemic outflow are difficult to manage and are probably best treated with a combined Stansel procedure and a shunt (see Chapter 28).

Management After the Neonatal Period

All patients should undergo routine cardiac catheterization at 6 months of age. If signs or symptoms of ventricular dysfunction, atrioventricular valve problems, or increased pulmonary vascular resistance are noted, the study should be performed earlier. These patients are prone to develop aortopulmonary collateral vessels. Therefore, during cardiac catheterization, a search for collateral vessels should be made, and, if present, they should be occluded with coils.

At this point, the goal is to minimize both the pressure and volume load on the single ventricle. Any aortic arch or subaortic obstruction that has not been dealt with previously must be corrected before proceeding with any other surgical interventions. Subaortic obstruction may require a Stansel procedure (see Chapter 28) or enlargement of the bulboventricular foramen. Aortic arch obstruction or discrete coarctation may respond to balloon angioplasty or may require surgical intervention (see Chapter 13).

Any situation that requires the single ventricle to pump blood to both the systemic and pulmonary circulations puts a so-called volume load on that ventricle. All single-ventricle complexes initially have an extra volume load on the ventricle. This is true whether the pulmonary blood flow is provided through a systemic to pulmonary artery shunt or through controlled forward flow from the single ventricle, as in patients with subpulmonary or pulmonary stenosis or after a pulmonary artery banding procedure. Many surgeons believe that this volume load should be removed as early as possible to preserve long-term ventricular function. For this reason, the Fontan procedure is nearly always staged. A bidirectional cavopulmonary artery anastomosis is performed at approximately 6 months of age. This procedure removes the volume load from the ventricle because all pulmonary blood flow is directly from the superior vena cava, and the ventricle provides forward flow only into the systemic circulation.

BIDIRECTIONAL CAVOPULMONARY ARTERY ANASTOMOSIS

The classic cavopulmonary shunt achieved by anastomosing the transected superior vena cava to the transected right pulmonary artery is rarely performed at present (Fig. 29-1). The bidirectional cavopulmonary artery anastomosis allows superior vena caval return to enter both the right and left pulmonary arteries. Because only 40% to 50% of the systemic venous return is presented to the pulmonary arterial bed, patients who would not be candidates for a full Fontan procedure may be able to undergo a bidirectional cavopulmonary shunt. This procedure is often used as a part of a staged approach for the patient with a single ventricle. A bidirectional cavopulmonary artery anastomosis removes the volume load and may allow ventricular remodeling. This allows the subsequent Fontan procedure to be performed with decreased operative risk and, it is hoped, better long-term ventricular function.

Incision

This procedure is routinely carried out through a median sternotomy.

Cannulation

A bidirectional cavopulmonary artery anastomosis can be carried out without cardiopulmonary bypass, using a shunt between the most proximal aspect of the superior vena cava and the right atrial appendage. In this case, two right-angled venous cannulae are selected, approximating the size of the superior vena cava. Purse-string sutures are placed at the superior vena cava–innominate vein junction and in the right atrial appendage. Systemic heparin is then administered, after which the superior vena caval cannula is placed. The cannula is allowed to fill with blood and clamped. A second cannula is then placed in the right atrial appendage. The blood from the right

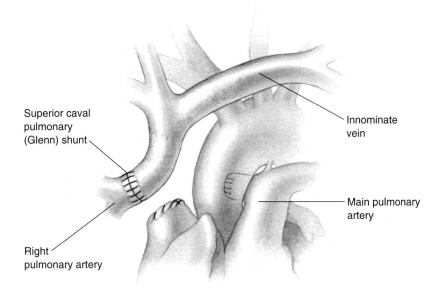

Superior caval pulmonary (Glenn) shunt

Right pulmonary artery

Innominate vein

Main pulmonary artery

FIG. 29-1. Classic Glenn shunt.

atrium is allowed to fill this cannula, which is then connected to the first cannula, making sure no air is trapped in the connector. The shunt is opened to allow flow from the superior vena cava into the right atrium. At this point, any previously placed Blalock-Taussig shunts or central shunts are dissected circumferentially. The azygos vein is doubly ligated with fine silk ties and divided between the ligatures to allow full mobilization of the superior vena cava. A tape around the superior vena caval cannula is now snared, and an angled vascular clamp is placed just above the right atrium–superior vena cava junction. The superior vena cava is then transected (Fig. 29-2). The right atrium–superior vena cava junction is oversewn with a running 6-0 Prolene suture, and the vascular clamp is removed.

 TORSION OF THE SUPERIOR VENA CAVA
To prevent twisting of the proximal superior vena cava after transection, the azygos vein may be simply ligated or occluded with a metal clip. This maintains the correct orientation of the superior vena cava during its anastomosis to the pulmonary artery.

The superior aspect of the right pulmonary artery is grasped with a curved clamp, and an opening on the superior aspect of the right pulmonary artery is made with a knife blade and Potts's scissors. The anastomosis of the superior vena cava to the right pulmonary artery is then accomplished with running 6-0 or 7-0 Prolene

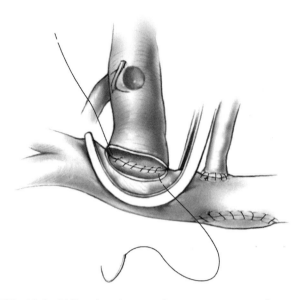

FIG. 29-3. Bidirectional cavopulmonary anastomosis: completing the posterior suture line.

sutures beginning at the most medial aspect of the pulmonary arteriotomy, completing the posterior row first with one needle and then the anterior aspect with the second needle (Fig. 29-3).

 TENSION ON THE SUPERIOR VENA CAVA–PULMONARY ARTERY ANASTOMOSIS
Tension on the anastomosis between the superior vena cava and right pulmonary artery must be avoided by leaving the superior vena cava as long as possible and placing the opening on the right pulmonary artery as close to the transected superior vena cava as feasible. This avoids any tension on the anastomosis that may lead to intraoperative bleeding from the suture line, dehiscence of the suture line, or long-term fibrosis and narrowing of the anastomosis.

Completing the Shunt

The clamp on the pulmonary artery is removed, and the anastomosis is inspected for bleeding and patency. The shunt is clamped, the superior vena caval cannula is taken out and the purse-string suture is secured. Any previously placed systemic to pulmonary artery shunt is occluded with metal clips.

If forward flow from the single ventricle into the pulmonary artery is present, the main pulmonary artery may be banded or ligated at this point. The right atrial cannula is removed, and protamine is administered.

 INJURY TO THE SINOATRIAL NODE
The sinoatrial node is located on the lateral aspect of the junction between the atrium and superior

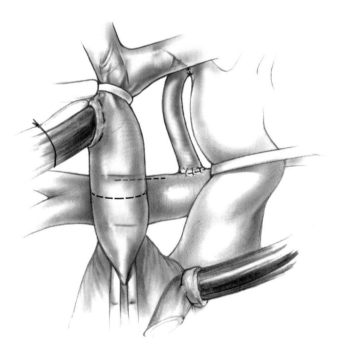

FIG. 29-2. Bidirectional cavopulmonary anastomosis: transection of the superior vena cava and a longitudinal opening on the superior aspect of the right pulmonary artery.

vena cava and is prone to injury. The surgeon should place the clamp well away from this area, and suturing should be carried out with this potential complication in mind.

 NB *DEVELOPMENT OF PULMONARY ARTERIOVENOUS MALFORMATIONS*

A group of patients develop pulmonary arteriovenous malformations after a bidirectional cavopulmonary artery anastomosis. Some surgeons believe that allowing for a small amount of antegrade pulsatile flow from the ventricle to the pulmonary artery may decrease the risk of developing these fistulae. If antegrade flow is maintained, the pulmonary artery pressure must be monitored.

 HIGH PULMONARY ARTERY PRESSURE

A pulmonary artery pressure greater than 20 mm Hg will not be tolerated, and this circumstance may necessitate interrupting forward flow into the pulmonary artery.

If superior vena cava pressures remain high, direct needle measurements of the pressure in the pulmonary artery and superior vena cava should be made to rule out an anastomotic problem.

If pulmonary artery pressures remain at 20 or above despite maneuvers to reduce pulmonary vascular resistance, the bidirectional cavopulmonary anastomosis must be taken down, the superior vena cava reanastomosed to the right atrium, and a systemic to pulmonary artery shunt performed.

 LEAVING A GORE-TEX SHUNT INTACT

If the previously placed shunt is simply occluded with a metal clip and not divided, the pulmonary artery may become distorted by upward traction at this site as the child grows. It is preferable to clip the shunt tubing proximally and distally and divide it.

NARROWING OF THE SUPERIOR VENA CAVA AT THE CANNULATION SITE

Simply tying down the purse-string suture at the superior vena caval cannulation site may result in significant distortion and obstruction to flow into the distal superior vena cava and pulmonary artery. If this occurs, the superior vena cava should be grasped with a shallow curved clamp, the purse-string suture removed, and the opening meticulously repaired with fine running or interrupted 7-0 Prolene sutures.

Performance on Cardiopulmonary Bypass

In some patients, it is safer to perform the bidirectional cavopulmonary shunt on cardiopulmonary bypass. This is particularly relevant when patients require some reconstruction of the pulmonary arteries or in patients with bilateral superior venae cavae who require bilateral bidirectional cavopulmonary shunts. In these cases, cannulation of the ascending aorta, very proximal superior vena cava, and right atrium is performed. Cardiopulmonary bypass is commenced, and previously placed systemic to pulmonary artery shunts are closed. The previously described procedure for anastomosis of the superior vena cava to the right pulmonary artery can then be performed with the heart decompressed. It is rarely necessary to cross-clamp the ascending aorta and arrest the heart.

 DISTALLY PLACED SHUNT

If the previous systemic to pulmonary shunt has been positioned close to the takeoff of the right upper lobe branch of the pulmonary artery, the bidirectional cavopulmonary anastomosis must be carried out on cardiopulmonary bypass. The shunt is clipped proximally and divided. The pulmonary artery end of the shunt is now removed, and the resultant opening in the pulmonary artery is enlarged and anastomosed to the superior vena cava.

Alternative Techniques

The bidirectional cavopulmonary artery anastomosis has the advantage of being relatively simple to carry out and can be accomplished without cardiopulmonary bypass or on cardiopulmonary bypass with a beating heart. It prepares the patient for an extracardiac conduit from the inferior vena cava to the pulmonary artery as complete Fontan procedure.

However, some patients who require extensive augmentation of the pulmonary arteries may be better served by a so-called hemi-Fontan procedure. Some surgeons use this operation routinely as the second-stage procedure in patients with hypoplastic left heart syndrome.

HEMI-FONTAN PROCEDURE

The hemi-Fontan procedure is an alternative technique that prepares the patient for a lateral tunnel intraatrial baffling of the inferior vena caval flow to the pulmonary artery as the completion Fontan operation. This procedure is especially useful if the main or branch pulmonary arteries are small or have discrete areas of stenosis.

Technique

A median sternotomy approach is used. The procedure may be carried out under hypothermic arrest or on cardiopulmonary bypass. The ascending aorta is cannulated in the usual fashion. A single right-angled cannula is placed in the right atrial appendage if hypothermic arrest is used. Alternatively, a right-angled cannula is placed at

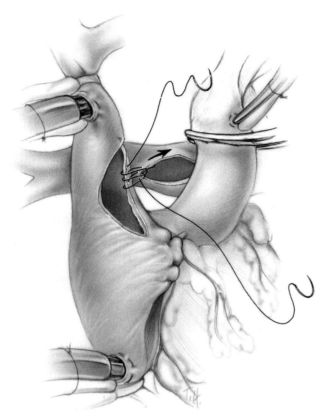

FIG. 29-4. Hemi-Fontan procedure: opening of the right atrium–superior vena cava junction and right pulmonary artery.

the superior vena cava–innominate artery junction and a second right-angled cannula is placed at the junction of the right atrium and inferior vena cava.

Cardiopulmonary bypass is initiated, and any previously placed shunt is mobilized and closed with a metal clip. If hypothermic arrest is to be used, cooling is carried out for at least 10 to 15 minutes to a rectal temperature of 18°C or lower. A single dose of cold blood cardioplegia is injected into the ascending aorta after the aorta is cross-clamped. The volume is emptied into the pump circuit, and the venous cannula is removed. If continuous bypass is used, cooling to 28°C is performed and intermittent cardioplegia is given every 15 to 20 minutes during the cross-clamp interval. Tapes are snugged down around both vena caval cannulae.

A longitudinal opening is made on the anterior surface of the right pulmonary artery and extended behind the aorta to the pulmonary artery confluence and rightward to a point directly behind the superior vena cava (Fig. 29-4).

NB *PREVIOUS SHUNT SITE*
Often a GORE-TEX tube graft has been anastomosed to the right pulmonary artery or pulmonary artery confluence. The tube graft should be mobilized, secured with two metal clips as far from the pulmonary artery as possible, and transected. The remaining GORE-TEX tube attached to the pulmonary artery should be removed and the resultant opening in the pulmonary artery incorporated into the longitudinal incision.

SMALL PULMONARY ARTERY CONFLUENCE
If the proximal right or left pulmonary artery is small or stenotic, the longitudinal incision should be extended to the hilum of the left lung.

An opening is made in the superior aspect of the right atrium and carried cephalad onto the medial aspect of the superior vena cava. The incision ends posteriorly on the superior vena cava 3 to 4 mm above the longitudinal incision in the pulmonary artery. A 6-0 Prolene suture is

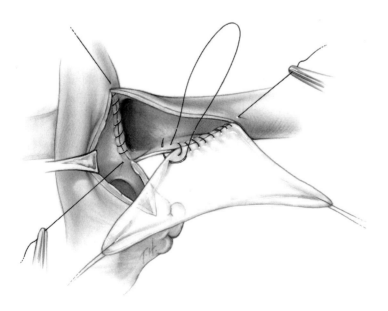

FIG. 29-5. Hemi-Fontan procedure: patching the pulmonary artery and superior vena cava with pericardium or piece of pulmonary homograft.

and superior vena cava. The suture line is begun at the leftward extent of the pulmonary artery opening and continued until the suture line meets the initial pulmonary artery–superior vena cava suture (Fig. 29-5). These sutures are tied securely together. The inferior aspect of the triangular patch is then sewn to the endocardium of the right atrium, extending from the right atrial opening posteriorly and up along the lateral aspect to meet the right atrial incision. The patch is then folded on itself and sewn to the remaining opening on the right atrium and superior vena cava (Fig. 29-6). This infolding creates a patch closure of the superior vena cava–right atrium junction (Fig. 29-7). When the completion Fontan procedure is undertaken, this pericardial or homograft patch is excised through the right atrial opening to reestablish flow through this junction.

 FORWARD PULMONARY ARTERY FLOW
The hemi-Fontan procedure is most often used for patients after stage I palliation for hypoplastic left heart syndrome. If there is forward flow through the pulmonary valve, the main pulmonary artery should be transected at the valve level and oversewn proximally with interrupted pledgeted 4-0 Prolene sutures incorporating valve tissue reinforced by a running 5-0 Prolene suture. The resultant opening in the pulmonary artery is then extended onto the right pulmonary artery.

COMPLETION FONTAN PROCEDURE

The full Fontan procedure can be accomplished when the child is approximately 2 years of age. Today, the Fontan procedure is usually performed as part of a staged approach in patients with a single ventricle after a bidirectional cavopulmonary artery anastomosis or a hemi-Fontan procedure.

Atrioventricular connection for hearts with a subpulmonary ventricular chamber is now rarely performed. The initial concept that incorporating the small ventricular chamber into the Fontan circulation improved the hemodynamics has proven false. The original Fontan procedure involved an atriopulmonary connection. The benefit of atrial contraction is greatly limited by the low resistance to backflow in the systemic veins. Today, a total cavopulmonary connection is performed to create the Fontan circulation. This consists of directing superior vena caval flow directly into the pulmonary artery and channeling inferior vena caval return through a straight conduit or baffle to the pulmonary artery. This connection is believed to provide improved flow patterns with presumed hemodynamic advantages, less stasis with decreased risk of thrombus formation, and fewer arrhythmias secondary to atrial distention.

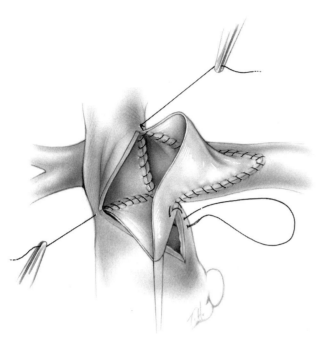

FIG. 29-6. Hemi-Fontan procedure: a folding patch to close a right atrium–superior vena cava junction.

used to anastomose the rightward extent of the pulmonary artery opening to the posterior edge of the superior vena cava (Fig. 29-4). A triangular patch of autologous pericardium or pulmonary homograft is used to augment the anterior opening of the pulmonary artery

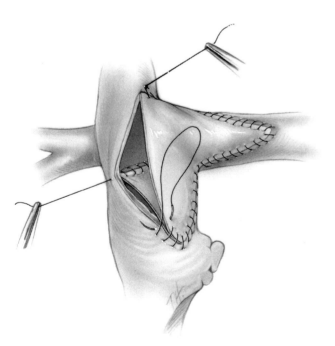

FIG. 29-7. Hemi-Fontan procedure: completing the anterior patch of the right pulmonary artery–superior vena cava anastomosis.

TOTAL CAVOPULMONARY CONNECTION

Incision

This is usually a reoperative procedure because the Fontan connection is usually staged. A standard median sternotomy provides excellent exposure.

Cannulation

Cannulation of the ascending aorta is carried out in the usual fashion. The superior vena cava should be cannulated near its junction with the innominate vein. The inferior vena caval cannula must be placed very low on the inferior vena cava itself or at the right atrium–inferior vena cava junction.

Technique for the Extracardiac Fontan Procedure

Patients who have undergone a previous bidirectional cavopulmonary artery anastomosis are ideally suited to have an extracardiac Fontan procedure. This can be performed on cardiopulmonary bypass without aortic cross-clamping. The potential advantages of this technique are improved flow dynamics through the conduit tubing into the pulmonary artery and decreased arrhythmias secondary to limited atrial suture lines and atrial distention.

On cardiopulmonary bypass with the heart decompressed and beating, the lateral aspect of the right atrium

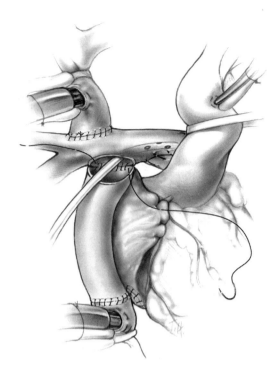

FIG. 29-9. Extracardiac Fontan procedure: an inferior vena caval anastomosis is completed. Sewing GORE-TEX conduit to the inferior aspect of the pulmonary artery. Note the vent in the pulmonary artery.

and inferior aspect of the right pulmonary artery are completely dissected. With the inferior caval tape tightened, a Satinsky clamp is placed 2 to 3 cm above the junction of the right atrium with the inferior vena cava (Fig. 29-8). The right atrium is divided approximately 1 cm from the edges of the clamp, and the edges are oversewn with a double running 4-0 Prolene suture.

An 18- or 20-mm GORE-TEX tube graft is cut straight transversely and anastomosed to the transected inferior vena caval cuff using a 6-0 or 5-0 Prolene suture. The graft is then measured to the appropriate length to lie posterolateral to the right atrium and meet the inferior edge of the right pulmonary artery (Fig. 29-9). The graft is trimmed, leaving the tube slightly longer medially. With the superior vena caval snare tightened, a longitudinal incision is made along the inferior aspect of the right pulmonary artery and extended medially toward the pulmonary artery confluence. The anastomosis of the GORE-TEX tube to the pulmonary artery opening is begun medially, passing the needle inside to outside the graft then outside to inside the arteriotomy with 6-0 Prolene (Fig. 29-9). The posterior anastomosis is completed, and the second needle is used to complete the anterior suture line.

The tapes are removed from the caval cannulae, and the heart is allowed to fill and eject while ventilation is begun. Cardiopulmonary bypass is then discontinued, and decannulation is carried out.

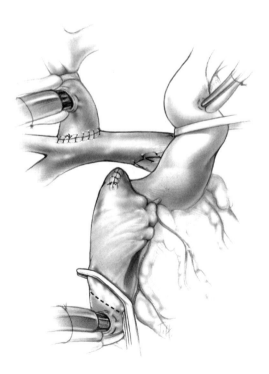

FIG. 29-8. Extracardiac Fontan procedure: a clamp placed on the wall of the right atrium 2 to 3 cm above the inferior vena cava.

LEAVING TOO SMALL A RIM OF TISSUE ON THE RIGHT ATRIUM
If the right atrial tissue slips out of the clamp, air embolism may result with devastating consequences. A 1-cm rim of tissue should be left beyond the clamp. In addition, beginning the suture line after cutting only 1 to 2 cm and continuing to cut 1 cm and then sew ensures that if the clamp should slip off, the right atrial opening will be controlled.

 INJURY TO THE CORONARY SINUS
Before and after placing the clamp on the right atrium, the heart should be inspected to ensure that the coronary sinus or right coronary artery is not included.

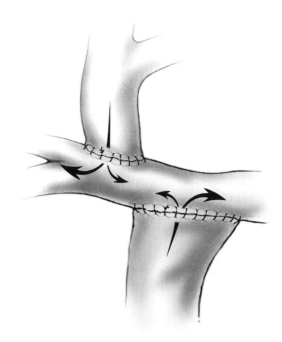

FIG. 29-10. Offset of superior and inferior vena caval flows.

FORWARD FLOW INTO THE PULMONARY ARTERY
If forward flow from the single ventricle into the pulmonary artery is present, the main pulmonary artery needs to be ligated or divided. To prevent the possible development of thrombus above the pulmonary valve and below the level of ligation owing to stasis, the preferred approach is to divide the pulmonary artery just above the valve and oversew the proximal end, incorporating valve tissue in the suture line. This requires a short period of aortic cross-clamping. The distal end can then be oversewn, patched, or used as the most medial aspect of the extracardiac conduit anastomosis.

 PULMONARY ARTERY STENOSIS
Any areas of pulmonary arterial narrowing must be addressed, usually with a longitudinal opening across the stenotic area and placement of a pulmonary homograft patch. Narrowing of the proximal right pulmonary artery can often be addressed by placing the GORE-TEX tube graft along this area.

NB *MAINTAINING LAMINAR FLOW INTO THE PULMONARY ARTERIES*
Many studies have suggested that the least disturbance to forward flow from the superior vena cava and inferior vena cava into the pulmonary arteries is achieved when the two flows are offset (Fig. 29-10). Therefore, every attempt should be made to place the GORE-TEX conduit as medially as possible to offset its opening to the left of the superior vena caval anastomosis.

 EXCESSIVE BACK FLOW FROM THE PULMONARY ARTERIES
A large amount of blood flow may be noted when the opening in the pulmonary artery is made. Plac-

ing a vent sucker into the pulmonary artery will control this backbleeding while the anastomosis is performed (Fig. 29-9).

Technique for a Lateral Tunnel Fontan Procedure

Patients who have previously undergone a hemi-Fontan procedure are good candidates for the lateral tunnel Fontan procedure. In these patients, the anastomosis of the top of the right atrium to the pulmonary artery has already been completed.

Bicaval cannulation and cardiopulmonary bypass with moderate hypothermia are used. The aortic cross-clamp is applied, and cold blood cardioplegic solution is infused into the aortic root.

A longitudinal right atriotomy is made starting at a point 0.5 to 1 cm anterior to and parallel with the sulcus terminalis after tightening the tape around the inferior vena caval cannula. Residual atrial septal tissue is excised to ensure unobstructed drainage of pulmonary venous return through the tricuspid valve. This is especially important when left-sided atrioventricular valve stenosis or atresia is present.

A piece of GORE-TEX tube graft, 10 to 12 mm in diameter, is cut to a length corresponding with the distance between the inferior vena cava–right atrium junction and the right superior vena cava–right atrium junction. The graft is cut in half lengthwise and its width adjusted as appropriate to the size of the patient to create an intraatrial baffle from the inferior vena cava to the superior vena cava. The baffle is placed inside the atrium,

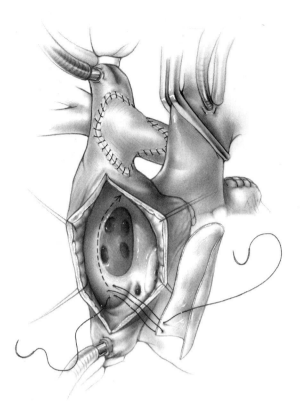

FIG. 29-11. Fontan procedure: intraatrial baffle.

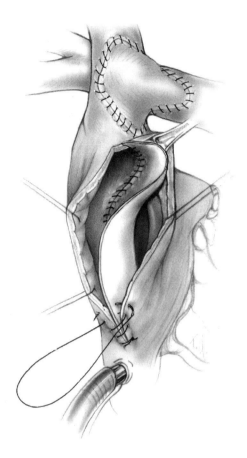

FIG. 29-12. Fontan procedure: completion of an intraatrial baffle.

and the posterior suture line is begun inferiorly using a running 5-0 Prolene suture (Fig. 29-11). The baffle is sutured in front of the opening of the right-sided pulmonary veins. The suture line is carried around the opening of the inferior vena cava into the right atrium, up to the right atriotomy where the suture is brought outside the right atrium. The remainder of the posterior suture line of the baffle is completed. At this point, if a previous hemi-Fontan procedure has been performed, the patch closing off the right atriopulmonary artery anastomosis is excised completely. The tape on the superior vena caval cannula must be tightened. Superiorly, the suture line is continued onto the crista terminalis, around the opening of the superior vena cava into the right atrium until the suture line meets the right atriotomy where, again, the suture is brought outside the right atrium. The baffle often needs to be trimmed in this area because the lateral distance between the inferior and superior venae cavae is shorter than the medial distance between the two structures. The baffle is completed by closing the right atriotomy including the polytetrafluoroethylene baffle in the suture line (Fig. 29-12). Just before this suture line is completed, a 16-gauge catheter can be placed through the suture line into the pulmonary venous side of the baffle to monitor pulmonary venous (left atrial) pressures in the postoperative period.

The anastomosis between the right atrial end of the transected superior vena cava and the pulmonary artery is

now performed if not previously accomplished. An incision is made on the inferior aspect of the pulmonary artery corresponding to the opening of the superior vena cava. The anastomosis is completed with a running suture of 6-0 or 5-0 Prolene.

Completing the Operation

Deairing maneuvers are carried out, and the aortic cross-clamp is removed. Ventilations are begun, and flow is allowed into the pulmonary arteries by removing the tapes from the caval cannulae. If a monitoring catheter has not been previously placed into the superior vena cava or inferior vena cava preoperatively, a second catheter should be placed into the baffle through the right atriotomy and secured with a pledgeted 5-0 Prolene suture for monitoring pulmonary arterial pressures. After systemic rewarming is completed, cardiopulmonary bypass is discontinued.

NB *PULMONARY ARTERY PRESSURE*
Pulmonary artery pressures are monitored, and if the pressure is persistently 20 mm Hg or higher,

efforts to identify correctable problems must be made.

Individual pressure measurements with a 25-gauge needle should be made in the superior vena cava, inferior vena cava, right atrial side of the baffle, and the pulmonary artery directly to rule out any anastomotic narrowing and pressure gradient. If pulmonary venous pressures are noted to be elevated, efforts to improve ventricular function and decrease ventricular end-diastolic pressure should be made. Transesophageal echocardiography may identify significant atrioventricular valve regurgitation. If this is present, repair or even replacement of the atrioventricular valve may be necessary.

NB In older children or young adults who do not require growth potential, a 16- or 18-mm GORE-TEX tube graft can be placed from the opening of the inferior vena cava to the opening of the superior vena cava into the right atrium rather than inserting a baffle.

NB Patients who have hepatic veins entering the base of the right atrium separately from the inferior vena cava require a more complicated intraatrial baffle to ensure that all systemic venous return is directed to the pulmonary artery.

NB Patients with bilateral superior venae cavae may be managed with a staged approach, performing bilateral bidirectional cavopulmonary anastomoses initially, followed by the intraatrial baffle technique as described previously. Alternatively, a one-staged Fontan procedure can be performed placing the intraatrial baffle around the coronary sinus if the left superior vena cava drains into the coronary sinus, thus including the left superior vena caval drainage in the baffle of systemic venous return to the pulmonary artery anastomosis.

🚫 *INJURY TO THE ATRIOVENTRICULAR NODE*
If the intraatrial baffle is sewn around the opening of the coronary sinus, care must be taken to avoid injury to the atrioventricular node. The suture line must be carried inside the medial aspect of the coronary sinus to avoid the conduction system.

NB Recently, patients who have undergone a previous hemi-Fontan procedure have had completion of the Fontan procedure performed in the cardiac catheterization laboratory. This is accomplished by placing a covered stent within the atrium extending from the opening of the inferior vena cava to the superior vena cava–right atrium junction and perforating and enlarging the opening in the patch closing off the right atrium–pulmonary artery anastomosis.

High-Risk Candidates for the Fontan Procedure

Staging the Fontan procedure by performing a bidirectional cavopulmonary artery anastomosis first may allow some patients who otherwise would not qualify for a full Fontan procedure to show improvement in ventricular function or decrease in pulmonary vascular resistance after removal of the volume load. Patients who have somewhat elevated pulmonary vascular resistance or mild to moderate ventricular dysfunction may be candidates for a Fontan procedure with the creation of a small fenestration between the extracardiac conduit and the right atrium or in the intraatrial baffle (Fig. 29-13). With the lateral tunnel Fontan procedure, an adjustable atrial septal defect can be performed. These techniques allow right-to-left shunting through the defect that allows increased filling of the single ventricle with maintenance of adequate cardiac output. The price to be paid for improved systemic perfusion and lower systemic venous pressure is a decrease in systemic arterial oxygen saturation.

Technique

For patients with an extracardiac conduit, the fenestration can be created while on cardiopulmonary bypass in borderline Fontan procedure candidates or after separation from cardiopulmonary bypass if the pulmonary artery pressures remain above 20 mm Hg. The GORE-TEX tube and right atrium are marked at a location where they are adjacent. Side-biting clamps are placed on the conduit and wall of the right atrium. A 4-mm aortic punch is used to create an opening in both structures, which are joined in a side-to-side fashion with a 6-0 Prolene suture (Fig. 29-13B). Deairing is carried out through the anastomosis as the clamps are removed. This defect can be later closed with an atrial septal defect closure device in the cardiac catheterization laboratory if necessary.

For patients undergoing a lateral tunnel Fontan procedure, either a fenestration must be created in the intraatrial baffle or an adjustable atrial septal defect fashioned during the period of aortic cross-clamping. The fenestration is created using a 4-mm aortic punch in the middle of the GORE-TEX baffle. This can be closed with an atrial septal defect closure device in the catheterization laboratory, although many close spontaneously.

An adjustable atrial septal defect is created by cutting a rectangular piece of GORE-TEX measuring 4 to 5 mm in diameter and 5 to 6 mm in length out of the posterior aspect of the polytetrafluoroethylene baffle (Fig. 29-13A). This defect is created directly over the opening of the right superior pulmonary vein into the pulmonary venous side of the baffle. A no. 1 Prolene suture is then passed through an autologous pericardial pledget, through the lateral wall of the right atrium near the junction of the right superior pulmonary vein, through the lat-

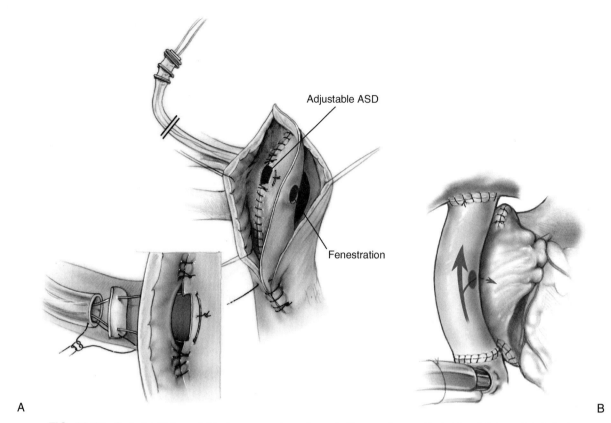

FIG. 29-13. A: Lateral tunnel Fontan procedure: fenestration and an adjustable atrial septal defect. **Inset:** Use of Prolene suture to control an adjustable atrial septal defect and chromic suture to prevent early closure. **B:** Extracardiac Fontan procedure with fenestration.

eral aspect of the defect in the GORE-TEX patch, back through the other side of the defect in the GORE-TEX patch, out through the free wall of the right atrium, and back through the pericardial pledget. The Prolene suture is secured to the edge of the defect in the GORE-TEX patch with a 5-0 Prolene suture. The no. 1 Prolene suture is then brought through an 8F polyethylene tube that is cut to a length so that the end can be placed beneath the linea alba when the sternotomy is closed. The polyethylene tubing is secured to the right atrial wall and the pericardial pledget with a chromic suture (Fig. 29-13A, inset). Thus, when the Prolene suture is pulled, the opening in the GORE-TEX baffle will close; when the heavy Prolene suture is pushed, the adjustable defect in the baffle will open. The distal end of the Prolene suture is looped back and secured with a metal clip. The atrial septal defect created in the GORE-TEX baffle can then be closed in stages by adding one metal clip at a time to the end of the 8F feeding tube. With the adjustable atrial septal defect, cardiopulmonary bypass can be discontinued and oxygen saturation and pulmonary arterial pressures monitored. If the oxygen saturation is too low, the atrial septal defect can be sequentially closed with one Ligaclip at a time, as long as the pulmonary artery pressure does not exceed 18 to 20 mm Hg. If the oxygen saturation is 85% or more, the atrial septal defect can be left open to allow for fluctuations in the pulmonary vascular resistance during the immediate postoperative period. This defect can be subsequently closed by opening the inferior aspect of the incision with the patient under local anesthesia, locating the feeding tube, and pulling on the heavy Prolene suture. This can be carried out 1 or 2 days after surgery or at any time during the postoperative period.

PREVENTING INFECTION
Leaving the feeding tube in the mediastinum and subcutaneous area does introduce the risk of infection. The tubing should be filled with dilute povidone iodine (Betadine) solution by piercing the tubing with a 25-gauge needle to inject the liquid.

CHAPTER 30

Coronary Artery Anomalies

Anomalies of the coronary arteries are rare and include left coronary artery origin from the pulmonary artery, coronary artery fistula, and aberrant origin of the left coronary artery.

ANOMALOUS LEFT CORONARY ARTERY FROM THE PULMONARY ARTERY

Origin of the left coronary artery from the pulmonary artery is the most common congenital coronary artery anomaly and occurs in one of every 300,000 livebirths. This anomaly is compatible with *in utero* life because of the presence of relatively high pulmonary artery pressure and oxygen saturation. However, over the first 1 to 3 months of life as the pulmonary vascular resistance decreases, the flow into the left coronary artery decreases, resulting in inadequate coronary perfusion. This may lead to progressive dilation of the left ventricle, myocardial infarction, and secondary mitral regurgitation. Lack of adequate perfusion stimulates the development of collateral circulation from the right coronary artery into the pulmonary artery. Significant left-to-right shunting may ensue. The clinical course of the patient depends on the relative dominance of the right and left coronary arteries and the rapidity and extent of collateral development.

Surgical Anatomy

The ostium of the anomalous left main coronary artery may be located anywhere in the main pulmonary artery or the proximal right or left pulmonary artery. Most commonly, it is found in the leftward posterior sinus of the pulmonary root.

Incision

An anomalous left coronary artery from the pulmonary artery is best approached through a median sternotomy with standard cardiopulmonary bypass.

Technique

Before commencing cardiopulmonary bypass, the right and left pulmonary arteries are dissected and encircled with snares. High cannulation of the ascending aorta with a single venous cannula is done. Immediately after starting cardiopulmonary bypass, the snares around the pulmonary arteries are tightened. A vent is placed into the left ventricle through the right superior pulmonary vein (see Chapter 4). Cooling to 28°C is carried out, and antegrade cardioplegic solution is delivered into the aortic root after the cross-clamp is applied.

A transverse incision is made on the pulmonary artery just above the sinotubular ridge. Snares around the right and left pulmonary arteries are removed. The ostium of the anomalous coronary artery is identified. It is often possible to administer cardioplegic solution directly into this vessel with an appropriately sized olive-tipped catheter for optimal myocardial protection. The main pulmonary artery is now transected, and the ostium of the anomalous left coronary artery is excised with a generous margin of tissue as a button or a U-shaped flap from within the pulmonary sinus (Fig. 30-1).

The anterior edge of the pulmonary artery root is pulled downward with a traction suture. This maneuver will improve visualization of the anomalous left coronary artery. It is mobilized and dissected free from the surrounding tissues with a low-current electrocautery. The coronary artery, now well mobilized, is brought up toward the left posterior aspect of the ascending aorta (Fig. 30-2). A small vertical or transverse incision is made on the aorta to identify the precise location of the aortic leaflets and commissures. Under direct vision, a slit is made on the posterior aspect of the aortic wall, taking meticulous care not to injure the aortic valve components. The opening is then enlarged appropriately to accommodate the left coronary using a 4-mm coronary aortic punch. The left coronary button or flap is then anastomosed to the aortic opening with 6-0 or 7-0 Prolene suture. The aortotomy is closed with continuous 6-0 Prolene suture. The

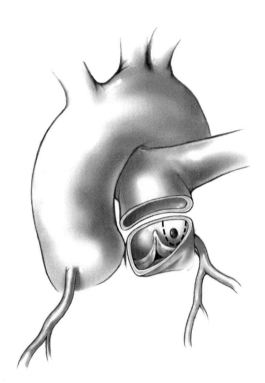

FIG. 30-1. Transected pulmonary artery. Dotted line demonstrates excision of the left main coronary artery.

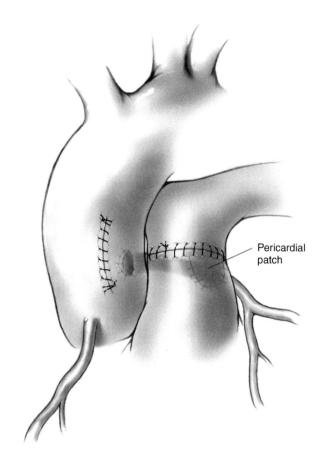

Pericardial patch

FIG. 30-3. Completed repair with autologous pericardial patch reconstruction of an excised pulmonary sinus and reanastomosis of the main pulmonary artery.

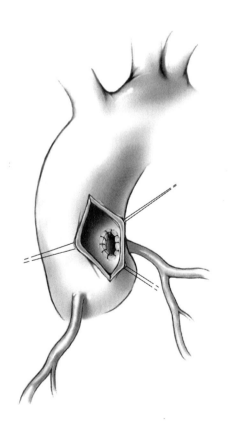

FIG. 30-2. Mobilizing the left main coronary artery for reimplantation into the posterolateral aspect of the aorta.

defect in the pulmonary root is filled with a patch of autologous pericardium using 6-0 or 7-0 Prolene suture. The pulmonary root is then reattached to the pulmonary artery confluence with a continuous suture of 5-0 Prolene (Fig. 30-3).

 CORONARY ARTERY STEAL
It is essential to occlude the right and left pulmonary arteries with the initiation of cardiopulmonary bypass. Otherwise, the right coronary artery flow may run off into the decompressed pulmonary artery through the coronary artery collaterals. This right coronary artery steal may cause global myocardial ischemia.

 LEFT VENTRICULAR DISTENTION
Most of these patients have dilated, compromised left ventricles and do not tolerate left ventricular distention. Snaring the pulmonary arteries helps to prevent a large volume of blood return through the

pulmonary veins into the left atrium. Venting through the right superior pulmonary vein provides excellent decompression of the left ventricle.

🚫 ### INADEQUATE LENGTH OF THE ANOMALOUS LEFT CORONARY ARTERY
It is usually possible to mobilize an adequate length of the left coronary artery to reach the aorta. When this does not appear to be feasible, an extension technique should be contemplated.

NB *EXTENSION OF THE LEFT ANOMALOUS CORONARY ARTERY*
Before excising the left coronary button or flap from the pulmonary artery, a judgment should be made regarding the ability to mobilize the left coronary for a tension-free direct anastomosis to the aorta. If the distance between the *in situ* left coronary artery and aorta is too great, the artery should be lengthened with an attached tongue of pulmonary artery wall (Fig. 30-4). The upper (superior) and lower (inferior) segments of the extension

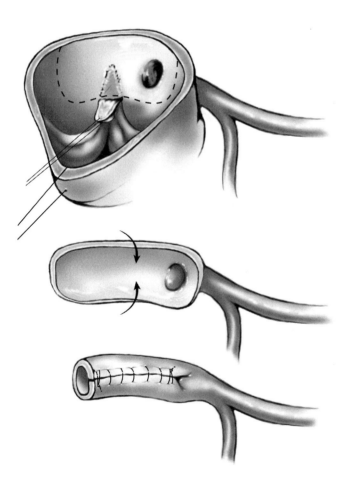

FIG. 30-4. Lengthening left main coronary artery an attached tongue of pulmonary artery wall to create a tube extension.

are sewn together with 6-0 or 7-0 Prolene suture to create a tube the same size or a little larger than the coronary artery. The end of this tube is anastomosed to the left side of the aorta. The defect in the pulmonary artery is patched with autologous pericardium. It may be necessary to detach the top of the posterior commissure of the pulmonic valve in excising the tongue of pulmonary wall. This commissure is then resuspended on the pericardial patch used to reconstruct the pulmonary root.

NB *CORRECT LIE OF THE LEFT CORONARY ARTERY*
It is useful to unclamp the aorta before reconstructing the pulmonary artery. This allows the surgeon to check the pressurized transferred coronary artery for distortion. If twisting of the artery is noted, the aortic anastomosis needs to be redone. Sometimes division of adventitial bands will compensate for minor degrees of torsion.

🚫 ### TENSION ON THE PULMONARY ANASTOMOSIS
Extensive mobilization of the main, right, and left pulmonary arteries and division of the ligamentum or ductus arteriosus allows a tension-free anastomosis.

NB Because many of these patients have very compromised left ventricular function, left ventricular support with a left ventricular assist device or extracorporeal membrane oxygenator may be required for a few days postoperatively.

CORONARY FISTULAE

It is very rare for coronary artery fistulae to be seen early in life. Many fistulae are small and cause no symptoms and no measurable left-to-right shunting. Patients who are symptomatic with angina from coronary steal or congestive heart failure owing to a significant left-to-right shunting should undergo surgery for an isolated coronary artery fistula. Not infrequently, patients undergoing coronary artery bypass surgery may be noted to have an incidental coronary artery fistula that can be closed at the time of the coronary artery bypass procedure.

Technique

A median sternotomy is used. The fistula may be directly oversewn without cardiopulmonary bypass. To avoid myocardial ischemia or infarction, the fistula should be ligated just at its entrance into the cardiac chamber while monitoring the electrocardiogram. Digital pressure to occlude the fistula before oversewing it may also be useful.

When the fistula drains into the right atrium or pulmonary artery, cardiopulmonary bypass is used to close the distal opening under direct vision. Often the fistula has multiple openings into the recipient chamber. When the fistula empties into the right atrium, bicaval cannulation is used. When the fistula opens into the pulmonary artery, a single atriocaval cannula is usually adequate. Through a standard oblique right atriotomy or a vertical pulmonary arteriotomy, the orifices of the fistula are identified. They are then oversewn with multiple pledgeted, horizontal mattress sutures. This can be accomplished on cardiopulmonary bypass without cross-clamping the aorta to allow blood flow through the fistula. Alternatively, if the aorta is clamped, the openings can be demonstrated during the antegrade administration of cardioplegia into the aortic root.

ABERRANT LEFT CORONARY ARTERY

When the left main artery arises from the anterior (right) Valsalva's sinus, it passes posteriorly and left-ward between the pulmonary artery and aorta before dividing into the left anterior descending and circumflex arteries. Increased cardiac output with exercise results in compression of the left coronary artery between the two great vessels and causes left ventricular ischemia. Because of the risk of sudden death, the identification of this anomaly warrants surgical intervention.

Technique

Although theoretically coronary transfer, mobilizing the left main coronary artery and reimplanting it posteriorly into the aorta, is possible, coronary artery bypass surgery is generally considered the appropriate treatment. Use of one or both internal mammary arteries to bypass the left anterior descending artery and a branch of the circumflex coronary artery is indicated (see Chapter 10).

SECTION VI

Miscellaneous

CHAPTER 31

Cardiac Tumors

Myxomas are primary cardiac tumors. Although they can occur in any chamber of the heart, 90% of myxomas arise from the interatrial septum and are seen most commonly in the left atrium. In approximately 10% of patients, the tumor arises from the atrial wall and less frequently from the right ventricular wall.

The diagnosis is suggested by the patient's symptoms, complemented by physical examination, and confirmed by echocardiography. Cardiac catheterization and coronary angiography are useful only in patients who may have concomitant coronary artery disease.

TECHNIQUE

The heart is exposed through a median sternotomy. The aorta is cannulated high in the usual fashion. The superior and inferior venae cavae are both directly cannulated (see Chapter 2). This is accomplished with great care to avoid excessive manipulation of the atrium.

 VENOUS CANNULATION THROUGH THE RIGHT ATRIUM
The introduction of large cannulae into the superior and inferior venae cavae through the right atrium may dislodge tumor fragments and occupy much needed space within both atrial cavities. Therefore, direct cannulation of both cavae is always preferred.

The aorta is clamped, and the heart is arrested with administration of cold blood cardioplegia into the aortic root (see Chapter 3). Previously placed snares around both venae cavae are snugged down on the venous cannulae. An oblique incision is begun on the right superior pulmonary vein with a long-handled no. 15 blade. The opening is extended obliquely across the right atrial wall. Two small retractors are placed on atriotomy edges to expose the right atrial cavity, interatrial septum, and any right atrial tumor that may exist (Fig. 31-1).

Right Atrial Myxomas

Myxomas occurring in the right atrium are usually bulky and may have a relatively wide base. The incision is now extended across the interatrial septum, encircling the base of the tumor with approximately a 5- to 8-mm margin of grossly normal septal wall. The tumor is excised and removed (Fig. 31-1, inset).

Left Atrial Myxomas

Myxomas occurring in the left atrium are usually pedunculated and have a relatively small base attached to the septum. The septal incision is extended across the septum under direct vision, and the base of the tumor is excised, leaving a 5- to 8-mm margin of normal septal tissue (Fig. 31-2).

 ARTERY TO THE SINOATRIAL NODE
The artery to the sinoatrial node traverses the atrial septum superiorly. Injury to this vessel may result in sick sinus syndrome. The base of a myxoma in this vicinity should be shaved off.

 INJURY TO THE ATRIOVENTRICULAR NODE
Dissection near the anterior aspect of the coronary sinus orifice may cause atrioventricular node injury with resultant heart block.

NB Myxomas can occasionally arise from the atrial wall. The base of the tumor is removed with a margin of normal atrial wall. The resection need not be full thickness. The defect, if any, is approximated with fine Prolene sutures or patched with a piece of autologous pericardium treated with glutaraldehyde.

The septal defect is now closed with a patch of autologous pericardium treated with glutaraldehyde or bovine pericardium using a continuous suture of 4-0 Prolene. The opening in the superior pulmonary vein and the right

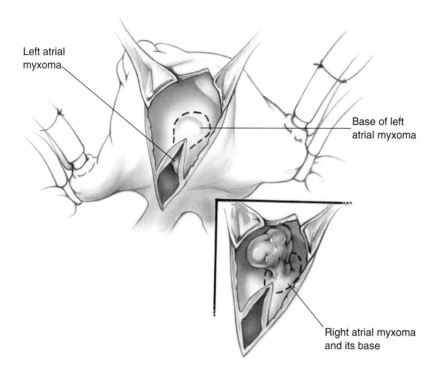

Left atrial
myxoma

Base of left
atrial myxoma

Right atrial myxoma
and its base

FIG. 31-1. Exposure of a left atrial myxoma and its base. **Inset:** Exposure of a right atrial myxoma and its base.

atriotomy are similarly closed with continuous suture of 4-0 Prolene (Fig. 31-3). Deairing is carried out, and the aortic clamp is removed.

 THICK ATRIAL SEPTUM

Occasionally, the atrial septum is thickened with hypertrophied muscle and fatty tissue. It is important to position the pericardial patch deep on the endothelial surface of the left atrial side of the septum to prevent a possible embolism of fatty tissue or thrombus formation (Fig. 31-4).

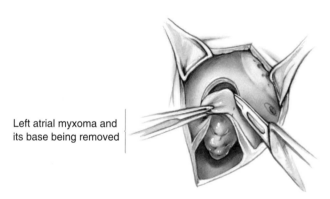

Left atrial myxoma and
its base being removed

FIG. 31-2. Excision of a left atrial myxoma and its base with a generous margin of septal wall.

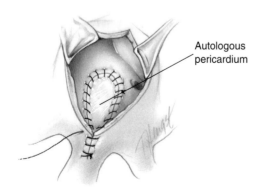

Autologous
pericardium

FIG. 31-3. Closure of a septal defect with autologous pericardium.

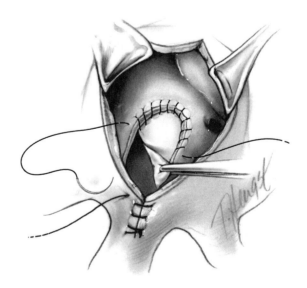

FIG. 31-4. Attaching a pericardial patch to the left atrial aspect of a thickened atrial septum.

CHAPTER 32

Surgery for Atrial Fibrillation

The Maze procedure was developed and modified by Dr. James Cox and has proven to be effective for treating atrial fibrillation associated with valvular heart disease and isolated atrial fibrillation refractory to medical therapy. The Maze III cut and sew technique is the gold standard against which modifications should be measured because of its greater than 95% cure of atrial fibrillation. However, this procedure adds significantly to the aortic clamp time and incurs the risk of serious bleeding from the back of the heart. Recently, several different energy sources have been used to effect the same or similar transmural lesions as the ones accomplished by the Maze III operation.

In our unit, we have used an irrigated radiofrequency probe, but the same lesion pattern can be accomplished with cryoablation, microwave energy, or laser. At present, we are not performing the radiofrequency Maze as an isolated procedure. Patients referred for mitral or multiple valve surgery are considered candidates if they have been in chronic atrial fibrillation for more than 6 months.

TECHNIQUE

A median sternotomy is used, and standard bicaval cannulation is performed. The initial right atrial incisions and lesions are accomplished on cardiopulmonary bypass with a beating heart. After tightening the caval tourniquets, the right atrial appendage is excised (Fig. 32-1). A lateral incision is made from the mid-portion of the base of the amputated appendage extending inferiorly 3 to 4 cm (Fig. 32-1).

The right atrium is incised beginning just anterior to the interatrial groove at the level of the right superior pulmonary vein. The incision is carried upward toward the atrioventricular groove, leaving at least 1 cm between this opening and the lateral incision from the base of the appendage (Fig. 32-2).

The irrigated radiofrequency probe is applied to the endocardial surface to create transmural lesions from the posterior aspect of the right atriotomy superiorly into the orifice of the superior vena cava and inferiorly into the inferior vena cava (Fig. 32-2). A retractor is placed under the superior edge of the atriotomy to expose the base of the amputated appendage, and a radiofrequency lesion is created from its medial aspect down to the annulus of the tricuspid valve (Fig. 32-3). Another lesion is made connecting the anterior extent of atriotomy to the tricuspid valve annulus (Fig. 32-3).

 PATENT FORAMEN OVALE
If a patent foramen ovale or small atrial septal defect is present, the right atrial lesions must be performed after the aorta is cross-clamped or with induced ventricular fibrillation to prevent an air embolism. The absence of a patent foramen ovale must be confirmed by transesophageal echocardiography in the operating room before instituting cardiopulmonary bypass.

 TRANSMURAL LESIONS
The irrigated radiofrequency probe must be drawn slowly over the tissue to be ablated to achieve a transmural lesion. The thicker the atrial wall is, the longer the ablation will take. Discoloration of the endocardium should be apparent.

The opening on the base of the atrial appendage and its inferior extension are closed with 5-0 or 4-0 Prolene suture. The aortic cross-clamp is applied, and antegrade cardioplegia is given. An incision is made in the right superior pulmonary vein and extended anteriorly to meet the right atriotomy. The atrial septum is opened into the fossa ovalis (Fig. 32-4). Retractors are placed underneath the atrial septum to expose the interior of the left atrium. Lesions are created around the left and right pulmonary vein orifices, and these two lesions are connected superiorly with a straight line (Fig. 32-5). The left atrial appendage can be amputated and its base oversewn with a

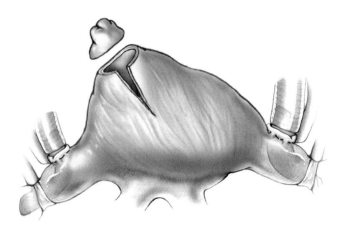

FIG. 32-1. Excision of the right atrial appendage and lateral incision from the base of the amputated appendage.

4-0 Prolene double-layer suture or a radiofrequency lesion is performed around the base of the appendage. An ablation line is then drawn from the left atrial appendage to the line surrounding the left pulmonary veins (Fig. 32-5).

An ablation line is created from the one encircling the left pulmonary veins to the posterior annulus of the mitral valve (Fig. 32-5). A curved clamp is placed into the coronary sinus from the right atrium to demonstrate the course of the coronary sinus, and a lesion is made with the radiofrequency probe extending from the mid-portion of the line connecting the pulmonary veins to the mitral annulus back to the atrial septum (Fig. 32-5).

 BLEEDING FROM THE BASE OF THE LEFT ATRIAL APPENDAGE
If the base of the appendage is ablated with the radiofrequency probe and then the appendage is amputated and oversewn, the ablated tissue may tear when the heart fills with blood and contracts.

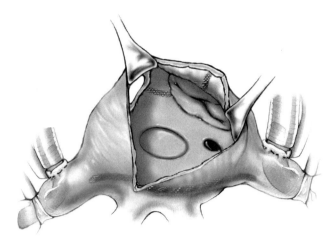

FIG. 32-3. Radiofrequency lesions from the amputated appendage to the tricuspid valve annulus and from the atrioventricular groove to the tricuspid annulus.

The appendage should be either surgically amputated or ablated with radiofrequency energy, not both, to avoid this complication.

 THROMBUS IN THE LEFT ATRIAL APPENDAGE
If a thrombus is present in the left atrial appendage, it is preferable to amputate the appendage rather than ablate it. Some surgeons believe that the appendage contributes to left atrial transport when sinus rhythm is restored, which may be an argument to preserve the left atrial appendage if a clot is not noted.

 STENOSIS OF THE PULMONARY VEIN ORIFICES
The healing process that takes place after radiofrequency ablation may lead to fibrosis and contraction of tissue. The lesions surrounding the orifices of the pulmonary veins should be well within the

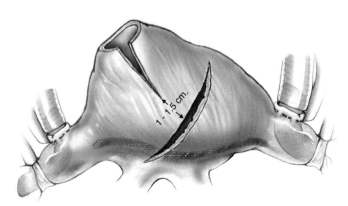

FIG. 32-2. Right atriotomy from just anterior to the right superior pulmonary vein to the atrioventricular groove. Radiofrequency lesions from the atriotomy into the orifices of the superior and inferior vena cava are indicated by shaded lines.

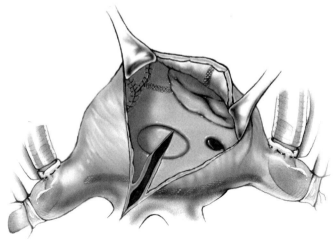

FIG. 32-4. Incision from the right superior pulmonary vein across the atrial septum to the fossa ovalis.

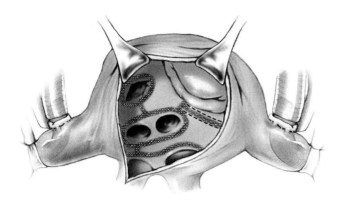

FIG. 32-5. Radiofrequency lesions within the left atrium (see text).

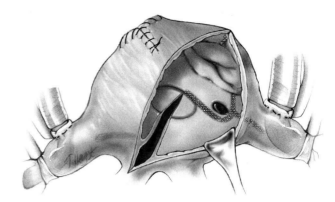

FIG. 32-6. Final ablation lines within the right atrium (see text).

left atrium to avoid subsequent scarring and pulmonary vein stenosis.

INJURY TO THE VALVE LEAFLET TISSUE

The radiofrequency energy will damage the valve leaflet tissue. Therefore, care must be exercised when creating lesions extending onto the tricuspid and especially the mitral valve annulus. Because of this concern, some surgeons prefer to use a cryoprobe to make these lesions because cryoablation does not permanently damage leaflet tissue. It is also important to carry out these lesions before any valve repair or replacement procedure.

INJURY TO THE CIRCUMFLEX CORONARY ARTERY

In performing the ablation from the left pulmonary veins to the mitral annulus, care must be taken because the circumflex coronary artery underlies this area. Transmural lesions may injure this artery. For this reason, cryoablation may be preferable in this location.

INJURY TO THE ESOPHAGUS

Although it has not occurred with the irrigated radiofrequency probe, esophageal injury has been seen with dry radiofrequency ablation of the posterior left atrial wall. The goal of any energy source used to create lines of ablation is to achieve transmural lesions to prevent electrical conduction without injuring adjacent tissues and structures.

THROMBOGENIC FOCI

Ablation lines created by some energy sources have been reported to result in thrombus forma-
tion within the left atrium. It may be prudent to anticoagulate all patients with Coumadin (warfarin) for at least 3 to 6 months even if they are in sinus rhythm to prevent this devastating complication.

The planned mitral valve procedure is now performed. The retractor beneath the atrial septum is removed, and the edges of the right atriotomy are retracted. Radiofrequency lesions are created from the end of the septal incision to the posterior aspect of the coronary sinus. Another ablation line is made from the coronary sinus inferiorly into the inferior vena cava. A final lesion is created from the coronary sinus to the posterior annulus of the tricuspid valve (Fig. 32-6).

The divided atrial septum is approximated with a continuous suture of 4-0 Prolene starting at the fossa ovalis and progressing toward the right superior pulmonary vein. Another suture is used to close the right superior pulmonary vein. This same suture can then be continued, or a third suture can be used to close the right atriotomy.

The tapes are removed from the caval cannulae, and the heart is allowed to fill. The aortic cross-clamp is removed, and deairing maneuvers are performed (see Chapter 4). Temporary epicardial atrial and ventricular pacing wires are applied.

Postoperative atrial arrhythmias are common and do not mean that the surgery has been unsuccessful. In general, these patients are maintained on sotalol or amiodarone for 3 to 6 months postoperatively. When irrigated radiofrequency ablation as described is used in patients in chronic atrial fibrillation undergoing mitral valve surgery, approximately 75% to 80% of patients will be in sinus rhythm at 1 year postoperatively.

Subject Index

Note: Page numbers followed by f indicate figures.